Clinical Cases in Nephrology

Clinical Cases in Nephrology

Editor: Braydon Butler

AMERICAN
MEDICAL PUBLISHERS
www.americanmedicalpublishers.com

AMERICAN
MEDICAL PUBLISHERS
www.americanmedicalpublishers.com

Cataloging-in-Publication Data

Clinical cases in nephrology / edited by Braydon Butler.
p. cm.
Includes bibliographical references and index.
ISBN 979-8-88740-630-5
1. Kidneys--Diseases. 2. Nephrology. 3. Clinical medicine. I. Butler, Braydon.
RC902 .C55 2023
616.61--dc23

American Medical Publishers,
41 Flatbush Avenue,
1st Floor, New York,
NY 11217, USA

ISBN 979-8-88740-630-5 (Hardback)

Contents

Preface

Nephrology is a medical specialty that focuses on the diagnosis, treatment, and management of kidney diseases and disorders. The kidneys play a vital role in filtering waste products, regulating fluid and electrolyte balance, and producing hormones that control blood pressure and stimulate red blood cell production. Nephrology covers a wide range of diseases and disorders, including glomerular diseases, hypertension-related kidney diseases, and kidney-related metabolic disorders. Glomerular diseases are a group of conditions that affect the glomeruli, the tiny blood vessels in the kidneys responsible for filtering waste and excess fluids. The treatment of hypertension-related kidney diseases involves controlling blood pressure to prevent or slow the progression of kidney damage. This book brings forth some of the most innovative concepts and elucidates the unexplored aspects of nephrology. It will provide comprehensive knowledge to the readers.

This book unites the global concepts and researches in an organized manner for a comprehensive understanding of the subject. It is a ripe text for all researchers, students, scientists or anyone else who is interested in acquiring a better knowledge of this dynamic field.

I extend my sincere thanks to the contributors for such eloquent research chapters. Finally, I thank my family for being a source of support and help.

Editor

1

Patiromer Acetate Induced Hypercalcemia: An Unreported Adverse Effect

Shreeyukta Bhattarai,[1,2] **Stephen Pupillo**,[1,2]
Gulshan Man Singh Dangol,[1,2] **and Erdal Sarac**[1,2,3,4]

[1]*Northeast Ohio Medical University, Department of Medicine, Rootstown, Ohio, USA*
[2]*St. Elizabeth Youngstown Hospital, Department of Internal Medicine, Youngstown, Ohio, USA*
[3]*Lake Erie College of Osteopathic Medicine, Erie, Pennsylvania, USA*
[4]*Ohio University Heritage College of Osteopathic Medicine, Athens, Ohio, USA*

Correspondence should be addressed to Shreeyukta Bhattarai; Shreeyukta135@gmail.com

Academic Editor: Yoshihide Fujigaki

Hyperkalemia, a potential life threating condition, is a commonly encountered problem in chronic kidney disease (CKD) patients. Patiromer acetate, a nonabsorbable cation exchange polymer, is a gastrointestinal agent for chronic therapy in patients with persistent hyperkalemia. Patiromer is generally well tolerated in patients; common side effects are gastrointestinal, such as diarrhea, constipation, flatulence, and vomiting. Hypercalcemia, although a theoretical possibility, has not been reported in any major clinical trials. We present a case of hypercalcemia associated with patiromer acetate used for treatment of hyperkalemia in a stage IV CKD patient. Clinicians should be aware of the possibility of hypercalcemia while taking patiromer.

1. Introduction

Patiromer acetate, a nonabsorbable cation exchange polymer, was recently approved for chronic management of hyperkalemia. Patiromer acetate decreases serum potassium by exchanging calcium for potassium in the intestine, especially the colon, resulting in gastrointestinal loss of potassium. It is considered safe and well tolerated; gastrointestinal side effects include diarrhea, constipation, flatulence, and vomiting. Other potential side effects include hypomagnesemia and hypokalemia. We present a case of a seventy-year-old man with diabetes, CKD stage IV, and hypertension with hypercalcemia on patiromer acetate for consistently elevated potassium.

2. Case

During routine follow-up, a 70-year-old Caucasian male with past medical history of type 2 diabetes mellitus, gout, chronic kidney disease (CKD) stage IV, anemia of chronic disease, vitamin D deficiency, and hypertension, managed with patiromer acetate for persistent hyperkalemia secondary to CKD, presented with hypercalcemia. Home medications included metformin, allopurinol, weekly erythropoietin, and vitamin D supplementation. Serum potassium was persistently above 5.5 mmol/L prior to treatment initiation. Estimated glomerular filtration rate (eGFR) was 24 ml/min/1.73 m^2, blood urea nitrogen (BUN) was 86 mg/dl, and creatinine was 2.6 mg/dl. Other labs included calcium (Ca), 9.2 mg/dl; potassium (K), 5.7 mmol/L; and parathyroid hormone (PTH), 86 pg/ml. BUN and creatinine were similar over the last year. Initial patiromer acetate dosing was 8.5 mg nightly. Symptomatically, the patient tolerated the medication very well. However, calcium at 30-day follow-up increased to 10.2 mg/dl, and potassium level decreased to 5.1 mmol/L. Since the patient was asymptomatic, he was advised to continue patiromer acetate and discontinue vitamin D supplementation. Repeat lab values after two months demonstrated higher calcium, 10.7 mg/dl, and unchanged potassium, 5.1 mmol/L.

At this point, secondary causes of hypercalcemia were investigated. See Table 1. Mild hyperparathyroidism of

Table 1

	Day 1	Day 30	Day 90	Day 120	Day 150
Potassium, mmol/L	5.7	5.1	5.1	4.6	5.3
eGFR, ml/min/m2	24	23	31	25	22
BUN, mg/dL	86	92	65	87	80
Creatinine, mg/dL	2.6	2.7	2.1	2.5	2.8
Calcium, mg/dL	9.2	10.2	10.7	11.6	8.4
PTH, pg/ml	86			10	204
25 OH vitamin D, ng/mL	31				34

86pg/ml before the initiation of therapy (normal 15-65pg/ml) was considered secondary to vitamin D deficiency. 25-hydroxy (OH) Vitamin D was 31 ng/ml (normal: 30-100ng/ml), and 1, 25-OH Vitamin D was 10.2 pg/ml (normal: 19.9-79.3pg/ml), suggesting insufficient 1-alpha hydroxylase enzyme secondary to CKD. Parathyroid hormone related peptide (PTHrP) was within the normal limit, 2.1 pmol/L (normal: 0.0-2.3pmol/L). Normal bone density was observed on dual energy X-ray absorptiometry (DEXA) scan; the lowest T score (– 1.2), was femoral. Urinalysis was negative for proteinuria; urine immunofixation demonstrated no light chains. Thyroid stimulating hormone (TSH) level was 0.874 uIU/mL (normal 0.27-4.2uIU/mL). Chest computed tomography (CT) scan showed multiple bilateral 2-3 mm calcified and noncalcified pulmonary nodules. Nodules were stable in size, compared to scan seven years before, and considered noncontributory to hypercalcemia. Angiotensin converting enzyme (ACE) level was 53 U/L (normal 9-67 U/L).

With no obvious secondary causes of hypercalcemia on laboratory assessment and imaging, patiromer was discontinued. Despite discontinuation, he continued the medication because of misunderstanding. On follow-up after an additional 30 days, calcium returned even higher, 11.6 mg/dL (Figure 1), and potassium even lower, 4.6 mmol/L (Figures 2 and 3). After additional patient education, he was advised again to stop taking patiromer acetate. One month after stopping medication, calcium normalized to 8.4 mg/dL. PTH level, suppressed at 10 pg/ml during the hypercalcemic state, returned to 66 pg/ml after calcium normalization and patiromer acetate cessation. BUN, 80 mg/dl; creatinine, 2.8 mg/dl; and GFR, 22 mL/min/1.73 m^2 remained stable. Potassium trended upward, 5.3 mmol/L.

3. Discussion

Prevalence of hyperkalemia in CKD patients is directly proportional to the residual renal function and increases from 13% in CKD stage II to 34% in CKD stage IV.[1] Gastrointestinal tract and renal systems are important regulators of potassium homeostasis. In patients with intact renal function, approximately 90 percent of potassium is excreted through the kidneys, the remaining 10 percent excreted through the gastrointestinal tract, especially the colon.[2] Renal potassium excretion is controlled by different physiologic signals, such as aldosterone, sodium delivery in

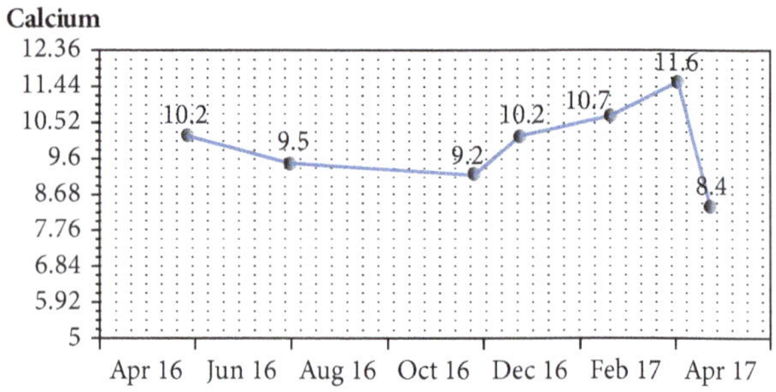

Figure 1: Trend in calcium level during the course of treatment with patiromer acetate.

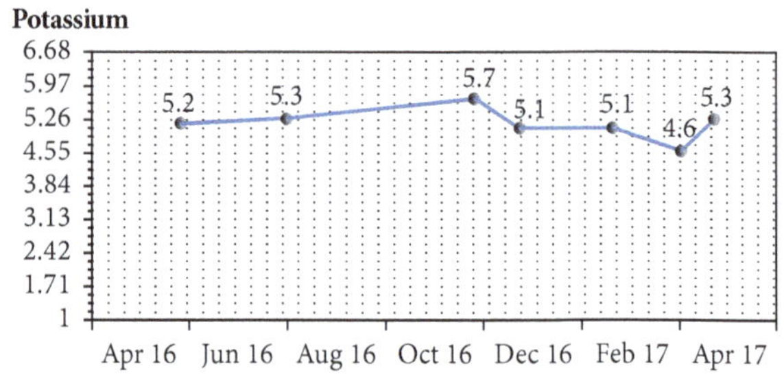

Figure 2: Trend in potassium level during the course of treatment with patiromer acetate.

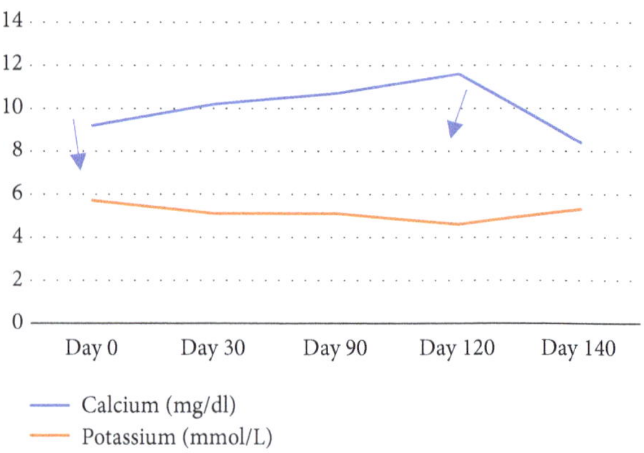

Figure 3: Trend in calcium and potassium level during the course of treatment with patiromer acetate. Arrows indicate start and stop date of patiromer acetate.

the distal tubule, urine output, dietary potassium, and acid base status. Additional potassium is processed by the colon through passive and active routes. Excretion occurs paracellularly through the passive route, whereas active secretion occurs through BK channels, also known as Big Potassium channels, present on the apical surface of colonic epithelial cells. When urinary potassium excretion is decreased in CKD patients, both active and passive mechanisms for colonic potassium excretion are upregulated, resulting in increased potassium excretion through the gastrointestinal tract.[3] However, adaptive responses may be insufficient to prevent hyperkalemia. Other contributing causes of hyperkalemia in CKD patients include use of angiotensin converting enzyme (ACE) inhibitors, angiotensin receptor blockers (ARBs), aldosterone antagonist, and renin inhibitors.

Patients with chronic mild to moderate hyperkalemia not requiring urgent lowering of serum potassium can be treated with dietary modification, diuretics, and discontinuation of offending medications. Cation exchange resins, such as sodium polystyrene sulfonate (SPS), approved for hyperkalemia more than 50 years ago, did not gain popularity because of side effects, such as fluid retention and bowel necrosis. [4] Patiromer acetate, a nonabsorbable cation exchange polymer, was recently approved as a gastrointestinal agent for chronic therapy in patients with persistent hyperkalemia. [5]

Patiromer acetate binds and exchanges potassium for calcium in the gastrointestinal tract, especially the colon. Potassium is the most abundant cation in the colon, and patiromer remains for the longest period in this segment of the gastrointestinal tract. Although potassium exchange can occur in the proximal gastrointestinal tract, colonic pH causes ionization of the patiromer molecule resulting in maximum ion exchange and increased potassium binding. Moreover, abundant colonic potassium, especially in CKD patients where BK channels are upregulated, makes patiromer more effective. Additionally, by binding potassium in the colonic lumen, patiromer creates a concentration gradient, increasing potassium secretion via BK channels.[3] Patiromer acetate demonstrates significant potassium lowering effect in patients with heart failure with concomitant renin-angiotensin-aldosterone inhibitor therapy, in diabetic nephropathy and in CKD patients. [6–8]

Bushinsky et al. studied the relationship between urinary excretion of ions and patiromer at various doses and suggested that any change in urinary ion excretion would reflect corresponding change in GI absorption of that ion. He noted a small, 73mg/day, increase in urinary calcium excretion, when healthy volunteers ingesting a normal 1000mg/day calcium containing diet used the maximum FDA approved dose of patiromer, 8.4 gm, three times daily. This suggested that only a small fraction of the calcium released from patiromer was absorbed.[9] Calcium released from patiromer in exchange for potassium can have multiple fates: it can bind to phosphorous and/or oxalate forming insoluble calcium phosphate and/or calcium oxalate salts and be excreted in the stool; it can rebind with patiromer; or it can be systematically absorbed. [9, 10] In a yearlong study of diabetic patients with GFR of 15- 59 ml/min/m2 treated with variable doses of patiromer, no clinically significant changes in serum calcium were noted.[7] At baseline calcium was 9.4-9.6 mg/dl across the patiromer dosing groups, and at weeks 4, 28, and 52, mean change in calcium from baseline was not statistically significant. The current patient, CKD stage IV and diabetic, was similar to patients studied by Bakris et al. but exhibited hypercalcemia with patiromer treatment and resolution on discontinuation. We suspect that patiromer use in this patient may have been associated with increased systematic calcium absorption, reduced renal calcium excretion, and/or a problem with systematic buffering of an exogenous calcium load in our patient. While there is no literature on drug-drug interaction, vitamin D supplementation with patiromer may play a role in hypercalcemia development. However, of note, serum calcium in the current patient continued to rise after vitamin D cessation. Although the mechanism remains unclear, some patients may be more prone to adverse effects. Discovery of these factors will require further investigation.

4. Conclusion

Although colonic excretion of potassium is increased in CKD patients, it may be inadequate to maintain normal levels. Patiromer is relatively safe and effective for hyperkalemia in CKD patients. Hypercalcemia has not been reported in any major clinical trials. Our case report of patiromer-induced hypercalcemia reminds clinicians of the importance of monitoring patient response in new treatment regimens, as well as the need for diligent investigations into urinary and serum calcium.

Acknowledgments

Authors wish to thank David Gemmel, PhD, for manuscript editing.

References

[1] C. Loutradis, P. Tolika, A. Skodra, A. Avdelidou, and P. A. Sarafidis, "Prevalence of Hyperkalemia in Diabetic and Non-Diabetic Patients with Chronic Kidney Disease: A Nested Case-Control Study," *American Journal of Nephrology*, vol. 42, no. 5, pp. 351–360, 2015.

[2] B. F. Palmer and D. J. Clegg, "Physiology and pathophysiology of potassium homeostasis," *Advances in Physiology Education*, vol. 40, no. 4, pp. 480–490, 2016.

[3] L. Li, S. D. Harrison, M. J. Cope et al., "Mechanism of Action and Pharmacology of Patiromer, a Nonabsorbed Cross-Linked Polymer That Lowers Serum Potassium Concentration in Patients with Hyperkalemia," *Journal of Cardiovascular Pharmacology and Therapeutics*, vol. 21, no. 5, pp. 456–465, 2016.

[4] R. H. Sterns, M. Grieff, and P. L. Bernstein, "Treatment of hyperkalemia: Something old, something new," *Kidney International*, vol. 89, no. 3, pp. 546–554, 2016.

[5] C. A. Thompson, "FDA approves patiromer for nonemergent hyperkalemia," *American journal of health-system pharmacy : AJHP : official journal of the American Society of Health-System Pharmacists*, vol. 72, no. 23, p. 2006, 2015.

[6] B. Pitt, S. D. Anker, D. A. Bushinsky, D. W. Kitzman, F. Zannad, and I.-Z. Huang, "Evaluation of the efficacy and safety of RLY5016, a polymeric potassium binder, in a double-blind, placebo-controlled study in patients with chronic heart failure (the PEARL-HF) trial," *European Heart Journal*, vol. 32, no. 7, pp. 820–828, 2011.

[7] G. L. Bakris, B. Pitt, M. R. Weir et al., "Effect of patiromer on serum potassium level in patients with hyperkalemia and diabetic kidney disease the AMETHYST-DN randomized clinical trial," *Journal of the American Medical Association*, vol. 314, no. 2, pp. 151–161, 2015.

[8] M. R. Weir, G. L. Bakris, D. A. Bushinsky et al., "Patiromer in patients with kidney disease and hyperkalemia receiving RAAS inhibitors," *The New England Journal of Medicine*, vol. 372, no. 3, pp. 211–221, 2015.

[9] D. A. Bushinsky, D. M. Spiegel, C. Gross et al., "Effect of patiromer on urinary ion excretion in healthy adults," *Clinical Journal of the American Society of Nephrology*, vol. 11, no. 10, pp. 1769–1776, 2016.

[10] M. Emmett and A. Mehta, "Patiromer–an oral calcium-loaded potassium binder: Kalirrhea with calciuresis," *Clinical Journal of the American Society of Nephrology*, vol. 11, no. 10, pp. 1723–1725, 2016.

2

Late-Onset Neutropenia after Rituximab Treatment for Adult-Onset Nephrotic Syndrome

Mayuko Yamazaki,[1,2] **Hidekazu Sugiura**,[1,2] **Yosuke Iwatani**,[1,2] **Mizuki Kyoda**,[1,2] **Hirohiko Nokiba**,[1,2] **Nobuyuki Amemiya**,[1,2] **Kosaku Nitta**,[2] **and Ken Tsuchiya**[2,3]

[1]*Department of Nephrology, Division of Medicine, Saiseikai Kurihashi Hospital, Saitama, Japan*
[2]*Department of Nephrology, Tokyo Women's Medical University, Tokyo, Japan*
[3]*Department of Blood Purification, Kidney Center, Tokyo Women's Medical University Tokyo, Japan*

Correspondence should be addressed to Mayuko Yamazaki; ymayuko@saikuri.org

Academic Editor: Władysław Sułowicz

A 41-year-old woman developed nephrotic syndrome at the age of 32 and was diagnosed with minimal change nephrotic syndrome based on a renal biopsy. Although remission was achieved with administration of prednisolone (PSL) and cyclosporine, the nephrotic syndrome recurred. She was also started on rituximab (RTX). She developed late-onset neutropenia after RTX treatment (R-LON) and improved 17 days later. Although the majority of R-LON cases undergo spontaneous remission, cases of death have been reported. This report is intended to warn about R-LON, since the use of RTX for adult-onset nephrotic syndrome is expected to increase in the future.

1. Introduction

Rituximab (RTX) binds to CD20 which is expressed on the surface of human B cells and produces complement-dependent cytotoxic and antibody-dependent cell-mediated cytotoxic effects [1]. RTX is used for B-cell non-Hodgkin's lymphoma but has been recently reported as an effective treatment for childhood-onset refractory nephrotic syndrome, adult-onset nephrotic syndrome [2–4], antibody-mediated rejection of ABO-incompatible kidney transplant, rheumatoid arthritis, and autoimmune diseases [5–10].

This report describes a case of grade 3 neutropenia that occurred after 188 days of RTX treatment for adult-onset nephrotic syndrome.

2. Case Report

Patient is a woman whose age is 41 years.

History of present illness is as follows: lower leg edema appeared 1.5 months after the delivery of her second child. The patient was hospitalized on the middle of October 2007 with a diagnosis of nephrotic syndrome. Severe edema and pleural effusion were observed, and the patient was started on hemodialysis and 500 mg/day of methylprednisolone for 3 days. After 3 days of administration, 60 mg/day of prednisolone (PSL) was initiated. Type I partial remission was achieved 24 days later, and the patient was taken off dialysis and discharged on the early November. After discharge, while the patient was being tapered off PSL, nephrotic syndrome recurred in June of 2008 when the PSL dosage was reduced to 17.5 mg/day. The PSL dosage was increased to 50 mg/day with the addition of 50 mg/day of cyclosporine, and the patient promptly tested negative for proteinuria. The PSL dose was gradually reduced again; however, the patient experienced a second recurrence of nephrotic syndrome when the dosage was decreased to 7.5 mg/day in August 2011. The patient underwent a renal biopsy and was diagnosed with minimal change nephrotic syndrome. Serology results (normal values for C3 at 102 mg/dL and C4 at 37 mg/dL and negative tests for antinuclear antibody and anti-dsDNA antibody) as well as negative immunostaining of the renal biopsy specimen (including for IgG, IgA, IgM, C3, C4, and C1q) excluded a diagnosis of lupus nephritis or other nephritis. The PSL dose was again increased to 50 mg/day, and complete remission

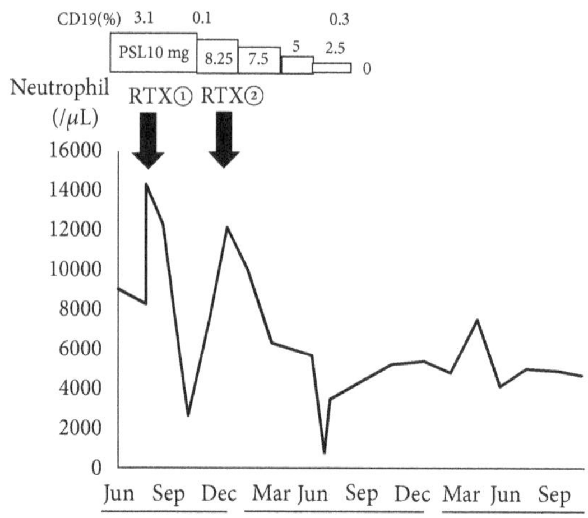

FIGURE 1: Clinical course. PSL: prednisolone. RTX: rituximab.

was rapidly achieved. The patient was being tapered off PSL when recurrent nephrotic syndrome occurred for the third time. Thus, the patient was deemed to have recurrent steroid-dependent nephrotic syndrome, in which PSL dose reduction is difficult.

In July of 2016, 500 mg of RTX was administered, after which a complete remission of nephrotic syndrome was maintained even with a reduced dose of PSL. Although mild neutropenia was noted (2,579/μL neutrophil count) on day 79 of RTX treatment, the neutrophil count rapidly increased to 12284/μl when steroids were administered (Figure 1). The second 500 mg dose of RTX was administered in December of 2016. In July of 2017, a further decrease in the neutrophil count of 619/μL was observed, which led to the patient's hospitalization.

Physical findings upon admission were height 155 cm, body weight 46.2 kg, blood pressure 90/58 mmHg, pulse 82/min, body temperature 36.3°C, no palpebral conjunctival anemia, no yellowing of the bulbar conjunctiva, clear lung sounds, no heart murmur, flat and soft abdomen, no abdominal tenderness, and no edema of the limbs.

Test findings upon admission (Table 1) were grade 3 neutropenia (neutrophil count < 500–1000/μL). CRP was negative at 0.05 mg/dL.

Course after hospitalization was as follows: despite the presence of neutropenia, no clear signs of infection were seen; thus, granulocyte-colony stimulating factor (G-CSF) treatment was not performed. After admission, the neutrophil count gradually increased and improved to 3,471/μL in the late July (Figure 1). The patient's nephrotic syndrome has remained in complete remission without medication for more than 18 months after the second RTX treatment. Therefore, there has not been an indication for further RTX.

3. Discussion

Commonly known adverse events of RTX include infusion reaction, infection, lymphocytopenia, progressive multifocal leukoencephalopathy, fulminant hepatitis caused by the hepatitis B virus, and exacerbation of hepatitis. Recent reports on R-LON occurring more than 4 weeks after the last dose of RTX exist. Although no widely accepted standard definition of R-LON has been established, the condition is defined as "otherwise unexplained grade ≥3 neutropenia (<1,000/μL) according to National Cancer Institute Common Toxicity Criteria occurring 3–4 weeks after the final RTX dose" [11].

R-LON is frequently reported in patients with B-cell lymphoma but has also been reported in cases of rheumatoid arthritis, systemic lupus erythematosus [9], overlap syndrome [8], renal transplantation [5, 7] and antineutrophil cytoplasmic antibody- (ANCA-) associated vasculitis [6]. The incidence is 3%-27% in B-cell lymphoma [11], 1.3%-2.3% in rheumatoid arthritis and autoimmune diseases [9], and 42%-70% in autologous stem cell transplantation [7]. The wide range of incidences is attributable to the diversity in patient backgrounds and treatments, inconsistent definitions of R-LON in the literature, and differences in the frequency of post-RTX administration blood sampling.

Although reports of R-LON in childhood-onset nephrotic syndrome exist [12], this is the first report of R-LON in a case of adult-onset nephrotic syndrome.

The median time interval between the final dose of RTX and R-LON onset is 38-175 days [11]. In the present case, neutropenia was observed 188 days after the final RTX dose. Furthermore, the neutrophil count 30 days after the first RTX dose was 12,284/μL but decreased to 2,579/μL 79 days after the first RTX dose. It is possible that more severe levels of neutropenia occurred but were undetected, as the patient was followed up at the outpatient clinic only every 7 weeks.

No consensus has been reached regarding the risks of R-LON onset. Arai et al. reported that stage ≥3 progressive B-cell lymphoma at the time of initiating treatment and age ≥60 years are risk factors [13]. Moreover, recent studies have reported that individuals with a specific IgG Fc receptor polymorphism (FCγRIIIa 158V/F) are at a higher risk for developing R-LON [13–16].

Although the precise mechanism underlying R-LON onset is yet to be established, the proposed hypothesis is one of two broadly classified options: (1) an immunological process or (2) a hematopoietic disorder [15]. Some B-cell

Table 1: Laboratory findings on admission.

Urinalysis		*Blood chemistry*	
Protein	(-)	TP	6.2 g/dL
Blood	(-)	Alb	4.0 g/dL
Glucose	(-)	Na	141 mEq/L
Keton	(-)	K	4.4 mEq/L
Blood cell count		Cl	108 mEq/L
		BUN	9 mg/dL
WBC	1770 /μL	Cr	0.66 mg/dL
Neut	35.0 %	AST	16 U/L
Lymp	11.7 %	ALT	15 U/L
Mono	8.6 %	LDH	151 U/L
Eosino	0.5 %	γGTP	17 U/L
Baso	0.5 %	CRP	0.05 mg/dL
Hb	14.1 g/dL	*Others*	
Ht	41.2 %	β-D glucan	<2.161 pg/mL
Plt	195×10^3 /μL	CD19	0.4 %
		Anti-Neutrophil antibody	(-)

clones can reportedly produce autoantibodies to neutrophils and myeloid progenitors during the recovery phase following an RTX-induced decrease of normal B-cell count [17, 18]. Other reports have described that the increase of stromal-derived factor-1, which plays an important role in B-cell count recovery, disturbs the migration of granulocytes from the bone marrow to the peripheral blood, among other actions [5, 13, 17]. The patient in the present case, however, tested negative for antineutrophil antibodies.

In the present case, the neutrophil count improved spontaneously. Although R-LON is generally asymptomatic and is known to spontaneously go into remission, reported cases of complicating infection that requires G-CSF or antibiotic treatment also exist [5, 6, 9–11, 13]. Deaths have also occurred due to severe infection [7, 19]. Caution is thus required to prevent R-LON onset. Although no consensus has been reached regarding G-CSF administration, G-CSF is commonly administered in grade 4 R-LON, regardless of infection. In many cases, myeloid progenitors with G-CSF receptors are maintained. Thus, prompt recovery of neutrophil count can be expected by administering G-CSF [18].

In cases of RTX readministration after the onset of R-LON [6, 9–11, 13, 19], reports of both R-LON recurrence and nonrecurrence exist. Since it is rare for cases of R-LON recurrence to become severe, RTX readministration is still considered possible. However, increasing the cumulative dose of RTX has also been reported to increase the risk of R-LON onset [20]. Many aspects of R-LON remain unknown, making it difficult to predict the risk or moment of onset. Thus, careful observation is required following RTX readministration.

4. Conclusions

We encountered a case of R-LON induced by administration of RTX for adult-onset nephrotic syndrome. Although spontaneous remission is frequently observed in R-LON, severe infection can also ensue. Patients should therefore be followed up carefully for signs of R-LON onset when RTX is administered for adult-onset nephrotic syndrome.

References

[1] T. Takei, Y. Iwabuchi, and K. Nitta, "Rituximab on steroid-dependent and steroid –resistant nephrotic syndrome in adult," *Jin To Touseki (Kidney and Dialysis)*, vol. 76, no. 1, pp. 91–95, 2014 (Japanese).

[2] H. Sugiura, T. Takei, M. Itabashi et al., "Effect of single-dose rituximab on primary glomerular diseases," *Nephron Clinical Practice*, vol. 117, no. 2, pp. c98–c105, 2011.

[3] Y. Iwabuchi, T. Takei, T. Moriyama, M. Itabashi, and K. Nitta, "Long-term prognosis of adult patients with steroid-dependent minimal change nephrotic syndrome following rituximab treatment," *Medicine (Baltimore)*, vol. 93, pp. 1–7, 2014.

[4] Y. Miyabe, T. Takei, Y. Iwabuchi, T. Moriyama, and K. Nitta, "Amelioration of the adverse effects of prednisolone by rituximab treatment in adults with steroid-dependent minimal-change nephrotic syndrome," *Clinical and Experimental Nephrology*, vol. 20, no. 1, pp. 103–110, 2016.

[5] K. Kabei, J. Uchida, T. Iwai et al., "Late-onset neutropenia and acute rejection in ABO-incompatible kidney transplant recipients receiving rituximab and mycophenolate mofetil," *Transplant Immunology*, vol. 31, no. 2, pp. 92–97, 2014.

[6] A. Knight, Y. Sundström, O. Börjesson, A. Bruchfeld, V. Malmström, and I. Gunnarsson, "Late-onset neutropenia after rituximab in ANCA-associated vasculitis," *Scandinavian Journal of Rheumatology*, vol. 45, no. 5, pp. 404–407, 2016.

[7] F. Ahmadi, S. Dashti-Khavidaki, M.-R. Khatami, M. Lessan-Pezeshki, H. Khalili, and M. Khosravi, "Rituximab-related late-onset neutropenia in kidney transplant recipients treated for antibody-mediated acute rejection," *Experimental and Clinical Transplantation*, vol. 15, no. 4, pp. 414–419, 2017.

[8] Q. Akram, M. Roberts, C. Oddis, A. Herrick, and H. Chinoy, "Oddis, Arianne Herrick, Hector Chinoy. Rituximab-induced neutropenia in a patient with inflammatory myopathy and systemic sclerisus overlap disease," *Reumatologia*, vol. 54, no. 1, pp. 35–37, 2016.

[9] J. H. Salmon, P. Cacoub, B. Combe et al., "Late-onset neutropenia after treatment with rituximab for rheumatoid arthritis and other autoimmune diseases: data from the autoimmunity and rituximab registry," *RMD Open*, vol. 1, Article ID e000034, 2015.

[10] O. Reitblat, A. Wechsler, and O. Reitvlat, "Rituximab-related late-onset neutropenia in patients with rheumatic diseases: successful re-challenge of the treatment," *American Journal of Case Reports*, vol. 16, pp. 211–214, 2015.

[11] O. Wolach, O. Bairey, and M. Lahav, "Late-onset neutropenia after rituximab treatment: case series and comprehensive review of the literature," *Medicine*, vol. 89, no. 5, pp. 308–318, 2010.

[12] R. Hiramoto, S. Matsumoto, H. Eguchi et al., "A case of a 7-year-old boy with steroid-dependent nephrotic syndrome who developed severe neutropenia three months after the administration of rituximab," *Nihon Shoni Jinzobyo Gakkai Zasshi (Japanese Journal of Pediatric Nephrology)*, vol. 22, no. 2, pp. 97–101, 2009 (Japanese).

[13] Y. Arai, K. Yamashita, K. Mizugishi et al., "Risk factors for late-onset neutropenia after rituximab treatment of B-cell lymphoma," *International Journal of Hematology*, vol. 20, no. 4, pp. 196–202, 2015.

[14] D. C. Moore, "Drug-induced neutropenia: A focus on rituximab-induced late-onset neutropenia," *P&T*, vol. 41, no. 12, pp. 765–768, 2016.

[15] D. Tesfa and J. Palmblad, "Late-onset neutropenia following rituximab therapy: Incidence, clinical features and possible mechanisms," *Expert Review of Hematology*, vol. 4, no. 6, pp. 619–625, 2011.

[16] C. Keane, J. P. Nourse, P. Crooks et al., "Homozygous FCGR3A-158V alleles predispose to late onset neutropenia after CHOP-R for diffuse large B-cell lymphoma," *Internal Medicine Journal*, vol. 42, no. 10, pp. 1113–1119, 2012.

[17] K. Chaiwatanatorn, N. Lee, A. Grigg, R. Filshie, and F. Firkin, "Delayed-onset neutropenia associated with rituximab therapy," *British Journal of Haematology*, vol. 121, no. 6, pp. 913–918, 2003.

[18] Y. Arai and K. Yamashita, "Characteristics and clinical significance of late-onset neutropenia after rituximab treatment," *Ketsueki Naika*, vol. 68, no. 4, pp. 529–533, 2014 (Japanese).

[19] D. Aguiar-Bujanda, M. J. Blanco-Sánchez, M. Hernández-Sosa et al., "Late-Onset Neutropenia after Rituximab-Containing Therapy for Non-Hodgkin Lymphoma," *Clinical Lymphoma, Myeloma & Leukemia*, vol. 15, no. 12, pp. 761–765, 2015.

[20] C. Cattaneo, P. Spedini, S. Casari et al., "Delayed-onset peripheral blood cytopenia after rituximab: Frequency and risk factor assessment in a consecutive series of 77 treatments," *Leuk Lymphoma*, vol. 47, no. 6, pp. 1013–1017, 2006.

3

Severe Hypocalcemia and Resulting Seizure Caused by Vitamin D Deficiency in an Older Patient Receiving Phenytoin: Eldecalcitol and Maxacalcitol Ointment as Potential Therapeutic Options for Hypocalcemia

Seishi Aihara,[1,2] Shunsuke Yamada,[2] Mika Kondo,[1] Hideaki Oka,[1] Taro Kamimura,[1] Atsumi Harada,[1] Toshiaki Nakano,[2] Kazuhiko Tsuruya,[3] and Takanari Kitazono[2]

[1]*Kidney Center, Matsuyama Red Cross Hospital, Japan*
[2]*Department of Medicine and Clinical Science, Graduate School of Medical Sciences, Kyushu University, Fukuoka, Japan*
[3]*Department of Nephrology, Nara Medical University, Nara, Japan*

Correspondence should be addressed to Atsumi Harada; haradaatumi@gmail.com

Academic Editor: Władysław Sułowicz

An 82-year-old man treated with phenytoin for the prevention of symptomatic epilepsy was hospitalized to treat consciousness disturbance, seizure, and hypocalcemia (serum calcium: 4.6 mg/dL). Serum 25-hydroxyvitamin D level was very low (5.4 ng/mL), whereas serum calcitriol level was normal (27 pg/mL) and serum intact parathyroid hormone level was increased (369 pg/mL). He was finally diagnosed with vitamin D deficiency associated with low sunlight exposure and long-term phenytoin use for symptomatic epilepsy: phenytoin is shown to accelerate catabolism of 25-hydroxyvitamin D. Combination treatment with eldecalcitol and maxacalcitol ointments successfully normalized corrected serum calcium level: both eldecalcitol and maxacalcitol are vitamin D receptor activators used for osteoporosis and psoriasis, respectively. Our case illustrates the importance of periodic serum calcium level monitoring in patients receiving anti-epileptic drugs and the usefulness of eldecalcitol and maxacalcitol ointment as a therapeutic option for hypocalcemia, especially in countries where native vitamin D and 25-hydroxyvitamin D are not available.

1. Background

Hypocalcemia is a lethal complication that can lead to arrhythmia, heart failure, and seizure [1–3]. Serum calcium (Ca) concentrations are normally maintained within a very narrow range that is required for optimal extracellular and intracellular function [4]. The major factors determining serum Ca concentration are parathyroid hormone (PTH), calcitriol, ionized Ca itself, vitamin D, and serum phosphate level [5]. Low serum Ca concentration, hypocalcemia, is most often caused by disordered regulation and metabolism of PTH and vitamin D axis [6]. For example, among medical conditions not caused by genetic disorders, primary hypoparathyroidism and vitamin D deficiency with or without chronic kidney disease (CKD) are the two major causes of hypocalcemia; patients with advanced CKD often have low serum calcitriol level, which is mediated by increased fibroblast growth factor 23 [7, 8].

Another factor related to vitamin D activity is disordered vitamin D metabolism associated with altered cytochrome P-450 activity [9]. A variety of drugs can affect cytochrome P-450 activity, which is a key enzyme metabolizing endogenous and exogenous substances in the human body. In vitamin D metabolism, anti-epileptic drugs (AEDs), including phenytoin, are known to interact with cytochrome P-450 activity. AEDs accelerate the rate of 25-hydroxyvitamin D and 1α-25-dihydroxyvitamin D catabolism to inactive metabolites, occasionally leading to vitamin D deficiency and hypocalcemia [10].

We present a case of an older patient with seizure and very severe hypocalcemia caused by vitamin D deficiency, which

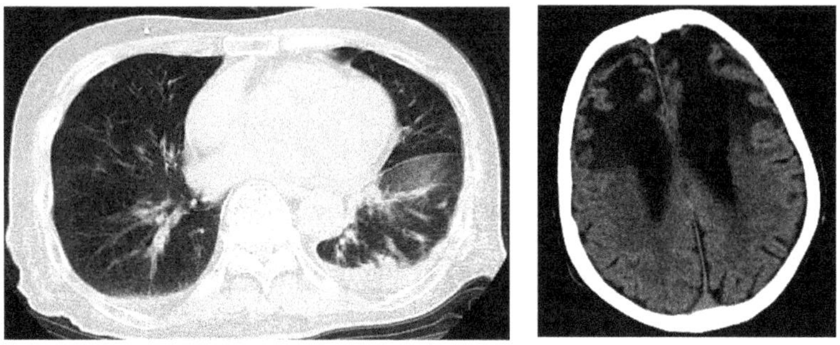

(a) (b)

FIGURE 1: Plain nonenhanced computed tomographic images of the lung and head. (a) Image shows a consolidation suspected as pneumonia at the bottom of the patient's left lung with concurrent interlobar pleural effusion and pleural effusion. (b) Although acute-phase lesions such as bleeding were not seen, frontal lobe atrophy and ventricular enlargement were confirmed.

was likely associated with long-term use of AEDs and lack of sunlight exposure, who was successfully treated with combined treatment with oral Ca supplement and vitamin D receptor activators (VDRAs), eldecalcitol, and maxacalcitol ointments. Our case also suggests the potential usefulness of eldecalcitol and maxacalcitol ointment in the management of hypocalcemia, especially in countries where native vitamin D or 25-hydroxyvitmin D is not available for the treatment of vitamin D deficiency-induced hypocalcemia.

2. Case Presentation

An 82-year-old man was hospitalized because of fever, seizure, and consciousness disturbance. He had a history of gastrectomy for gastric ulcer when he was young. At age 74 years, he developed subarachnoid hemorrhage and secondary symptomatic epilepsy, and was treated with phenytoin, an AED. With progressive disuse syndrome after the brain event, he had been bedridden for the last 8 years under insufficient sunlight exposure. Two weeks before hospitalization, he suffered an acute seizure, followed by consciousness disturbance. Thereafter, food intake and oral dosing were insufficient. Three days before hospitalization, he developed a fever >38°C. Because of concurrent respiratory failure, he was transferred to our hospital for further treatment.

On admission, the patient showed impaired consciousness with closed eyes. Verbal response was incomprehensible, and the best motor response was a response to localized pain (Glasgow coma scale score: E1V2M5). His vital signs were: blood pressure, 84/52 mmHg; heart rate, 84 bpm; body temperature, 40.0°C; and arterial blood oxygen saturation measured by pulse oximetry of 94% with supplemental oxygen at 8 L/min. His height was 161 cm, his weight was 48.5 kg, and his body mass index was 18.7 kg/m^2. He showed neither jolt accentuation of headache nor spastic rigidity. A coarse crackle was heard in his left lung. Importantly, Chvostek and Trousseau signs indicative of tetany were positive.

Laboratory data on admission are shown in Table 1. Briefly, the following results were obtained: white blood cell count (10 390/μL), serum albumin (3.1 g/dL), blood urea nitrogen (13.8 mg/dL), creatinine (0.44 mg/dL), estimated glomerular filtration rate (134.5 mL/min/1.73 m^2), phosphate (1.6 mg/dL), Ca (3.7 mg/dL), ionized Ca (0.55 mmol/L), magnesium (2.97 mg/dL), intact PTH (386.8 pg/mL), and serum C-reactive protein (1.67 mg/dL). Although blood phenytoin concentration was low (<0.8 μg/mL), this value was plausible because phenytoin has a half-life of 20–30 h, and it was not being administered sufficiently at the time of hospitalization over the last few days. An electrocardiogram showed a sinus rate of 93 beats per minute with long QT interval (0.398 s) and corrected QT-T interval (0.398 second).

At the bottom of his left lung, a consolidation was visible that was suspected pneumonia, and interlobar pleural effusion was also identified on non-contrast-enhanced computed tomography (Figure 1(a)). Although acute-phase lesions such as bleeding were not observed, frontal lobe atrophy and ventricular enlargement were confirmed by head computed tomography (Figure 1(b)). Based on these results, he was diagnosed as having bacterial pneumonia and its related sepsis. Because the patient showed neither jolt accentuation of headache nor spastic rigidity, meningitis was ruled out as a cause of seizure.

At that point, several differential diagnoses were considered for the hypocalcemia. The serum Ca level corrected for serum albumin was 4.6 mg/dL, and ionized Ca was 0.55 mmol/L, indicating true hypocalcemia, not pseudo-hypocalcemia. CKD was also excluded as a possible cause based on his kidney function. There was also no evidence of severe hypomagnesemia to cause decreased secretion of PTH, although serum magnesium level was slightly low (1.6 mg/dL). In addition, serum intact PTH level on admission was very high. Accordingly, we considered that parathyroid gland was normally functioning because intact PTH appropriately increased in response to hypocalcemia. Bone formation was slightly increased in response to increased serum intact PTH, whereas bone resorption was decreased judging from the serum tartrate-resistant acid phosphatase-5b level. At that point, the differential diagnosis of hypocalcemia still included pancreatitis and sepsis. Pancreatitis was ruled out based on the normal serum amylase and lipase levels and absence of pancreas enlargement by imaging. Although the mechanism of hypocalcemia in septic patients is complex and not well understood, previous studies showed that kidneys are reported to increase urinary Ca excretion in sepsis [11]. However, fractional excretion of Ca was remarkably low (0.13%), indicating

Table 1: Patient's laboratory data on admission.

		Reference range
Complete blood count		
White blood cells	10 390/μL	
Neutrophils	90.6%	
Red blood cells $\times 10^4$	342/μL	
Hemoglobin	10.8 g/dL	
Platelets $\times 10^4$	26.5/μL	
Serum biochemistry		
Total protein	6.2 g/dL	
Albumin	3.1 g/dL	
Blood urea nitrogen	13.8 mg/dL	
Creatinine	0.44 mg/dL	
Uric acid	1.9 mg/dL	
Total bilirubin	0.3 mg/dL	
Aspartate aminotransferase	74 U/L	
Alanine aminotransferase	36 U/L	
Alkaline phosphatase	463 U/L	
γ-Glutamyl transpeptidase	33 U/L	
Lactate dehydrogenase	729 U/L	
Total cholesterol	186 mg/dL	
Amylase	158 U/L	
LDL-cholesterol	96 mg/dL	
Sodium	131 mEq/L	
Potassium	3.1 mEq/L	
Chloride	92 mEq/L	
Calcium	3.7 mg/dL	
Phosphate	1.6 mg/dL	
Magnesium	2.97 mg/dL	
Hemoglobin A1c (NGSP)	5.6%	
Coagulation		
PT-INR	1.20	
APTT	32.1 sec	
Immunological testing		
C-reactive protein	1.67 mg/dL	
Procalcitonin	0.52 mg/dL	
Endocrinology		
Intact PTH	386.8 pg/mL	10–65
Calcitriol	27 pg/mL	20–60
25-hydroxyvitamin D	5.4 ng/mL	9.0–33.9
TRACP-5b	116 mU/mL	120–420
BAP	31.3 μg/L	3.8–22.6
Osteocalcin	10.2 ng/mL	*N*; 2.5–13
Calcitonin	<0.5 pg/mL	26.2–49.0
Arterial blood gas		
pH	7.458	
PaO_2	81.7 mmHg	
$PaCO_2$	33.9 mmHg	
HCO_3^-	23.7 mmol/L	
Ca^{2+}	0.55 mmol/L	
Urinary biochemistry		
Urinary creatinine	121.7 mg/dL	
Urinary calcium	0.8 mg/dL	
Urinary phosphate	22.6 mg/dL	

Abbreviations: APTT, activated partial thrombin time; BAP, bone-type alkaline phosphatase; Ca^{2+}, ionized calcium; HCO_3^-, hydrogen carbonate; LDL, low-density lipoprotein; NGSP, national glycohemoglobin standardization program; $PaCO_2$, partial pressure of arterial carbon dioxide; PaO_2, partial pressure of arterial oxygen; PT-INR, prothrombin time-international normalized ratio; PTH, parathyroid hormone; TRACP-5b, tartrate-resistant acid phosphatase 5b.

Ca resorption enhancement across renal tubules. Taken together, sepsis-related hypocalcemia was not regarded as the primary cause of the hypocalcemia in the present case.

Another potential mechanism for the severe hypocalcemia was decreased Ca absorption from the gastrointestinal tract. Because he had been in a nursing home, which was an environment with extremely low sunlight exposure, vitamin D_3 generally produced in the skin was potentially lacking. Notably, he was on long-term treatment with phenytoin, which is shown to accelerate conversion of 25-hydroxyvitamin D to 24,25-dihydroxyvitamin D [9, 12]. The low level of 25-hydroxyvitamin D (5.4 ng/mL), which is an indicator of vitamin D status in the body, strongly indicated that he had been suffering from 25-hydroxyvitamin D deficiency, probably caused by combination of low sunlight exposure and long-term use of phenytoin.

The patient's clinical course is shown in Figure 2. He received intravenous hydration for sepsis and antibiotics to target anaerobes (sulbactam + ampicillin 4.5 g/day) for possible aspiration pneumonia. He was treated with intravenous Ca gluconate (8.5% 10–20 mL, 3.9–7.8 mEq/day) and trans-gastric tube administration of Ca lactate/phosphate hydrate (3–6 g/day) and we discontinued phenytoin from the first hospital day. Administration of 0.25 μg/day of calcitriol by nasal gastric tube was performed between the first and second hospital days. From the third hospital day, we exchanged calcitriol with 0.75 μg/day of eldecalcitol, a VDRA often used for osteoporosis in Japan [13], because eldecalcitol is shown to have a higher binding ability to vitamin D binding protein (DBP) than calcitriol: binding ability of eldecalcitol to DBP is 4.4 times higher than that of calcitriol [14]. Indeed, previous studies have shown that vitamin D analogues that have a higher affinity for DBP show a longer half-life. Although the mechanism remains unclear, vitamin D analogue that binds tightly to the DBP may be less catalyzed by the cellular 24-hydroxylase activity, which is expressed in the target cells of vitamin D [15]. After treatment with effective antibiotics, inflammatory markers decreased steadily, and oxygen support was discontinued. His consciousness recovered after improvements in the pneumonia and hypocalcemia. Glasgow coma scale score on the 8th hospital day was E4V4M6, and he was able to eat orally. Intravenous Ca gluconate was continued until his serum Ca level increased to within the reference

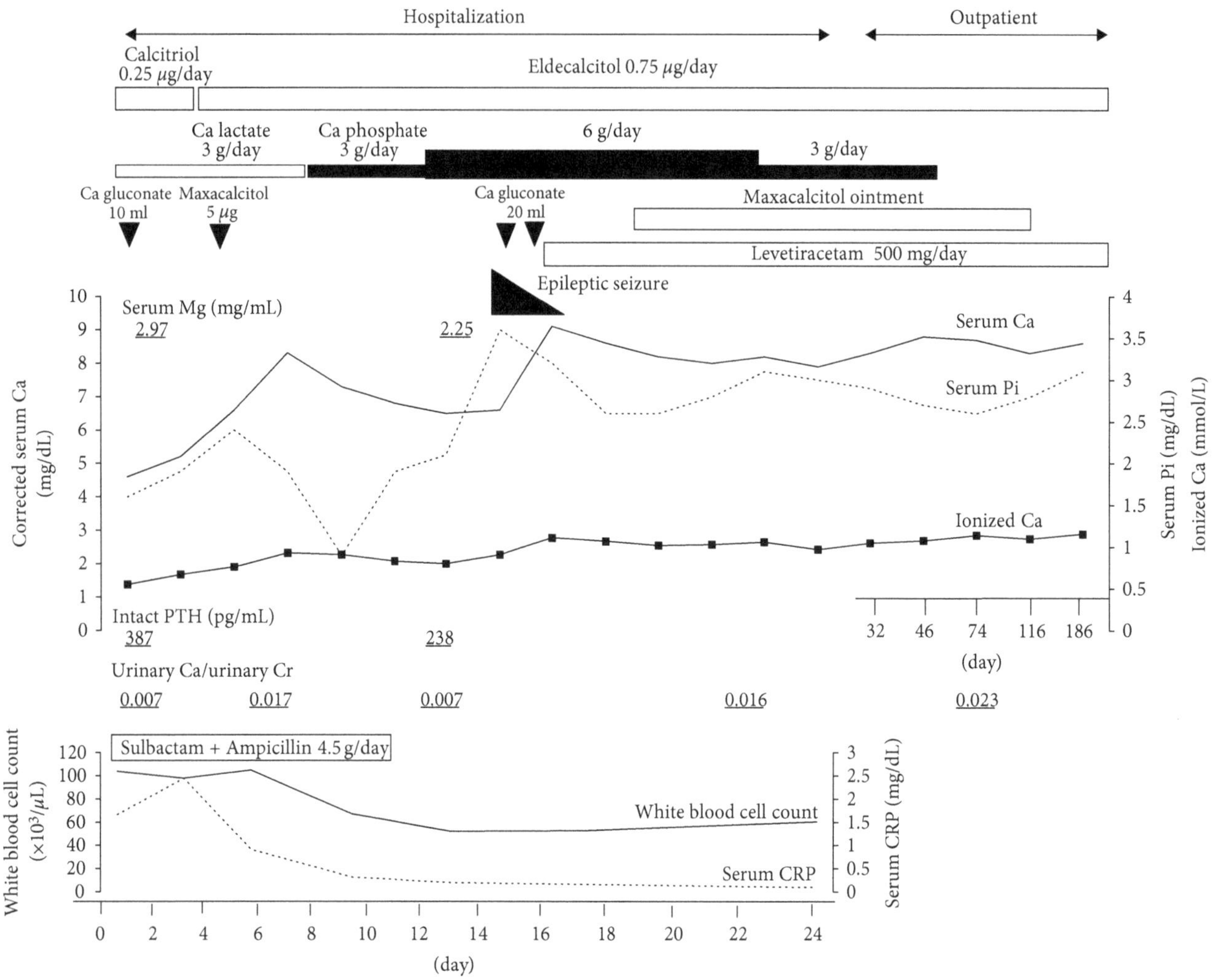

FIGURE 2: Patient's clinical course before and after the combined medical treatment. Ca, calcium; Cr, creatinine; CRP, C-reactive protein; PTH, parathyroid hormone; Pi, phosphate; Mg, magnesium.

range. While continuing intravenous Ca gluconate and oral administration of calcitriol and Ca supplement, we administered maxacalcitol ointment, another VDRA used for psoriasis. Maxacalcitol was applied to trunk and limbs twice daily with less than 10 g/day. The absorption rate, maximum drug concentration time, and biological half-life of maxacalcitol ointment are 83.1%, 3 h, and 2–4 h, respectively. An epileptic seizure occurred on the 15th hospital day when his serum Ca level was still below the lower reference limit. The seizure episode might also have been caused by his prolonged hypocalcemia or might have been related to his history of traumatic subarachnoid hemorrhage. Thereafter, oral administration of levetiracetam was started.

After those combined treatment, his serum corrected Ca level finally increased up to 8.2 mg/dL, and his serum phosphate level increased from 1.6 mg/dL to 3.1 mg/dL. After his serum Ca and phosphate levels were stabilized, he was discharged on the 24th hospital day. At 3 months after discharge, he was in the nursing home without relapse of hypocalcemia, followed by discontinuation of maxacalcitol ointment. With continuous eldecalcitol administration only, his serum Ca level remained stable after 5 months.

3. Discussion

In the present case, we successfully treated vitamin D deficiency-induced hypocalcemia and seizure associated with phenytoin use and lack of sunlight exposure in an older patient without CKD, who had a history of traumatic subarachnoidal hemorrhage. Our treatment protocol included administering Ca preparations, oral eldecalcitol, and maxacalcitol ointments, and discontinuation of phenytoin. After 24 days of these combined treatments, the patient's serum Ca level normalized, and no further seizures occurred.

Hypocalcemia has many causes and results primarily from inadequate PTH secretion or PTH resistance, vitamin D deficiency or vitamin D resistance, abnormal magnesium metabolism, and extravascular deposition of Ca salts, which can occur with several medical conditions [16, 17]. In our patient, serum levels of PTH and alkaline phosphatase were elevated and fractional excretion of Ca was very low, while serum levels of magnesium and calcitriol were within the reference ranges, indicating that the parathyroid gland was functioning normally in response to the hypocalcemia, and that the kidneys were acting to enhance tubular Ca reabsorption. Bone formation was slightly increased in response to increased serum intact PTH, whereas bone resorption was decreased judging from the serum tartrate-resistant acid phosphatase-5b. Importantly, serum 25-hydroxyvitamin D level was extremely low, indicating that 25-hydroxyvitamin D deficiency was the primary cause of the hypocalcemia in our patient, and that all other changes in the serum and urine mineral markers were secondary.

There were two possible reasons for the 25-hydroxyvitamin D deficiency. One is the long-term use of phenytoin to prevent seizure secondary to the previous traumatic subarachnoid hemorrhage, because AEDs including phenytoin accelerate 24-hydroxylase activity and thereby decrease serum 25-hydroxyvitamin D level, inducing hypocalcemia [18, 19]. There are no past reports about other effects of AEDs on Ca metabolism; however, AEDs may have other potential influence on Ca metabolism, such as decreasing Ca absorption from the gastrointestinal tract or reducing cellular sensitivity to PTH in the parathyroid gland. Another factor affecting the low serum calcitriol level might have been that our patient was bedridden and had less opportunity for sunlight exposure; 25-hydroxyvitamin D is partially derived from vitamin D_3 produced in the skin in response to sunlight exposure. Because older patients with histories of stroke or other brain disorders are often bedridden and treated with AEDs to prevent symptomatic epilepsy, these patients are at increased risk of 25-hydroxyvitamin D deficiency-induced hypocalcemia. Because today's population is aging rapidly, leading to increased numbers of older people in nursing homes who are experiencing decreased activity, the chances of a similar clinical scenario are also increased in clinical practice. Our case highlights the importance of periodic monitoring of serum Ca levels to prevent the severe hypocalcemia induced by vitamin D deficiency.

Treatment strategies for hypocalcemia differ depending on the severity and mode of onset of hypocalcemia. As a replacement therapy for vitamin D deficiency, we selected eldecalcitol, which has a higher binding ability to vitamin D binding protein (DBP) [13, 14]. Because non-protein-bound vitamin D is easily catabolized locally or in the liver, complex of 25-hydroxyvitamin D and DBP is resistant to degradation. Generally, eldecalcitol is usually used for osteoporosis and potentially increases serum Ca level; 0.88% of patients treated with eldecalcitol for osteoporosis developed hypercalcemia during the course of treatment [20]. Actually, based on our previous study, we think that patients treated with eldecalcitol are likely to develop hypercalcemia and acute kidney injury more frequently than has been reported, especially female patients with lower body weight [21]. Therefore, eldecalcitol may be more useful than calcitriol when treating patients with hypocalcemia. Using concurrent maxacalcitol ointment, we successfully controlled serum Ca levels within the reference range. As for maxacalcitol ointment, hypercalcemia is a potential side effect because it is absorbed through skin and increases Ca absorption from the gastrointestinal tract [22]. In this regard, this maxacalcitol-related hypercalcemia may be wisely used to treat hypocalcemia, in some special conditions where oral administration of native vitamin D or 25-hydroxyvitamin D is not an option.

Our treatment strategy to treat vitamin D deficiency-induced hypocalcemia with VDRAs may not be accepted by some physicians. Actually, phenytoin-induced hypocalcemia should be treated with native vitamin D or 25-hydroxyvitamin D administration and discontinuation of phenytoin. However, both native vitamin D and 25-hydroxyvitamin D are not available as official drugs in Japan: only native vitamin D is available as supplement. Accordingly, we administered VDRAs instead of native vitamin D or 25-hydroxyvitamin D. In this regard, our strategy to use VDRAs for vitamin D deficiency-induced hypocalcemia could be justified in countries where native vitamin D and 25-hydroyvitamin D are not available. We also warn against the potential danger that VDRAs can induce hypercalcemia and hyperphosphatemia and should be cautiously used with a close monitoring of serum levels of Ca and phosphate.

Hypocalcemia might have contributed to the seizure that occurred 2 weeks prior to hospitalization and/or on the 15th hospital day. Unfortunately, the patient was in a nursing home at 2 weeks prior to the hospitalization and his attending physician did not examine his serum Ca level. Therefore, we were unable to know his serum Ca levels before hospitalization. This is a limitation of the present case. Importantly, hypocalcemia can cause seizures without concomitant tetany because low ionized Ca concentrations in the cerebrospinal fluid are associated with increased excitability in the central nervous system [2, 3]. In our case, vitamin D deficiency was probably a chronic condition due to the long history of phenytoin use and lack of sun exposure. Hence, we thought that there must have been some factors that triggered hypocalcemia-induced seizure. It is plausible that his excitability of the motor area was enhanced by superimposing metabolic factors such as infection-related fever on the vulnerable cerebral cortex, ultimately leading to the seizure episodes. Importantly, patients with a history of symptomatic epilepsy commonly receive AEDs and are at increased risk of AED-associated hypocalcemia, which may in turn lower the seizure threshold. Therefore, we must be aware that vitamin D deficiency-induced hypocalcemia could be caused by AEDs and consider this an old but very important differential diagnosis, especially when we encounter hypocalcemic older patients receiving AEDs.

In summary, we presented a case of severe symptomatic hypocalcemia caused by vitamin D deficiency, which was likely associated with the long-term use of phenytoin and lack of sunlight exposure in a nonCKD patient. Although the best strategy to treat phenytoin-induced hypocalcemia would be treatment with native vitamin D replacement and discontinuation of phenytoin, it is a treatment option to administer vitamin D receptor activators such as eldecalcitol and maxacalcitol ointment for severe hypocalcemic patients, especially in countries where native vitamin D or 25-hydroxyvitamin D is not available as treatment option. Besides, periodic monitoring of serum Ca levels is necessary to prevent severe symptomatic hypocalcemia induced by vitamin D deficiency in patients treated with AEDs.

Consent

Written informed consent was obtained from the patient for publication of this case report and accompanying images.

Acknowledgments

We thank Edanz Group (https://www.edanzediting.com) for editing a draft of this manuscript.

References

[1] J. F. Tohme and J. P. Bilezikian, "Hypocalcemic emergencies," *Endocrinology and Metabolism Clinics of North America*, vol. 22, no. 2, pp. 363–375, 1993.

[2] P. Han, B. J. Trinidad, and J. Shi, "Hypocalcemia-induced seizure: demystifying the calcium paradox," *ASN Neuro*, vol. 7, no. 2, pp. 1–9, 2015.

[3] E. C. Zuckermann and G. H. Glaser, "Anticonvulsive action of increased calcium concentration in cerebrospinal fluid," *Archives of Neurology*, vol. 29, no. 4, pp. 245–252, 1973.

[4] E. W. Moore, "Ionized calcium in normal serum, ultrafiltrates, and whole blood determined by ion-exchange electrodes," *Journal of Clinical Investigation*, vol. 49, no. 2, pp. 318–334, 1970.

[5] D. Riccardi and E. M. Brown, "Physiology and pathophysiology of the calcium-sensing receptor in the kidney," *American Journal of Physiology-Renal Physiology*, vol. 298, no. 3, pp. 485–499, 2010.

[6] A. S. Dusso, A. J. Brown, and E. Slatopolsky, "Vitamin D," *American Journal of Physiology-Renal Physiology*, vol. 289, no. 1, pp. 8–28, 2005.

[7] M. Cozzolino, A. Galassi, M. Apetrii, and A. Covic, "What would we like to know, and what do we not know about fibroblast growth factor 23?," *Journal of Nephrology*, vol. 24, no. 6, pp. 696–706, 2011.

[8] A. S. Dusso and M. Tokumoto, "Defective renal maintenance of the vitamin D endocrine system impairs vitamin D renoprotection: a downward spiral in kidney disease," *Kidney International*, vol. 79, no. 7, pp. 715–729, 2011.

[9] J. M. Pascussi, A. Robert, M. Nguyen et al., "Possible involvement of pregnane X receptor-enhanced CYP24 expression in drug-induced osteomalacia," *Journal of Clinical Investigation*, vol. 115, no. 1, pp. 177–186, 2005.

[10] M. S. Cooper and N. J. Gittoes, "Diagnosis and management of hypocalcaemia," *BMJ*, vol. 336, no. 7656, pp. 1298–1302, 2008.

[11] A. Kelly and M. A. Levine, "Hypocalcemia in the critically ill patient," *Journal of Intensive Care Medicine*, vol. 28, no. 3, pp. 166–177, 2013.

[12] K. G. Tolman, W. Jubiz, J. J. Sannella et al., "Osteomalacia associated with anticonvulsant drug therapy in mentally retarded children," *Pediatrics*, vol. 56, no. 1, pp. 45–50, 1975.

[13] S. Hatakeyama, S. Nagashima, N. Imai et al., "Synthesis and biological evaluation of a 3-positon epimer of 1alpha, 25-dihydroxy-2beta-(3-hydroxypropoxy) vitamin D3 (ED-71)," *The Journal of Steroid Biochemistry and Molecular Biology*, vol. 103, no. 3–5, pp. 222–226, 2007.

[14] H. Kawate, Y. Noguchi, M. Nomura, and R. Takayanagi, "Eldecalcitol for the treatment of osteoporosis," *Clinical Interventions in Aging*, vol. 8, pp. 1312–1321, 2013.

[15] A.-M. Kissmeyer, I. S. Mathiasen, S. Latini, and L. Binderup, "Pharmacokinetic studies of vitamin D analogues: relationship to vitamin D binding protein (DBP)," *Endocrine*, vol. 3, no. 4, pp. 263–266, 1995.

[16] F. M. Hannan and R. V. Thakker, "Investigating hypocalcaemia," *BMJ*, vol. 346, no. 1, pp. f2213–f2213, 2013.

[17] J. Fong and A. Khan, "Hypocalcemia: updates in diagnosis and management for primary care," *Canadian Family Physician*, vol. 58, no. 2, pp. 158–162, 2012.

[18] M. Kawaguchi, Y. Mitsuhashi, and S. Kondo, "Iatrogenic hypercalcemia due to vitamin D3 ointment (1,24(OH)2D3) combined with thiazide diuretics in a case of psoriasis," *Journal Dermatology*, vol. 30, no. 11, pp. 801–804, 2003.

[19] G. Nseir, D. Golshayan, and F. Barbey, "Phenytoin-associated severe hypocalcemia with seizures in a patient with a TSC2-PKD1 contiguous gene syndrome," *Renal Failure*, vol. 35, no. 6, pp. 866–868, 2013.

[20] H. Saito, H. Kakihata, Y. Nishida et al., "The safety and effectiveness profile of eldecalcitol in a prospective, post-marketing observational study in Japanese patients with osteoporosis: interim report," *Journal of Bone and Mineral Metabolism*, vol. 35, no. 4, pp. 456–463, 2017.

[21] S. Aihara, S. Yamada, H. Oka et al., "Hypercalcemia and acute kidney injury induced by eldecalcitol in patients with osteoporosis: a case series of 32 patients at a single facility," *Renal Failure*, vol. 41, no. 1, pp. 88–97, 2019.

[22] S. Ohigashi, I. Tatsuno, D. Uchida et al., "Topical treatment with 22-oxacalcitriol (OCT), a new vitamin D analogue, caused severe hypercalcemia with exacerbation of chronic renal failure in a psoriatic patient with diabetic nephropathy; a case report and analysis of the potential for hypercalcemia," *Internal Medicine*, vol. 42, no. 12, pp. 1202–1205, 2003.

4

Acute Kidney Injury Secondary to Necrotizing Sarcoid Granulomatosis

Varun Mamidi, Manikantan Shekar, Jaiju James Chakola, Vamsi Krishna Makkena, and Jayakumar Matcha

Department of Nephrology, Sri Ramachandra Institute of Higher Education and Research, Chennai, India

Correspondence should be addressed to Manikantan Shekar; dr_manishekar@yahoo.com

Academic Editor: Ricardo Enríquez

Background. Sarcoidosis is a chronic disease characterized by noncaseating lesions involving any organ and tissue in the body. Hypercalcemia and acute kidney injury is a common renal presentation of sarcoidosis. Necrotizing sarcoid granulomatosis (NSG) is a granulomatous disease entity which presents with nodular masses of sarcoid like granuloma which primarily effects the lungs. It is a rare necrotizing variant of sarcoidosis. Extra pulmonary presentation of NSG is very rare. *Case presentation.* We present a 36-year-old female with hypercalcemia and acute kidney injury refractory to treatment. Whole body Flourine-18-fluorodeoxyglucose positron emission tomography computed tomography (18F-FDG PET/CT) showed increased metabolic uptake with ill-defined lesions in the liver, spleen, and pelvic lymph nodes. Biopsy of the ill-defined lesions in the liver showed necrotizing granulomatous lesions without angiitis. All the markers of tuberculosis were negative and angiotensin converting enzyme levels were elevated. Patient improved with 1 mg/kg/day oral steroid therapy and is on regular follow-up with minimal dose of steroids. *Conclusion.* Necrotizing sarcoid granulomatosis (NSG) is a rare systemic granulomatous disease. Due to its rarity and diagnostic difficulty, treatment is challenging for clinicians, pathologists and radiologists. Treatment of choice for symptomatic patients is steroid therapy. Prognosis is good with complete recovery.

1. Introduction

Renal manifestations in sarcoidosis includes acute interstitial nephritis, altered calcium metabolism, and rarely caused by glomerular disease and obstructive uropathy. The prevalence of hypercalcemia in sarcoidosis is variable with an accepted range of 10–20% and clinically has a wide spectrum of presentations [1]. Hypercalcemia is defined as serum calcium concentration more than two standard deviations above the mean values found in individuals with normal calcium levels [2]. The two most common causes of hypercalcemia seen in about 90% of all cases are malignancy and primary hyperparathyroidism. The remaining 10% incidence is due to other disorders such as familial hypocalciuric hypercalcemia, tertiary hyperparathyroidism, hyperthyroidism, drug effects, sarcoidosis, tuberculosis, and immobilization [3]. Sarcoidosis, characterized by noncaseating granulomas, can affect any organ and tissue in the body and is a chronic multisystem disorder. Necrotizing sarcoid granulomatosis (NSG) is a granulomatous disease entity which presents with nodular masses of sarcoid like granuloma with necrosis and granulomatous angiitis which primarily effects the lungs with rare extra pulmonary involvement. Approximately, only 200 cases of NSG have been reported after its first description [4]. Here, we report a case of a middle age female presenting with hypercalcemia causing acute kidney injury secondary to this rare variant of granulomatous disease.

2. Case Presentation

A 36-year-old female with history of diabetes and hypertension presented with complaints of pain in the abdomen and fatigue for a duration of one month. She denied history of vomiting, diarrhoea, fever, chills, rashes, haematuria, cough, weight loss, chest pain, and shortness of breath. On examination, vitals were stable. General and systemic examination was also normal.

Laboratory investigations revealed the total serum calcium of 13.2 mg/dl, with corrected calcium of 14.4 mg/dl and a low

Table 1: Laboratory values.

Test name	Result	Normal range
Hemoglobin (gm/dl)	9.8	12.0–15.0
Total count (cells/cumm)	10800	4000–11000
Polymorphs	78.6%	45%–70%
Lymphocytes	8.3%	25% –40%
Eosinophils	3.7%	1%–6%
Basophils	0.2%	0%–1%
Platelet count (lakhs/cumm)	4.35	1.5–4.5
Blood urea nitrogen (mg/dl)	22	5–21
Serum creatinine (mg/dl)	2.4	0.60–1.10
Serum sodium (mmol/l)	134	136–146
Serum potassium (mmol/l)	3.6	3.5–5.1
Serum chloride (mmol/l)	98	101–109
Serum bicarbonate (mmol/l)	26	21–31
Serum calcium (mg/dl)	13.2	8.8–10.6
Serum phosphorus (mg/dl)	4.0	2.5–4.5
Serum uric acid (mg/dl)	11.1	2.6–6.0
Serum intact parathyroid hormone (IPTH) (pg/ml)	6.8	12–88
Serum vitamin D (25OH) (ng/ml)	9.9	<20
Serum vitamin D3 (125OH) (ng/ml)	37.6	19.6–54.3
Random plasma glucose (mg/dl)	109	70–140
Urine colour	Straw yellow/ clear	
Urine pH	6.0	4.6–8
Urine specific gravity	1.005	1.001–1.035
Urine glucose	Negative	Negative
Urine protein	Negative	Negative
Urine bilirubin	Negative	Negative
Urine ketone	Negative	Negative
Urine urobilinogen (Eu/dl)	0.2	0.2–1.0
Urine pus cells (cells/hpf)	2–3	<5 cells
Urine RBC (cells/hpf)	Nil	0–2
Urine epithelial cells (cells/hpf)	2–3	0–4
Urine casts (cells/hpf)	Nil	Nil
Urine crystals (cells/hpf)	Nil	Nil
Urine protein creatinine ratio (mg/mmol)	0.90	<0.3
24 h Urine calcium (mg/day)	160	<250 mg/day
Urine bence jones protein	Negative	Negative
Total bilirubin (mg/dl)	0.67	0.3–1.2
Direct bilirubin (mg/dl)	0.20	<0.2
SGOT (U/L)	19	<35
SGPT (U/L)	16	<35
Total protein (gm/dl)	6.8	6.6–8.3
Albumin (gm/dl)	2.8	3.5–5.2
Globulin (gm/dl)	4.0	2.0–3.5
Alkaline phosphatase (U/L)	286	30–120

Table 1: Continued.

Test name	Result	Normal range
ANA	Negative	Negative
C3 (mg/dl)	164.0	90–180
C4 (mg/dl)	55.70	10–40
PR3–ANCA by ELISA	<1:40	<1:40–Negative
MPO – ANCA by ELISA	<1:40	<1:40–Negative
FT3 (pmol/l)	2.92	2.5–3.9
FT4 pmol/l)	1.38	0.56–1.50
TSH (mU/L)	1.660	0.34–5.60
Carcino embryonic antigen (CEA) (mcg/l)	1.3	<3.0
Alpha feto protein (mcg/l)	1.15	<0.9
Angiotensin converting enzyme levels (ACE) (nmol/ml)	119	
HIV	Nonreactive	Nonreactive
HBSAG	Nonreactive	Nonreactive
HCV	Nonreactive	Nonreactive
Peripheral smear	Normocytic Normochromic Anemia	

intact parathyroid hormone level (IPTH) of 6.8 pg/dl, and serum creatinine of 2.4 mg/dl. She denied to a history of calcium supplements intake. The serum vitamin D3 (125OH) levels are 37.6 ng/ml and vitamin D (25OH) levels are 9.9 ng/ml. The PTHrP levels could not be tested due to unavailability of the test. Work up for multiple myeloma, thyrotoxicosis, and tumor markers were negative. Table 1 shows the relevant laboratory investigations performed. Ultrasound of the abdomen showed increased echotexture of liver, normal kidney, and no other abnormalities. The patient was treated conservatively for hypercalcemia, hyperuricemia, and renal failure.

Since hypercalcemia and renal failure persisted even after treatment with intravenous fluids, diuretics, and calcitonin, a whole body flourine-18-fluorodeoxyglucose positron emission tomography computed tomography (18F-FDG PET/CT) was done which showed lesions with increased metabolic activity in the liver, spleen, and left internal iliac, left external iliac, right internal iliac lymph nodes as shown in Figure 1. Hence, CT—guided percutaneous biopsy of the liver lesions was done which showed necrotizing granulomatous inflammation with no features suggestive of vasculitis as shown in Figure 2.

Biopsy stain for fungi, AFB, TB PCR and blood TB QuantiFERON gold test was negative, but angiotensin converting enzyme (ACE) levels were elevated (119 mcl, Normal range: 8–53 mcl).

The patient was diagnosed with sarcoidosis of liver with necrotizing granulomatous lesions which is a rare variant of sarcoidosis. The patient was started on 1 mg/kg/day prednisolone. After one month follow up the patient was symptomatically better with normal calcium levels (8.6 mg/dl), reduced ACE levels (<50 mcl) and with serum creatinine of 0.9 mg/dl (eGFR- 82 ml/min/1.73m2). Steroids were tapered after one month and presently she is on a regular follow up with minimal dose of steroids.

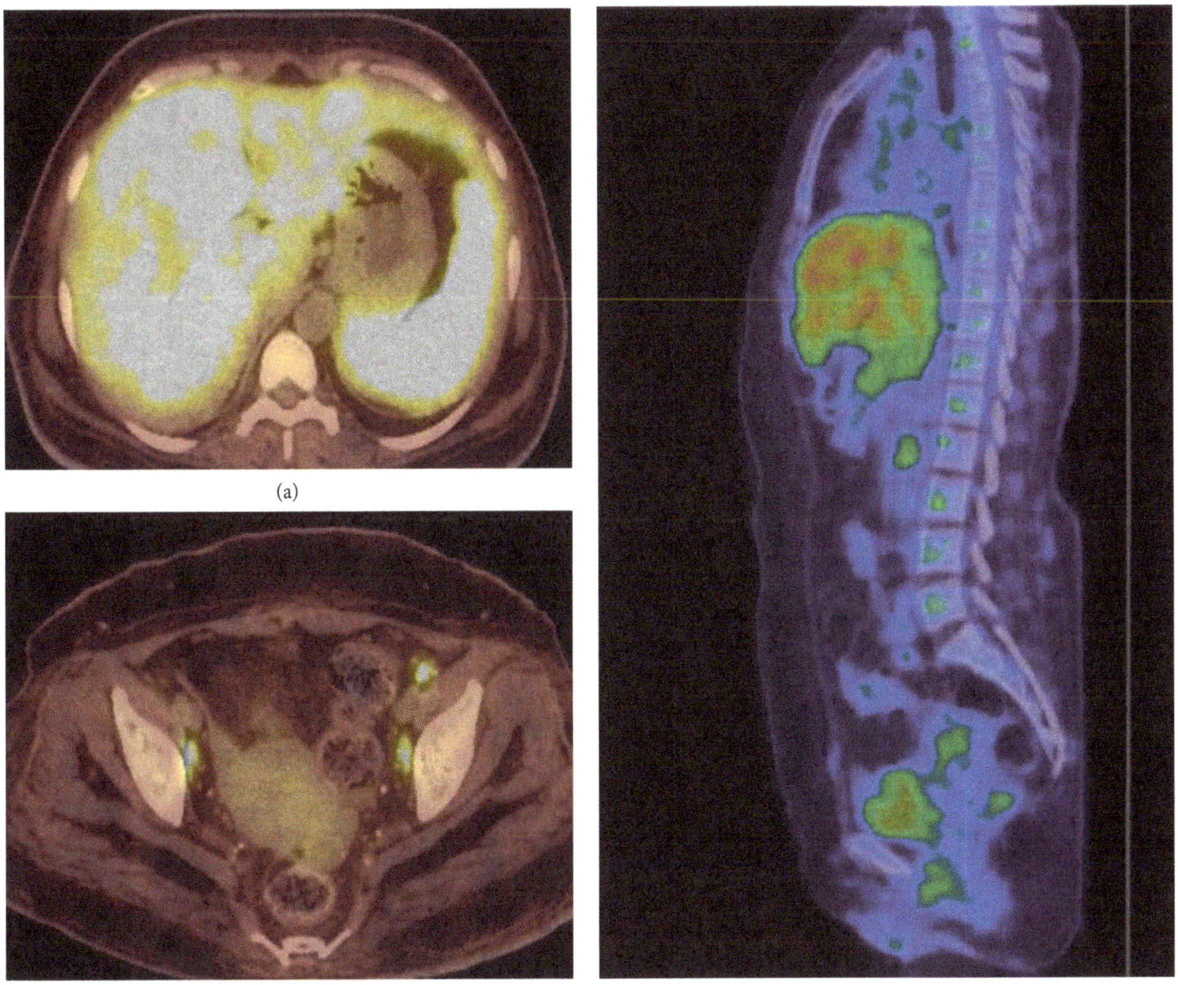

(a) (b) (c)

FIGURE 1: Whole body Flourine-18-fluorodeoxyglucose positron emission tomography/computed tomography (18F-FDG PET/CT). (a) Coronal PET/CT abdomen showing enlarged liver and spleen with multiple ill-defined FDG avid lesions. (b) Coronal PET/CT abdomen showing FDG avidity in few small pelvic lymph nodes. (c) Whole body sagittal PET/CT showing FDG avidity in the liver, spleen and pelvic lymph nodes.

3. Discussion

Granulomatous disease can either be due to infectious or a noninfectious aetiology and it commonly affects the lungs. Infectious aetiology can be due to tuberculosis, nontuberculous mycobacteria, fungi, some bacteria, and parasites (dirofilaria). Noninfectious causes include sarcoidosis, hypersensitivity pneumonitis, berylliosis, aspiration pneumonia, Wegener's granulomatosis, churg-strauss syndrome or other systemic diseases [5]. Well-formed nonnecrotizing granulomas are seen in sarcoidosis, whereas presence of necrosis signifies infection or Wegener granulomatosis [6].

Necrotizing sarcoid granuloma (NSG) is a rare controversial entity showing features that lie in between sarcoidosis and Wegener granulomatosis. These are sarcoid like granulomas with extensive necrosis and vasculitis. It was first reported by Dr. Averill A. Liebow in a series of 11 patients in 1973 [7]. He speculated that NSG may be a form of angiocentric granulomatosis showing a far better prognosis, in contrast to the other forms, or that it may be a variant of sarcoidosis [6].

There are around 200 reported cases of NSG in the last 43 years [4]. There are only 3 case reports of extrapulmonary NSG involving the liver [8–10] and only one case report with NSG liver presenting with hypercalcemia [8]. According to Karpathiou et al., median age at diagnosis was 42 years with female predominance. Clinical manifestations in NSG are mild compared to other necrotizing granulomatous diseases such as tuberculosis. The usual clinical manifestations are cough, fever, dyspnoea, weight loss, night sweats, and fatigue. About 40% can be asymptomatic at presentation. Usually it affects the lungs, the subcutaneous tissue of the skin, the kidney, the gastrointestinal tract, the liver, and the spinal cord may also be involved. Extrapulmonary manifestations are seen in 30% of the patients and involvement of the liver is very rare. Histologically, it shows a triad of sarcoid granulomas, vasculitis, and large areas of necrosis. On imaging a solitary mass, hyperfixating in PET scan is often seen. Differential diagnosis includes nodular sarcoidosis, Wegener's granulomatosis, and tuberculosis [6]. In our case, it was a 36-year-old female with pain in the abdomen and fatigue. Patient had extra pulmonary

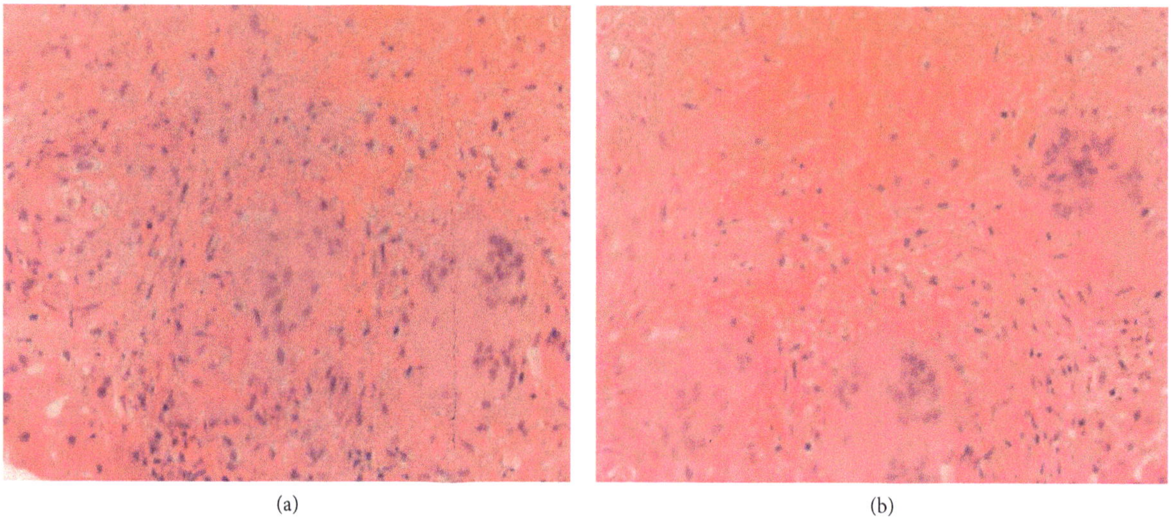

FIGURE 2: Histopathology findings. (a and b) Liver biopsy showing multifocal nodular granulomatous inflammation with central necrosis and giant cells.

TABLE 2: Teaching points.

(1) Necrotizing sarcoid granuloma (NSG) is a rare controversial entity showing features that lie in between sarcoidosis and Wegener granulomatosis with sarcoid like granulomas and extensive necrosis.
(2) The usual clinical manifestations are cough, fever, dyspnea, weight loss, night sweats, fatigue. About 40% can be asymptomatic at presentation. Extra pulmonary manifestations are seen in 30% of the patients and involvement of liver is very rare.
(3) Histologically, it shows a triad of sarcoid granulomas, vasculitis and large areas of necrosis. On Imaging a solitary mass hyperfixating in PET Scan is often seen. Differential diagnosis includes nodular sarcoidosis, Wegener's granulomatosis and tuberculosis.
(4) Corticosteroids are mainstay of treatment. Prednisone (1 mg/kg/day) tapered over several weeks to months is recommended. In steroid resistant cases azathioprine, methotrexate and hydroxychloroquine may be used.
(5) Due to its rarity and diagnostic difficulty, treatment is challenging for clinicians, pathologists and radiologists. Prognosis is good, but relapse is common.

involvement with NSG in the liver diagnosed by 18F-FDG PET-CT and histology.

The key histopathologic features of NSG includes vasculitis, granuloma with necrosis, and giant cell infiltrations [4]. Very rarely it may lack these features [6]. In the histopathology of the present case vasculitis was not apparent. However, features such as biopsy of liver showing granulomas with necrosis and giant cells, hypercalcemia, elevated ACE levels, response to steroids, negative workup for other causes for hypercalcemia, and renal failure clench the diagnosis of NGS in this case.

Mechanism of hypercalcemia in sarcoidosis is due to increased 1α-hydroxylase activity in the alveolar macrophages. Hence there is excessive calcitriol synthesis resulting in increased intestinal calcium absorption. Hypercalcemia is rare in extra pulmonary involvement. Our patient had no pulmonary involvement and had low 25-OH vitamin D levels and normal calcitriol levels with possibility suggesting increased calcitriol production in extra pulmonary granulomatous tissue such as the liver. Possibility of occult pulmonary disease should be considered even though work up for pulmonary involvement was negative [8].

Regardless of the aetiology, the clinical features of hypercalcemia are the same. Hypercalcemia can present with symptoms involving many organ systems such as dehydration, nausea, vomiting, abdominal pain, and mental confusion. Several mechanisms involved with acute kidney injury in the context of hypercalcemia include prerenal involvement, direct alterations in vascular tone, and glomerular permeability. Due to this direct vasoconstrictive effect of calcium the renal consequences that occur are: arteriolar vasoconstriction, reduction in glomerular ultrafiltration coefficient (Kf), reduction in tubular sodium reabsorption, nephrogenic diabetes insipidus, prerenal azotaemia, acute tubular necrosis, nephrocalcinosis, and tubulointerstitial fibrosis [11]. This intrarenal vasoconstriction is also one of the mechanism of renal toxicity in rhabdomyolysis [12]. In the present case both prerenal involvement or direct vasoconstrictive effect of the calcium ion on vascular smooth muscle can be the probable mechanism of AKI secondary to hypercalcemia.

According to literature ACE level is used to monitor the disease activity in sarcoidosis. With hypercalcemia as a major clinical manifestation, calcitriol level may be useful in guiding therapy. According to a case report by Priyadarshini B et al., patient presenting with hypercalcemia as major clinical manifestation and has persistently elevated ACE level, calcitriol level monitoring can help guide steroid dose and provide the potential to prevent symptomatic hypercalcemia. In acute setting calcitriol level monitoring will help to guide steroid therapy whereas ACE levels may be useful for chronic disease monitoring rather than treatment guidance when sarcoidosis is associated with hypercalcemia [8].

Corticosteroids are mainstay of treatment. Prednisone (1 mg/kg/day) tapered over several weeks to months is recommended. In steroid resistant cases azathioprine, methotrexate, and hydroxychloroquine may be used (Table 2). There are no gold standard tests to monitor therapy. Over all prognosis for NSG is good and depends on gender, race, age, organ involvement, and presenting clinical manifestations.

4. Conclusion

Necrotizing sarcoid granulomatosis (NSG) is a rare systemic granulomatous disease. Histologically NSG is defined by sarcoid-like granulomas, granulomatous vasculitis and necrosis superimposed on confluent granulomas [13]. Clinical presentation is nonspecific. Due to its rarity and diagnostic difficulty, treatment is challenging for clinicians, pathologists, and radiologists (Table 2). Treatment of choice is steroids. Prognosis is good, but relapse is common.

Abbreviations

NSG: Necrotizing sarcoid granulomatosis
18F-FDG PET/CT: Flourine-18-fluorodeoxyglucose positron emission tomography computed tomography
IPTH: Intact parathyroid hormone level
AFB: Acid fast bacilli test
TB: Tuberculosis
TB PCR: Tuberculous polymerase chain reaction
ACE: Angiotensin converting enzyme
eGFR: Estimated glomerular filtration rate.

Consent

The patient has been informed about the publication of case report and his written consent for publication of case report has been taken.

References

[1] A. R. Berliner, M. Haas, and M. J. Choi, "Sarcoidosis: the nephrologist's perspective perspective," *American Journal of Kidney Diseases*, vol. 48, no. 5, pp. 856–870, 2006.

[2] S. Minisola, J. Pepe, and S. Piemonte, "The diagnosis and management of hypercalcemia," *BMJ*, vol. 350, p. h2723, 2015.

[3] F. W. Lafferty, "Differential diagnosis of hypercalcemia," *Journal of Bone and Mineral Research*, vol. 6, no. S2, pp. S51–S59, 1991.

[4] T. Shibata, K. Takahashi, M. Uchida, F. Yamasaki, M. Kawashima, and A. N. Sueoka, "Necrotizing sarcoid granulomatosis with natural resolution after a surgical lung biopsy," *Internal Medicine*, vol. 57, no. 11, pp. 1625–1629, 2018.

[5] S. Mukhopadhyay and A. A. Gal, "Granulomatous lung disease: an approach to the differential diagnosis," *Archives of Pathology & Laboratory Medicine*, vol. 134, no. 5, pp. 667–690, 2010.

[6] G. Karpathiou, A. Batistatou, and P. Boglou, "Necrotizing sarcoid granulomatosis: A distinctive form of pulmonary granulomatous disease," *The Clinical Respiratory Journal*, vol. 12, pp. 1313–1319, 2018.

[7] A. A. Liebow, "The J. Burns Amberson lecture—pulmonary angiitis and granulomatosis," *American Review of Respiratory Disease*, vol. 108, no. 1, pp. 1–18, 1973.

[8] P. Balasubramanian, D. K. Kadayakkara, and G. Soloway, "Calcitriol mediated hypercalcemia due to necrotizing sarcoid granuloma of liver," *International Journal of Case Reports and Images*, vol. 8, no. 7, pp. 458–461, 2017.

[9] N. Momah, A. Otesile, and R. Pawa, "Sarcoidosis presenting as necrotizing sarcoid granulomatosis of liver, sclerosing cholangitis, and gastric ulcer," *ACG Case Reports Journal*, vol. 1, no. 3, pp. 164–166, 2014.

[10] F. Binesh, H. Halvani, and H. Navabii, "Systemic sarcoidosis with caseating granuloma," *BMJ Case Reports*, vol. 2012, p. brc0520114278, 2012.

[11] M. Moyses-Neto, F. M. Guimaraes, F. H. Ayoub, O. M. Vieira-Neto, J. A. C. Costa, and M. Dantas, "Acute renal failure and hypercalcemia," *Ren Failure*, vol. 28, no. 2, pp. 153–159, 2006.

[12] V. Mamidi, E. Indumathi, M. Shekar et al., "Pigment nephropathy in a patient with *PYGM* gene mutation," *Kidney International Reports*, vol. 4, no. 5, pp. 740–744, 2019.

[13] J. Yeboah, M. Afkhami, and C. Lee, "Necrotizing sarcoid granulomatosis granulomatosis," *Current Opinion in Pulmonary Medicine*, vol. 18, pp. 493–498, 2012.

5

A Case of Rheumatoid Arthritis Presenting with Renal Thrombotic Microangiopathy Probably due to a Combination of Chronic Tacrolimus Arteriolopathy and Severe Hypertension

Fumika Honma,[1] Yoshihide Fujigaki,[1] Yoshikazu Nemoto,[1] Hirotoshi Kikuchi,[1] Michito Nagura,[1] Shigeyuki Arai,[1] Kenichi Ishizawa,[1] Osamu Yamazaki,[1] Yoshifuru Tamura,[1] Fukuo Kondo,[2] Ryuji Ohashi,[3] Shunya Uchida,[1] and Shigeru Shibata[1]

[1]*Department of Internal Medicine, Teikyo University School of Medicine, Itabashi-ku, Tokyo, Japan*
[2]*Department of Pathology, Teikyo University Hospital, Itabashi-ku, Tokyo, Japan*
[3]*Department of Diagnostic Pathology, Nippon Medical School Musashikosugi Hospital, Kawasaki, Kanagawa, Japan*

Correspondence should be addressed to Yoshihide Fujigaki; fujigaki@med.teikyo-u.ac.jp

Academic Editor: Rumeyza Kazancioglu

A 51-year-old woman with rheumatoid arthritis presented with mild hypertension 20 months after tacrolimus treatment and developing proteinuria 24 months after the treatment. Tacrolimus was discontinued 27 months after the treatment, followed by heavy proteinuria, accelerated hypertension, and deteriorating renal function without ocular fundus lesions as a clinical sign of malignant hypertension. Renal biopsy revealed malignant nephrosclerosis characterized by subacute and chronic thrombotic microangiopathy (TMA), involving small arteries, arterioles, and glomeruli. Focal segmental glomerulosclerosis, probably secondary to chronic TMA, was identified as a cause of heavy proteinuria. The zonal tubulointerstitial injury caused by subacute TMA may have mainly contributed to deteriorating renal function. The presence of nodular hyalinosis in arteriolar walls was indicative of tacrolimus-associated nephrotoxicity. Together with other antihypertensive drugs, administration of aliskiren stabilized renal function with reducing proteinuria. Owing to the preexisting proteinuria prior to severe hypertension and the complex renal histopathology, we postulated that chronic TMA, which was initially triggered by tacrolimus, was aggravated by severe hypertension, resulting in overt renal TMA.

1. Introduction

Thrombotic microangiopathy (TMA) is a pathologic term where vascular and glomerular lesions due to endothelial damage and vascular occlusion can be observed and is characterized by a clinical presentation with thrombocytopenia, hemolytic anemia, and organ injuries, including acute kidney injury (AKI) [1]. However, localized renal TMA without systemic manifestation of TMA exists and can be diagnosed only by renal biopsy.

Severe hypertension can induce TMA within the renal vasculature typically associated with fibrinoid necrosis of arterioles and the glomerular capillary tufts [2]. The exact mechanism remains to be established, but TMA may occur when vascular autoregulation cannot accommodate the severe hypertension-induced shear stress. Severe hypertension-induced TMA showed a low incidence of thrombocytopenia and hemolytic anemia [2]. Renal function may improve or stabilize in about 50 to 80% of patients of severe or malignant hypertension with or without biopsy-proven TMA upon adequate blood pressure (BP) control [2, 3].

Calcineurin inhibitor (cyclosporine and tacrolimus)-associated TMA is a rare but well documented cause of AKI [4, 5]. Calcineurin inhibitor-associated TMA is attributed to the endothelial injury secondary to vasoconstriction, which induces ischemia, increases platelet aggregation, and activates prothrombotic factors [6]. Calcineurin inhibitor-associated TMA may often localize to the renal graft in posttransplant

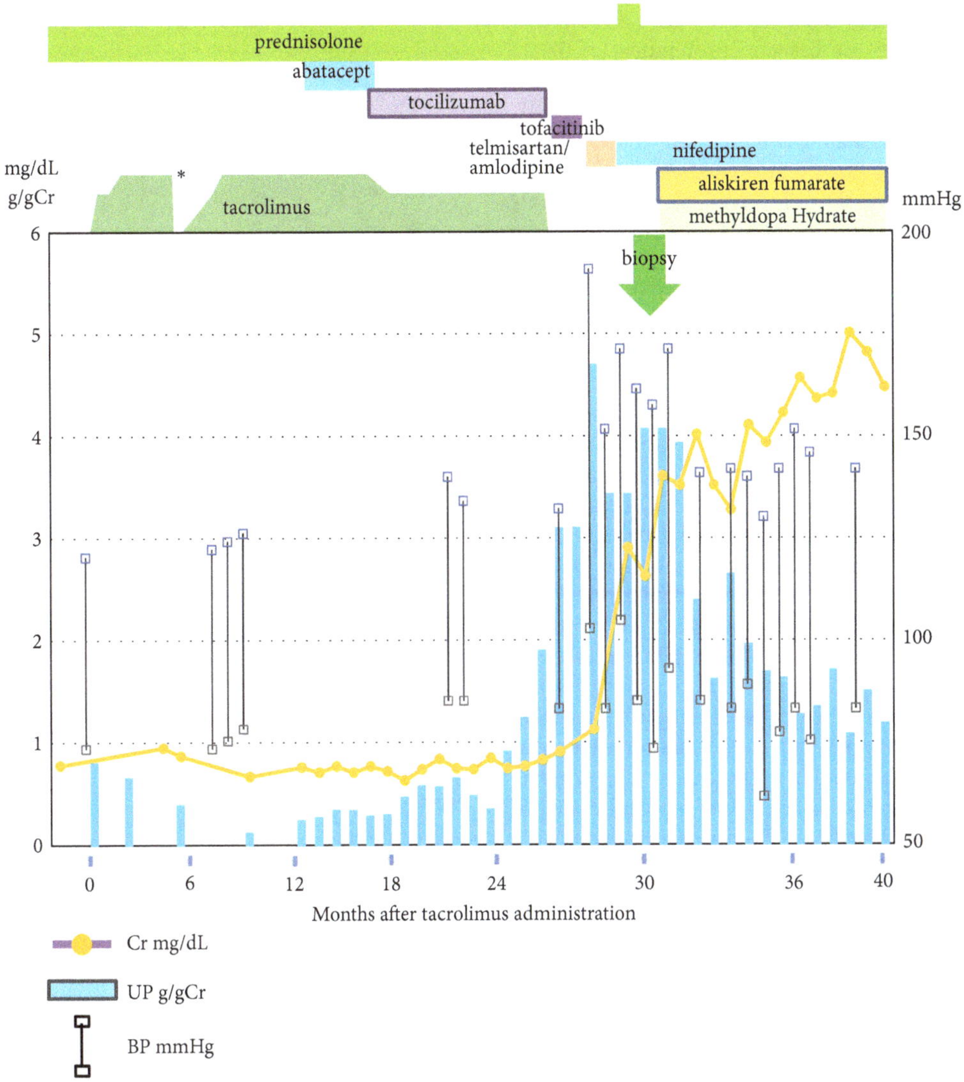

FIGURE 1: Clinical course of the patient after introduction of tacrolimus treatment. ∗: surgical operation, Cr; creatinine, UP; proteinuria, and BP; blood pressure.

patients and show AKI or delayed graft function with few or no systemic manifestations of TMA [6]. Discontinuation or reduced dose of calcineurin inhibitor is the main treatment of calcineurin inhibitor-associated TMA [7].

Severe hypertension may be either a cause of TMA or a manifestation of renal involvement from an underlying TMA. About 20-40% of patients with severe/malignant hypertension presented with TMA and/or microangiopathic hemolysis [3, 8]. Thus, concomitant renal TMA and severe hypertension could raise the differential diagnosis of TMA and lead to a vicious cycle.

Here, we describe a patient of rheumatoid arthritis (RA) with a most recent history of long-term tacrolimus use, who presented with localized renal TMA in association with clinical feature of developing heavy proteinuria and severe hypertension, subsequently deteriorating renal function. We assumed that renal TMA in our case may be caused by a combination of chronic tacrolimus arteriolopathy and subsequent severe hypertension.

2. Case Report

A 51-year-old Japanese woman was admitted to our hospital for the evaluation of heavy proteinuria, deteriorating renal function, and severe hypertension. She had a medical history of RA at the age of 42 and left vitrectomy for retinal detachment and bilateral femoral head replacement following fracture at the age of 49. Since she had drug allergies to many drugs, various treatments for RA were tried to introduce including methotrexate, infliximab, etanercept, salazosulfapyridine, leflunomide, bucillamine, tacrolimus, abatacept, and/or tocilizumab in addition to prednisolone (PSL) and nonsteroidal anti-inflammatory drugs. She was treated with the dosage of 2 to 3 mg/day of tacrolimus, standard dose for RA in addition to PSL 8 mg/day from the age of 48 for 2 years and 3 months. Clinical course after introduction of tacrolimus is shown in Figure 1. BP was increased from 120/70 mmHg to 140/80 mmHg 20 months after tacrolimus treatment, trough levels of tacrolimus fell within acceptable ranges between 5 and 10 ng/dL during the course. Proteinuria began to increase from the baseline proteinuria of 0.3 to 0.5 g/g creatinine 24 months after tacrolimus treatment, but serum creatinine level was sustained around 0.8 mg/dL. Tacrolimus and tocilizumab were changed to tofacitinib citrate 27 months after tacrolimus treatment because of uncontrolled arthritis of RA. However, tofacitinib citrate was discontinued 2 months after the treatment because of allergic reaction. Proteinuria was further increased after discontinuation of tacrolimus and tocilizumab, and then severe hypertension 190/100 mmHg and progressive renal dysfunction developed. 40 mg telmisartan/5 mg amlodipine besilate combination tablet was introduced 2 months after tacrolimus discontinuation. Her renal function was further deteriorated to creatinine of 2.63 mg/dL; thus she was admitted to our hospital 3 months after tacrolimus discontinuation.

On admission, body temperature was 36.5°C, height 154.0 cm, weight 44.9 kg, BP 170/102 mmHg, and pulse rate 88/min. Physical examination showed numbness in hands, pain in the elbows, wrists, knees, and metacarpophalangeal (MP) joint of the right thumb finger, swelling of MP joint in the right second finger, and mild pitting edema in bilateral legs but no abdominal bruit. She had no focus of infection and sclerotic skin lesion and no experience of Raynaud's phenomenon. The laboratory data on admission are shown in Table 1. Urinary examination showed heavy proteinuria and microscopic hematuria. Urinary low-molecular-weight proteins and urinary N-acetyl-β-D-glucosaminidase were elevated. Blood examination showed anemia, hypoalbuminemia, renal dysfunction, and hypocalcemia. Immunological examination indicated normocomplementemia, normal tests for anti-DNA antibody, anticardiolipin antibody, and myeloperoxidase and proteinase 3-anti-neutrophil cytoplasmic antibodies, but positive tests for RA-associated factors including rheumatoid factor, matrix metalloproteinase-3, and anti-SS-A antibody. Repeated peripheral smears showed no evidence of hemolysis. Serum renin activity and aldosterone concentration were of high value. Her hypocalcemia could be explained by use of denosumab for the treatment of steroid-induced osteoporosis.

The electrocardiogram showed voltage criteria of left ventricular hypertrophy. Chest X-ray showed no apparent cardiomegaly and lung edema. Abdominal ultrasound detected normal shape and size in the kidneys and multiple hemangioma in the liver. Echocardiography revealed ejection fraction 56% Simpson method, ratio of E to e' 22.6, and left ventricular wall thickening. Fundoscopy did not show exudate hemorrhage and papilledema.

With a clinical suspicion of secondary amyloidosis, focal segmental glomerulosclerosis (FSGS), or malignant nephrosclerosis, renal biopsy was performed. A renal biopsy showed 5 glomeruli with adhesive lesions and segmental sclerosis or global sclerosis and 8 glomeruli with ischemic shrinkage of glomerular tufts out of 22 obtained glomeruli (Figures 2(a), 2(b), and 2(c)). Some of the remaining glomeruli showed collapse of capillary tufts (Figures 2(a) and 2(b)), FSGS (Figure 2(a)), and segmental thickening of capillary walls showing double contour (Figure 2(d)). There were extensive tubular atrophy and interstitial edema to fibrosis involving 70% of renal parenchyma, accompanied by chronic and acute inflammatory cell infiltration (Figures 2(a) and 2(b)). Distribution of the tubulointerstitial

Table 1: Laboratory data on admission.

Urinalysis
Gravity 1.014
pH 6.0
Protein 3+
Glucose (-)
Occult blood trace
Sediments
Red blood cell 1-4 /high power field
Wight blood cell 10-19 /high power field
Urine chemistry
Protein 245 mg/dL
Creatinine 60.2 mg/dL
N-acetyl-β-D-glucosaminidase 12.5 U/L
β2-microglobulin 40,066 μg/L
Complete blood count
WBC 15,000 /μL
Hb 10.6 g/dL
Platelet 36.8×10^4/μL
Blood chemistry
Albumin 2.7 g/dL
Lactate dehydrogenase 385 IU/L
Urea nitrogen 46.9 mg/dL
Creatinine 2.86 mg/dL
Uric acid 6.9 mg/dL
Na 139 mEq/L
K 3.4 mEq/L
Cl 103 mEq/L
Ca 6.8 mg/dL
Pi 1.8 mg/dL
Estimated GFR 14.7 ml/min/1.73m^2
Serology
HBs antigen 0.1 C.O.I
HCV antibody 0.1 C.O.I
IgG 621 mg/dL
IgA 251 mg/dL
IgM 152 mg/dL
CH50 60< U/mL
C3 110 mg/dL
C4 30 mg/dL
C-reactive protein 2.87 mg/dL
Rheumatoid factor 24.2 U/mL
MMP-3 413.8 ng/mL
Antinuclear antibody ×160 speckled
Anti-DNA antibody 0.6 IU/mL (<9.0)
Anti-SS-A antibody 89.7 U/ml (<6.0)
MPO-ANCA 1.0 U/mL (<3.4)
PR3-ANCA 1.0 U/mL (<3.4)
Anti-cardiolipin antibody (IgM) <8 U/mL

GFR; glomerular filtration rate, MMP-3; matrix metalloproteinase-3, MPO-ANCA; myeloperoxidase-anti-neutrophil cytoplasmic antibody, PR3-ANCA; proteinase 3-anti-neutrophil cytoplasmic antibody. The values in the parentheses show the normal range.

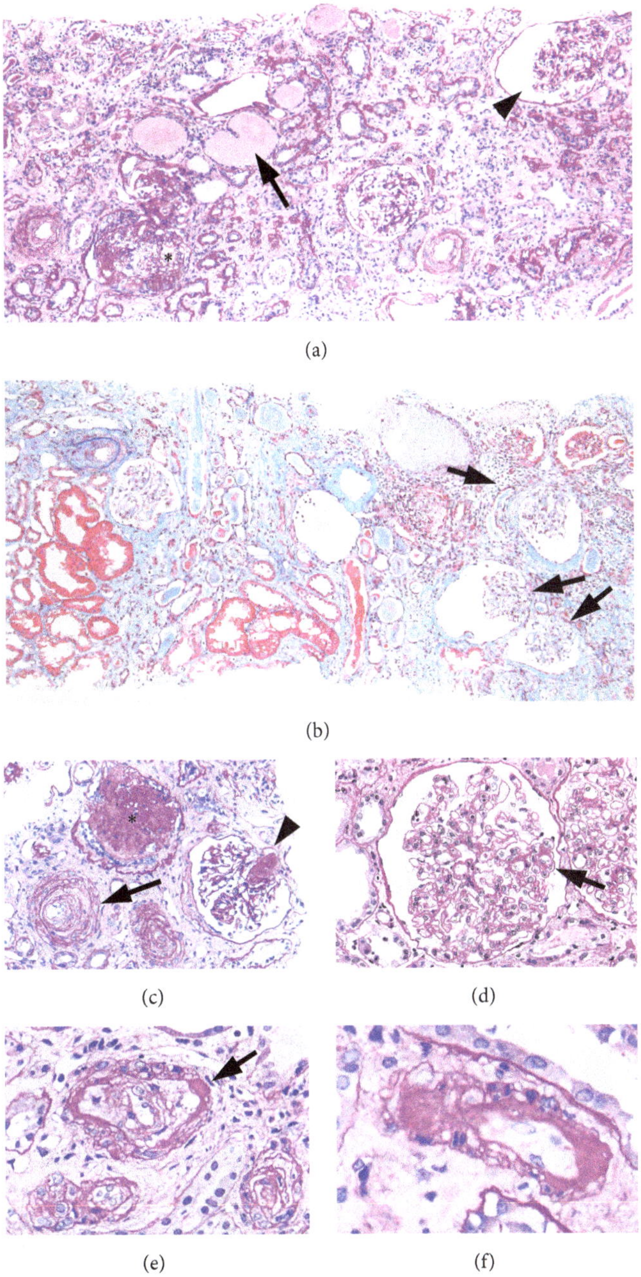

Figure 2: Light micrographs of renal tissues. (a) A glomerulus (asterisk) is mildly enlarged, showing focal segmental glomerulosclerosis while another glomerulus exhibits collapsed capillary tuft (arrowhead). Dilated tubules with flattened epithelial cells containing proteinaceous casts are present (arrow) (periodic acid-Schiff stain; original magnification x200). (b) Several glomeruli have collapsed capillary tufts (arrows). There is an extensive striped pattern of interstitial fibrosis and tubular atrophy (Elastica–Masson staining; original magnification x200). (c) A glomerulus is globally sclerotic (asterisk). There is organized thrombus formation within an afferent arteriolar lumen (arrowhead). Concentric intimal hyperplasia of arterioles forming "onion skin" lesion is noted (arrow) (periodic acid-Schiff stain; original magnification x200). (d) Glomerular capillary wall is segmentally thickened showing double contour (arrow) (periodic acid-Schiff stain; original magnification x400). (e) Arteriolar lumina are occluded by fibrous intimal thickening with recanalization. Nodular hyalinosis of arterial walls is noted (arrow) (periodic acid-Schiff stain; original magnification x400). (f) An arteriolar wall shows circumferential and transmural hyalinosis forming peripheral nodules (periodic acid-Schiff stain; original magnification x400).

damage was zonal, indicative of ischemic injury following vascular compromise (Figure 2(b)). The afferent arteriole of the glomerulus was occluded by an organized thrombus, and the arterioles showed concentric intimal hyperplasia forming "onion skin" lesion (Figure 2(c)). Some of the small arterial and arteriolar lumina were markedly narrowed by thickened fibrous intima (Figure 2(e)). Of note, some arteriolar walls exhibited circumferential and transmural nodular hyalinosis (Figures 2(e) and 2(f)). An immunofluorescence study showed nonspecific segmental staining of IgM, C1q, and C3 in glomeruli, and IgA and IgM in tubular casts. Electron microscopy revealed swollen glomerular endothelial cells with loss of fenestrations, irregularly thickened lamina rara interna, and foot process effacement involving 30% of podocytes (Figure 3). No electron dense deposit was identified. Collectively, these histological findings are suggestive of malignant nephrosclerosis and tubulointerstitial damage, represented by subacute/chronic TMA.

Severe hypertension and tacrolimus use were considered to be causes of TMA in our patient. Since tacrolimus had already been withdrawn, we tried to manage blood pressure on an appropriate level. It is reported that hypertension is highly prevalent among patients with RA, and use of anti-inflammatory analgesics and disease-modifying drugs with hypertensive potential, and yet to be determined inflammatory pathways, and genetic factors may synergistically lead to hypertension [9]. Nonsteroidal anti-inflammatory drugs and tofacitinib citrate [10] might have contributed to severe hypertension in our patient. However, it is more likely that her severe hypertension may have been caused by renal parenchymal damage with marked activation of renin-angiotensin-aldosterone system. To control severe hypertension, amlodipine besilate was changed to nifedipine. In addition, methyldopa and also aliskiren to inhibit renin-angiotensin system were introduced, then BP was gradually decreased. After aliskiren was administered, renin activity was reduced from 12 to 0.6 ng/mL/h and aldosterone concentration from 242 to 69.4 pg/mL in one week. Blood pressure and renal function eventually stabilized with gradual reduction of proteinuria. One year after renal biopsy, serum creatinine was 4.03 mg/dL and proteinuria was 1.0 g/g creatinine (Figure 1).

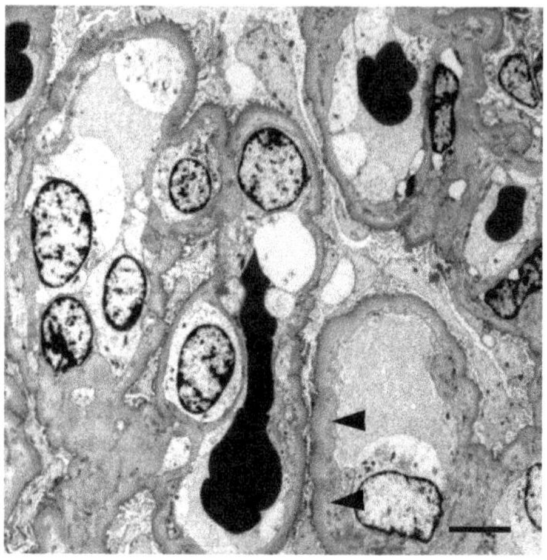

Figure 3: Electron micrograph of a glomerulus. Swollen glomerular endothelial cells with loss of fenestrations, irregularity thickened lamina rara interna with small remnants in the subendothelial spaces (arrowheads), and partial foot process effacement are seen. Bar=5.0 μm.

3. Discussion

Causes of TMA including hemolytic uremic syndrome, thrombotic thrombocytopenic purpura, and atypical hemolytic uremic syndrome, which were almost uniformly include thrombocytopenia and hemolytic anemia, were excluded in our patient. Thus, we did not examine ADAMTS13 (a disintegrin and metalloprotease with thrombospondin-1-like domains) activity. As for secondary TMA, she had no clinical evidence of infection. She had no skin lesion, and anti-SCL-70 and anti-centromere antibodies were negative 2 and a half years ago. This may support the fact that scleroderma renal crisis is excluded. Our patient had conditions including RA, tacrolimus use, and severe hypertension which could raise TMA. However, we postulated that renal TMA in our patient was not caused by severe hypertension alone but by a combination of chronic tacrolimus arteriolopathy and severe hypertension. This could be explained as follows.

First, our patient had severe hypertension, but the absence of fundus lesion, which did not fulfill the diagnosis of accelerated/malignant hypertension. Renal histology of accelerated/malignant hypertension shows TMA involving intrarenal fibrinoid necrosis of arterioles, containing the necrotic remnants of the smooth muscle cells as well as fibrin and platelet deposits [11]. Another type of lesion is a proliferative endarteritis of medium and small sized arteries and arterioles, containing proliferated smooth muscle cells and myofibroblasts. This lesion is called "onion skin" [11]. Though hyaline thrombus in one arteriole and onion skin in arterioles were observed in our patient, fibrinoid necrosis of renal arterioles, which is often observed in the acute phase of malignant hypertension-associated TMA, was not found. Signs of nephritis due to severe renal ischemia usually appear in parallel with severe hypertension in patients with malignant hypertension [11]. Unlike this clinical manifestation, our patient showed the development of proteinuria before severe hypertension occurred. These facts suggest that renal TMA was not merely caused by severe hypertension, but also by other exacerbating factors in the current case.

Second, the renal biopsy showed features of chronic TMA, characterized by double contours of glomerular capillary walls, and fibrous thickening of arterial walls with organized or recanalized thrombi, and nodular hyalinosis of arteriolar walls. Given the clinical course of the patient, the presence of these chronic changes cannot be explained by short-term severe hypertension alone. As these chronic lesions can reportedly be induced by calcineurin-associated nephrotoxicity [6, 12], it is probable that the chronic lesions of our case may have appeared as part of tacrolimus-associated TMA. It is reported that chronic calcineurin inhibitor nephrotoxicity is clinically characterized by hypertension, progressive renal insufficiency, and variable degree of proteinuria. Histologically, hyaline arteriolopathy, striped interstitial fibrosis with proportional tubular atrophy, and glomerulosclerosis are often found [12] like the present case. In calcineurin inhibitor-associated TMA among postrenal transplant patients, it is emphasized that TMA is confined to the kidney with little or no systemic evidence of the thromboangiopathic process, underscoring the importance of the graft biopsy in making the diagnosis [6]. Secondary FSGS in our patient could be caused by chronic calcineurin inhibitor nephrotoxicity and/or severe/malignant hypertension [13, 14]. It is noteworthy that normal donor kidneys of kidney-pancreas transplant recipients during tacrolimus based therapy with tacrolimus concentration averaged 7.9 ± 3.9 ng/dL showed chronic arteriolar toxicity in 4.3%, 33.6%, and 77.2% after 1-, 5-, and 10-year treatment, respectively [15]. The authors suggested that cumulative nephrotoxicity from prolonged tacrolimus exposure over years-to-decades remains the best explanation in their cohort. Earlier increasing proteinuria, raising BP, and subsequently deteriorating renal function may rather suspect that TMA lesions were made possibly by a contribution of chronic, smoldering tacrolimus arteriolopathy [16] and severe hypertension. Though nodular hyalinosis is not specific for calcineurin inhibitor nephrotoxicity, it is conceivable that nodular hyalinosis in our patient may indicate chronic tacrolimus nephrotoxicity [17].

Lastly, since our patient suffered from RA, secondary TMA associated with RA should be considered. Except for rheumatoid vasculitis only a few cases with RA were reported to be associated with systemic TMA not localized renal TMA [18, 19], all which were thought to be caused by severe deficiency of ADAMTS13 due to autoantibodies that alter its function [20]. Since there were no renal vasculitic lesions, RA-associated TMA was excluded in our patient.

Taken together, since glomerular and tubulointerstitial lesions in our patient were too severe and chronic for her recorded BP to explain the lesions, we postulated that long-term tacrolimus arteriolopathy with smoldering renal TMA caused at least in part secondary FSGS with heavy proteinuria and hypertension [13]. Subsequently, even after discontinuation of tacrolimus, severe hypertension, not malignant hypertension level due to developing renal parenchymal damage further damaged arteriolar endothelium, resulting in overt renal TMA with deteriorating renal function. The zonal tubulointerstitial injury caused by subacute TMA may have mainly contributed to deteriorating renal function. Interestingly JAK3-STAT pathway has been claimed to be a responsible pathway in some forms of glomerulonephritis. Targeting of this pathway has been reported to be effective in the treatment of experimental lupus nephritis [21]. On the other hand disturbances of renal function have been reported with use of tofacitinib, a first-generation JAK inhibitor [22]. Therefore, increase in serum creatinine was also concerned in our patient with RA using tofacitinib; however, recent clinical trial reported that slightly decrease in measured glomerular filtration rate 6 weeks after tofacitinib treatment retuned towards baseline after tofacitinib discontinuation with no significant difference versus placebo [23]. Accordingly, it is conceivable that BP control with renin-angiotensin system inhibition could not ameliorate renal dysfunction due to the preexistence of chronic renal damage but stabilize renal function with reducing proteinuria in our patient.

In summary, some subsets of patients who receive tacrolimus for a long time may be suffered from heavy proteinuria, severe hypertension associated with progressive deterioration of renal function due to renal TMA even after withdrawal of tacrolimus. Severe hypertension must act as a subsequent aggressor to intensify damage of endothelial cells in small arteries, arterioles, and glomeruli, which had been already injured by tacrolimus arteriolopathy, leading to overt renal TMA. Physician should keep in mind that tacrolimus can insidiously evoke chronic smoldering renal TMA.

Consent

Written informed consent was obtained from the patient.

Disclosure

This article does not contain any studies with human participants performed by any of the authors.

Acknowledgments

We would like to thank Ms. Hiromi Yamaguchi for her technical assistance.

References

[1] V. Brocklebank, K. M. Wood, and D. Kavanagh, "Thrombotic microangiopathy and the kidney," *Clinical Journal of the American Society of Nephrology*, vol. 13, no. 2, pp. 300–317, 2018.

[2] B. Zhang, C. Xing, X. Yu, B. Sun, X. Zhao, and J. Qian, "Renal thrombotic microangiopathies induced by severe hypertension," *Hypertension Research*, vol. 31, no. 3, pp. 479–483, 2008.

[3] B. J. H. Van Den Born, U. P. F. Honnebier, R. P. Koopmans, and G. A. Van Montfrans, "Microangiopathic hemolysis and renal failure in malignant hypertension," *Hypertension*, vol. 45, no. 2, pp. 246–251, 2005.

[4] P.-T. T. Pham, A. Peng, A. H. Wilkinson et al., "Cyclosporine and tacrolimus-associated thrombotic microangiopathy," *American Journal of Kidney Diseases*, vol. 36, no. 4, pp. 844–850, 2000.

[5] M. T. Herman, D. T. Lugan, B. Stephen, M. G. Juan, and N. S. Wadi, "FK506-associated thrombotic microangiopathy," *Transplantation*, vol. 67, no. 4, pp. 539–544, 1999.

[6] A. Zarifian, S. Meleg-Smith, R. O'Donovan, R. J. Tesi, and V. Batuman, "Cyclosporine-associated thrombotic microangiopathy in renal allografts," *Kidney International*, vol. 55, no. 6, pp. 2457–2466, 1999.

[7] G. Thölking, H. U. Gerth, K. Schuette-Nuetgen, and S. Reuter, "Tacrolimus metabolism rate on renal function after solid organ transplantation," *World Journal of Transplantation*, vol. 7, pp. 26–33, 2017.

[8] T. Akimoto, S. Muto, C. Ito et al., "Clinical features of malignant hypertension with thrombotic microangiopathy," *Clinical and Experimental Hypertension*, vol. 33, no. 2, pp. 77–83, 2011.

[9] V. F. Panoulas, G. S. Metsios, A. V. Pace et al., "Hypertension in rheumatoid arthritis," *Rheumatology*, vol. 47, no. 9, pp. 1286–1298, 2008.

[10] J. A. Gomez-Puerta and A. Mócsai, "Tyrosine kinase inhibitors for the treatment of rheumatoid arthritis," *Current Topics in Medicinal Chemistry*, vol. 13, no. 6, pp. 760–773, 2013.

[11] A. Shantsila and G. Y. H. Lip, "Malignant hypertension revisited - Does this still exist?" *American Journal of Hypertension*, vol. 30, no. 6, pp. 543–549, 2017.

[12] J. R. Chapman, "Chronic calcineurin inhibitor nephrotoxicity-lest we forget," *American Journal of Transplantation*, vol. 11, no. 4, pp. 693–697, 2011.

[13] V. D. D'Agati, A. B. Fogo, J. A. Bruijn, and J. C. Jennette, "Pathologic classification of focal segmental glomerulosclerosis: a working proposal," *American Journal of Kidney Diseases*, vol. 43, no. 2, pp. 368–382, 2004.

[14] K. Fukuda, A. Shimizu, T. Kaneko et al., "A case of secondary focal segmental glomerulosclerosis associated with malignant hypertension," *CEN Case Reports*, vol. 2, no. 1, pp. 68–75, 2013.

[15] B. J. Nankivell, C. H. P. Ng, P. J. O'Connell, and J. R. Chapman, "Calcineurin inhibitor nephrotoxicity through the lens of longitudinal histology: Comparison of cyclosporine and tacrolimus eras," *Transplantation*, vol. 100, no. 8, pp. 1723–1731, 2016.

[16] S. Sreedharanunni, K. Joshi, R. Duggal, R. Nada, M. Minz, and V. Sakhuja, "An analysis of transplant glomerulopathy and thrombotic microangiopathy in kidney transplant biopsies," *Transplant International*, vol. 27, no. 8, pp. 784–792, 2014.

[17] M. A. Lusco, A. B. Fogo, B. Najafian, and C. E. Alpers, "AJKD atlas of renal pathology: calcineurin inhibitor nephrotoxicity," *American Journal of Kidney Diseases*, vol. 69, no. 5, pp. e21–e22, 2017.

[18] E. M. Kfoury Baz, R. A. Mahfouz, and A. F. Masri, "Thrombotic thrombocytopenic purpura in a patient with rheumatoid arthritis treated by plasmapheresis," *Therapeutic Apheresis*, vol. 3, no. 4, pp. 314–316, 1999.

[19] R. Sakthirajan, J. Dhanapriya, T. Dineshkumar, N. Gopalakrishnan, S. Murugan, and T. Balasubramaniyan, "Thrombotic microangiopathy. An unusual cause of renal failure in rheumatoid arthritis," *Indian Journal of Nephrology*, vol. 27, no. 1, pp. 81–83, 2017.

[20] S. Tateno and Y. Kobayashi, "Renal thrombotic microangiopathy in a patient with rheumatoid arthritis and antiphospholipid syndrome: successful treatment with cyclophosphamide pulse therapy and anticoagulant," *Internal Medicine*, vol. 33, no. 8, pp. 484–487, 1994.

[21] È. Ripoll, L. de Ramon, J. Draibe Bordignon et al., "JAK3-STAT pathway blocking benefits in experimental lupus nephritis," *Arthritis Research & Therapy*, vol. 18, no. 1, p. 136, 2016.

[22] J. D. Isaacs, A. Zuckerman, S. Krishnaswami et al., "Changes in serum creatinine in patients with active rheumatoid arthritis treated with tofacitinib: Results from clinical trials," *Arthritis Research & Therapy*, vol. 16, no. 4, article no. R158, 2014.

[23] J. M. Kremer, A. J. Kivitz, J. A. Simon-Campos et al., "Evaluation of the effect of tofacitinib on measured glomerular filtration rate in patients with active rheumatoid arthritis: Results from a randomised controlled trial," *Arthritis Research & Therapy*, vol. 17, p. 95, 2015.

6

High Lyso-Gb3 Plasma Levels Associated with Decreased miR-29 and miR-200 Urinary Excretion in Young Non-Albuminuric Male Patient with Classic Fabry Disease

Sebastián Jaurretche[1,2] **Germán R. Perez,**[3,4] **and Graciela Venera**[5]

[1] *Physiology Department, School of Medicine, Instituto Universitario Italiano de Rosario, Rosario, Argentina*
[2] *Los Manantiales, Neurosciences Center, Rosario, Argentina*
[3] *School of Biochemical and Pharmaceutical Sciences, National University of Rosario, Rosario, Argentina*
[4] *Gammalab Grupo Gamma, Rosario, Argentina*
[5] *Research Department, School of Medicine, Instituto Universitario Italiano de Rosario, Rosario, Argentina*

Correspondence should be addressed to Sebastián Jaurretche; sebastianjaurretche@hotmail.com

Academic Editor: John A. Sayer

Renal involvement is associated with a greater morbidity and mortality in Fabry disease. Pathological albuminuria, the first Fabry nephropathy clinical manifestation, can occur from early childhood, although histological lesions such as tubulo-interstitial fibrosis and glomerulosclerosis are present or may precede the onset of pathological albuminuria. In renal cells, exposure to Lyso-Gb3 is correlated with increased expression of Transforming Growth Factor-βeta (TGF-β). miR-21, miR-192, and miR-433 that promote fibrosis are activated by TGF-β, and miR-29 and miR-200 that suppress fibrosis are inhibited by TGF-β. A 23-year-old male was diagnosed with FD. αGalA decreased enzyme activity: 0.1 nmol/hour/liter; genotype: [c.317T>G (p.L106R)]; GFR: 104.4 mL/min/m^2; urinary albumin excretion: 6.00 mg/day; plasma Lyso-Gb3: 124.5 nmol/L. A decrease urinary excretion of miR-29 and miR-200 was found ($p < 0.005$) compared to controls. In addition to its usefulness as a phenotype marker, Lyso-Gb3 has been proposed as an indicator of therapeutic response. We detect an association of high Lyso-Gb3 plasma values with decreased urinary excretion of miRNAs with known antifibrotic effect (miR-29 and miR-200). Although the present work is a case report, it could be hypothesized that one of the harmful Lyso-Gb3 effects could be the miRNAs regulation through changes in TGF-β expression.

1. Introduction

Fabry disease (FD) is an X-linked α-galactosidase-A (αGalA) deficiency which results in the failure of glycosphingolipids catabolism, particularly globotriaosylceramide (Gb3) and globotriaosylsphingosine (Lyso-Gb3) [1]. The progressive glycosphingolipids storage in lysosomes of different cells starts in fetal life [1] and leads to deteriorated cellular and tissue function which cause FD clinical manifestations [1].

Nephropathy is a major FD complication and mainly includes proteinuria and progressive decreased glomerular filtration rate (GFR) [1, 2]. Renal involvement is associated with a greater morbidity and mortality when it is present in affected patients both males and females [1, 3]. Over the last years, research has shown that females carrying mutated allele also develop symptoms, demonstrating a wide range of disease severity, from a virtually asymptomatic to more classical phenotype, with cardiac, renal, and cerebrovascular manifestations. This variable expression in females is thought to be influenced by the process of X-chromosome inactivation (Lyon hypothesis) [1]. Males with classical GLA gene mutations develop overt proteinuria and progressive renal impairment by the second-to-fifth decade of life, while in women the renal involvement has been described to be milder and later than in men [1].

Pathological albuminuria, which is long considered the first clinical manifestation of Fabry nephropathy, can occur from early childhood [1, 4], although it is well known that

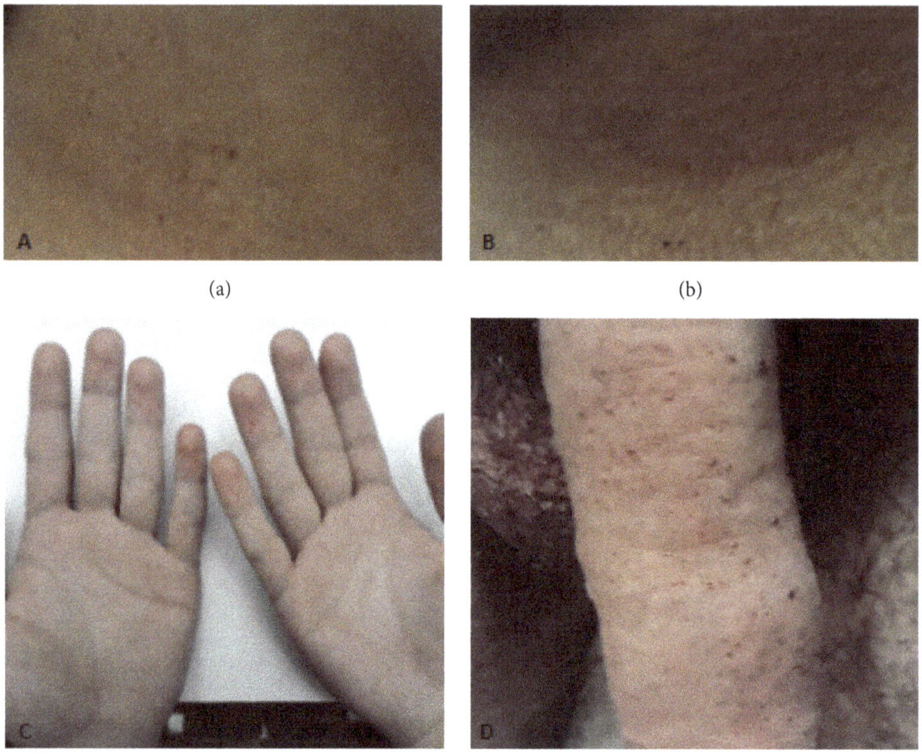

(a) (b) (c) (d)

FIGURE 1: **Typical skin lesions (angiokeratomas) of Fabry disease.** (a) and (b) Angiokeratomas in lower abdomen skin. (c) Angiokeratomas in skin of hands. (d) Angiokeratomas in penile skin.

morphological changes, even irreversible, such as tubulointerstitial fibrosis and glomerulosclerosis, are present or may precede the onset of pathological albuminuria [5, 6].

In Fabry nephropathy, glycolipids deposit in glomerular, tubular, and vascular cells leading to glomerulosclerosis, tubular atrophy, interstitial fibrosis, and inflammation [5, 7].

Lyso-Gb3, a deacylated Gb3, increases in plasma of FD patients [1]. The highest Lyso-Gb3 plasma concentrations have been observed in males affected by most severe FD form ("Classic" or "Type I" FD) [8]. The Lyso-Gb3 deleterious effects on podocytes and renal tubular cells have been demonstrated in both animal and human models of Fabry nephropathy [9, 10]. In podocytes, exposure to Lyso-Gb is correlated with increased Transforming Growth Factor-βeta (TGF-β) and extracellular matrix components expression, both mechanisms associated with renal fibrosis development [9]. In renal tubular cells exposed to Lyso-Gb3, epithelial-mesenchymal transition has been described as another mechanism related to renal fibrosis [10].

TGF-β also regulates several microRNAs (miRs; miRNAs) during renal fibrosis, suggesting that they play essential roles in this process. miR-21, miR-192, and miR-433 that promote fibrosis are activated by TGF-β, and miR-29 and miR-200 that suppress fibrosis are inhibited by TGF-β [11]. miRNAs are small, endogenous, non-coding RNAs that regulate various cellular processes. Several studies suggest the potential role of miRNAs in kidney physiology [11].

We have recently demonstrated that young FD patients present a miRNAs urinary profile excretion indicative of renal fibrosis in correlation with decreased αGalA activity, even in non-albuminuric patients [12]. This work includes the study of miRNAs families regulated by TGF-β. We have observed that, in comparison with the control group, the relative excretion levels of miR-29 and miR-200 families were decreased, while miR-21, miR-192, and miR-433 were not [12].

The aim of this work is to describe the clinical case of a young FD patient without nephropathy manifestations, high Lyso-Gb3 plasma levels, decreased αGalA enzyme activity, and relative urinary excretion levels of miR-29 and miR-200 diminished.

2. Case Presentation and Methods

A 23-year-old male who suffered from acroparesthesias, decreased sweating, exercise intolerance, and frequent episodes of diarrhea and abdominal discomfort was diagnosed with FD. Physical examination: angiokeratomas on palms and genitals were found (Figure 1). The αGalA test in dried blood spot disclosed decreased enzyme activity, 0.1 nmol/hour/liter (normal > than 4 nmol/hour/liter). A mutation [c.317T>G (p.L106R)] was identified in the GLA gene, by sequential analysis. The laboratory results were unremarkable, with a GFR of 104.4 mL/min/m^2 estimated by the CKD-EPI equation, 24-hour urinary albumin

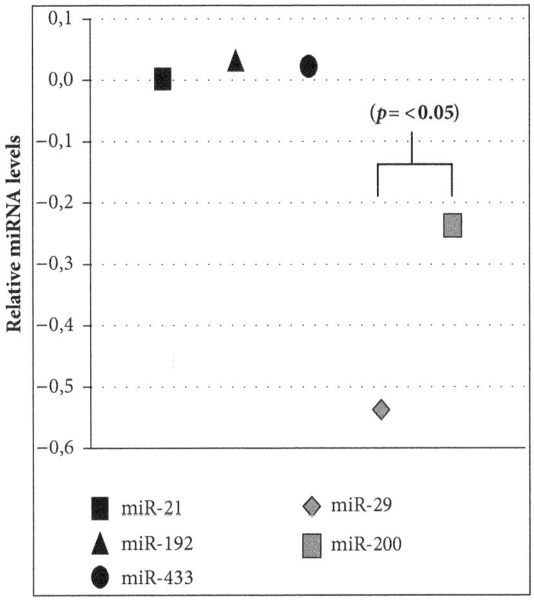

Figure 2: **Relative expression levels of miRNAs in urinary sediment versus controls:** Y axis represents $2^{-\Delta\Delta Ct}$ miRNAs values calculated by Delta-Delta Ct (ΔΔCt) method versus control. Expression was normalized to U6, and data are represented as means ± SEM.

excretion 6.00 mg/day. A renal ultrasound and DOPPLER echocardiogram were normal. A plasma Lyso-Gb3 value of 124.5 nmol/L was found, determined by tandem mass spectrometry method. To detect the relative excretion urinary levels of miR-21, miR-29, miR-192, miR-200, and miR-433, reverse transcription reaction with a stem-loop primer was used. The resulting cDNA was amplified using a miRNA-specific forward primer and the universal reverse primer [12]. Relative miRNAs expression levels were calculated using the $2^{-\Delta\Delta Ct}$ method as previously described [13] (Figure 2).

After the FD diagnostic confirmation enzyme replacement therapy with agalsidase-beta at a dose of 1 mg/Kg/every other week was indicated.

3. Discussion and Conclusion

The mechanisms that lead to renal fibrosis in FD patients are not completely understood. However, it is well known that Fabry nephropathy progresses to renal fibrosis and that fibrotic lesions may precede pathological albuminuria, the first clinical manifestation of renal involvement in affected patients [1, 2, 4, 5].

The origin of excessive plasma accumulation of Lyso-Gb3 in affected patients is not clearly identified. It has been proposed that it comes from the deacylation of abnormally accumulated Gb3 molecules due to the deficit of αGalA [9, 10, 14]. Elevated plasma Lyso-Gb3 is a hallmark of classical FD in males although in Fabry females it is relatively lower [15]. In addition to its usefulness as a phenotype marker, Lyso-Gb3 has been proposed as an indicator of therapeutic response. It has been reported that ERT is capable of decreasing or stabilizing plasma Lyso-Gb3 levels, mainly in patients treated with high doses of ERT [15]. Lyso-Gb3 has been associated with some FD clinical manifestations in various organs. In the present report, pain was the most prominent clinical manifestation and also motivated the consultation. In animal models a direct correlation between the administration of Lyso-Gb3 and allodynia has been demonstrated [14]. In certain circuits of sensory neurons, lyso-Gb3 induces an increase in intracellular calcium by a functional upregulation of voltage-dependent Ca^{2+} channels [14].

Gb3 and lyso-Gb3 are involved with various cellular mechanisms implying renal fibrosis [9, 10]. Glycolipids, mainly Gb3 are deposited in all types of kidney cells [5, 6]. The abnormal deposit of Gb3 has been associated with tissue ischemia due to microvascular occlusion and its final result, the renal fibrosis [1].

Sanchez Niño et al. have described that lyso-Gb3 dose- and time-dependently increased the TGF-β1expression, extracellular matrix proteins (fibronectin and type IV collagen), and CD74, in human podocytes [9]. Jeon et al. (2015) described that FD renal tubular cells treated with Gb3 and lyso-Gb3 showed a transition from epithelial to mesenchymal cells, a key event in the development of renal fibrosis of any cause [10]. Both groups described that this Gb3 and lyso-Gb3 effect is mediated by TGF-β.

We report for the first time that young FD patients with classical GLA gene mutations and mild or absent nephropathy presented a miRNAs urinary excretion profile indicative of renal fibrosis, even in pre-albuminuric stage. This profile was produced by a decrease of miRNAs downregulated by TGF-β (miR-29 and miR-200) and significantly correlated with decreased αGalA activity [12].

In the presented case, plasma Lyso-Gb3 levels within the mean values of patients with the classic FD were found [8]. We detect an association of high plasma Lyso-Gb3 values with decreased urinary excretion of miRNAs that suppress fibrosis (miR-29 and miR-200). On the other hand, normal values of miRNAs miR-21, miR-192, and miR-433 with recognized profibrotic effect were observed. Although the present work is a case report, it could be assumed that one of harmful Lyso-Gb3 effects could be the miRNAs regulation through changes in TGF-β expression.

Acknowledgments

The present work was carried out with the financial support of SANOFI-Genzyme Argentina, for the purchase of medical supplies used in the laboratory.

References

[1] D. P. Germain, "Fabry disease," *Orphanet Journal of Rare Diseases*, vol. 5, article 30, 2010.

[2] S. Jaurretche, N. Antongiovanni, and F. Perretta, "Prevalence of chronic kidney disease in fabry disease patients: multicenter cross sectional study in Argentina," *Molecular Genetics and Metabolism Reports*, vol. 12, pp. 41–43, 2017.

[3] S. Waldek, M. R. Patel, M. Banikazemi, R. Lemay, and P. Lee, "Life expectancy and cause of death in males and females with Fabry disease: Findings from the Fabry Registry," *Genetics in Medicine*, vol. 11, no. 11, pp. 790–796, 2009.

[4] D. A. Laney, D. S. Peck, A. M. Atherton et al., "Fabry disease in infancy and early childhood: a systematic literature review," *Genetics in Medicine*, vol. 17, no. 5, pp. 323–330, 2015.

[5] A. B. Fogo, L. Bostad, E. Svarstad et al., "Scoring system for renal pathology in Fabry disease: report of the international study group of fabry nephropathy (ISGFN)," *Nephrology Dialysis Transplantation* , vol. 25, no. 7, pp. 2168–2177, 2010.

[6] C. Tøndel, L. Bostad, A. Hirth, and E. Svarstad, "Renal biopsy findings in children and adolescents with fabry disease and minimal albuminuria," *American Journal of Kidney Diseases*, vol. 51, no. 5, pp. 767–776, 2008.

[7] J. Alroy, S. Sabnis, and JB. Kopp, "Renal pathology in Fabry disease," *American Society of Nephrology*, vol. 13, pp. S134–S138, 2002.

[8] T. Togawa, T. Kodama, T. Suzuki et al., "Plasma globotriaosylsphingosine as a biomarker of Fabry disease," *Molecular Genetics and Metabolism*, vol. 100, no. 3, pp. 257–261, 2010.

[9] M. D. Sanchez-Niño, A. B. Sanz, S. Carrasco et al., "Globotriaosylsphingosine actions on human glomerular podocytes: implications for Fabry nephropathy," *Nephrology Dialysis Transplantation* , vol. 26, no. 6, pp. 1797–1802, 2011.

[10] Y. J. Jeon, N. Jung, J.-W. Park, H.-Y. Park, and S.-C. Jung, "Epithelial-mesenchymal transition in kidney tubular epithelial cells induced by globotriaosylsphingosine and globotriaosylceramide," *PLoS ONE*, vol. 10, no. 8, Article ID e0136442, 2015.

[11] A. C. K. Chung and H. Y. Lan, "MicroRNAs in renal fibrosis," *Frontiers in Physiology*, vol. 6, p. 50, 2015.

[12] S. Jaurretche, G. Venera, N. Antongiovanni, F. Perretta, and G. R. Perez, "Urinary Excretion of microRNAs in Young Fabry Disease Patients with Mild or Absent Nephropathy," *Open Journal of Nephrology*, vol. 8, no. 3, p. 71, 2018.

[13] K. J. Livak and T. D. Schmittgen, "Analysis of relative gene expression data using real-time quantitative PCR and the $2^{-\Delta\Delta C_T}$ method," *Methods*, vol. 25, no. 4, pp. 402–408, 2001.

[14] L. Choi, J. Vernon, O. Kopach et al., "The Fabry disease-associated lipid lyso-Gb3 enhances voltage-gated calcium currents in sensory neurons and causes pain," *Neuroscience Letters*, vol. 594, pp. 163–168, 2015.

[15] M. J. van Breemen, S. M. Rombach, N. Dekker et al., "Reduction of elevated plasma globotriaosylsphingosine in patients with classic Fabry disease following enzyme replacement therapy," *Biochimica et Biophysica Acta (BBA) - Molecular Basis of Disease*, vol. 1812, no. 1, pp. 70–76, 2011.

7

Multiple Faces of Chronic Lymphocytic Leukaemia: A Patient with Renal, Cardiac and Skeletal Complications

Zay Myo Htet,[1] Cesar Gomez,[2] Ahsan Ali,[3] Sunil Nair,[4] and Mahzuz Karim[1]

[1]*Department of Renal Medicine, Norfolk and Norwich University Hospital, Norwich, UK*
[2]*Department of Haematology, Norfolk and Norwich University Hospital, Norwich, UK*
[3]*Department of Cellular Pathology, Norfolk and Norwich University Hospital, Norwich, UK*
[4]*Department of Cardiology, Norfolk and Norwich University Hospital, Norwich, UK*

Correspondence should be addressed to Mahzuz Karim; mkarim@doctors.org.uk

Academic Editor: Ricardo Enríquez

We describe a patient who had chronic lymphocytic leukaemia (CLL) Binet stage A at presentation with further evidence of disease at multiple sites but who initially required no treatment. However, several years later, her peripheral blood lymphocyte count started to increase, and soon after that she suffered an acute myocardial infarct (in the absence of coronary atheroma) together with proteinuric renal failure due to membranoproliferative glomerulonephritis. Her renal function improved markedly following anti-CLL chemotherapy. We postulate that her cardiac and renal disease were both complications of her CLL. In patients with CLL who develop new clinical signs or symptoms (even if apparently unrelated), consideration should be given as to whether these may be disease complications as this may serve as an indication to commence anti-CLL therapy; close liaison between different specialties is vital.

1. Case History

A 55-year-old woman was referred to the renal clinic in February 2016 with heavy proteinuria and deteriorating renal function. She had had a diagnosis of chronic lymphocytic leukaemia (CLL) for 6 years. This was first detected in August 2010 when a screening mammogram revealed right axillary lymphadenopathy. Core biopsy (Figure 1) demonstrated abnormal lymphoid tissue with small- to medium-sized lymphocytes with irregular nuclei. These cells stained positively for CD5, CD20, and CD23 but were negative for CD10 and cyclin D1. The proliferation index (Ki-67) was 5-10%. She had a staging computed tomography scan with contrast: this showed multiple enlarged cervical, axillary, and inguinal lymph nodes, but no mediastinal, abdominal, or pelvic lymphadenopathy and no hepatomegaly or splenomegaly. As she was asymptomatic and her full blood count was normal (including lymphocyte count 2.3×10^9/L, reference range 1-3 $\times 10^9$/L), she required no active treatment but was kept under review.

Two years later (April 2012), she developed a right breast mass. Excision biopsy showed an intraductal papilloma. A few months later, in November 2012, she noted some lumps in her left axilla; core biopsy was performed, and this was again consistent with CLL. Management remained conservative. In July 2013, she presented to the orthopaedic surgeons with a painful left shoulder. Plain radiography showed an ill-defined lucency projected over the lateral aspect of the left humeral head (Figure 2(a)), and magnetic resonance imaging (MRI, Figure 2(b)) revealed extensive marrow infiltration of the humeral head and shaft, shoulder girdle, and ribs, together with axillary lymphadenopathy. Bone biopsy confirmed infiltration by CLL but no evidence of high-grade transformation. Her peripheral blood lymphocyte count remained normal (6.57×10^9/L). A serum IgG λ paraprotein was detected and quantified at 1.8g/L. During 2014, her lymphocyte count rose, and by early 2015 it was 22.6×10^9/L (Figure 3).

In November 2015, she presented with acute onset ischaemic chest pain. Although her ECG showed no acute changes, troponin I level was 44.5ng/L (0-15.6), climbing

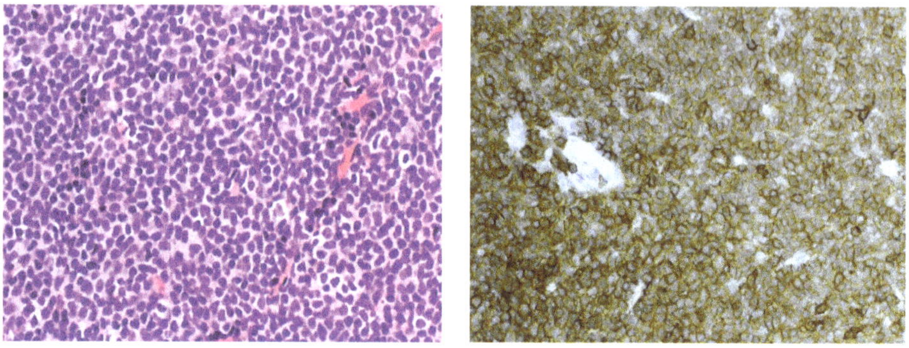

(a) (b)

FIGURE 1: Axillary lymph node: (a) Haematoxylin and eosin stain showing monomorphic proliferation of small lymphocytes in keeping with CLL. (b) Immunoperoxidase stain showing positive staining of lymphocytes for CD5.

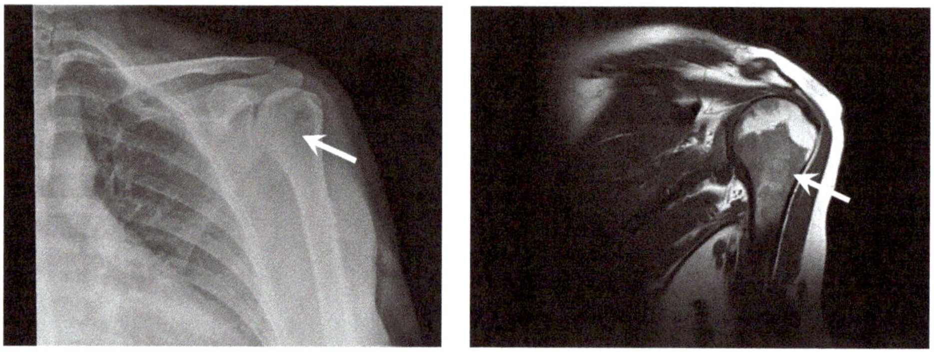

(a) (b)

FIGURE 2: Imaging of left shoulder: (a) Plain radiograph showing lucency of humeral head. (b) MRI scan showing marrow infiltration of humeral head and shaft.

to 350.5ng/L two hours later; her lymphocyte count had also continued to rise (39.9×10^9/L). Coronary angiography showed no significant stenosis or thrombus within the coronary arteries (Figures 4(a) and 4(b)). Antiplatelet therapy was commenced. Cardiac MRI demonstrated full-thickness enhancement in the midseptum with associated hypokinesia, consistent with an infarct (Figures 4(c) and 4(d)); left ventricular ejection fraction was well maintained at 72%. She underwent echocardiography to investigate the possibility of a paradoxical embolus as the cause for this infarct; this confirmed an area of hypokinesis in the mid-interventricular septum, but with no evidence of an atrial septal defect or patent foramen ovale. She had no further cardiac symptoms.

Referral to the renal clinic in February 2016 was prompted by a decline in renal function (Figure 3). Her serum creatinine had risen progressively from 66 μmol/L (45-84) two years earlier (April 2014) to 182 μmol/L. Lymphocyte count was 56.5×10^9/L, without anaemia or thrombocytopaenia. Serum albumin was low at 24 g/L (35-50). Urine dipstick testing showed 3+ blood and 4+ protein, with microscopy showing red cells but no casts; urine protein:creatinine ratio was elevated at 1574 mg/mmol (0-20). Her serum IgG λ paraprotein level remained low at 1.0g/L, with serum free λ chains 96.5mg/L (5.7-26.3), serum free κ chains 24.4mg/L (3.3-19.4), and κ:λ ratio 0.25 (0.26-1.65). Other normal investigations included anti-nuclear antibodies 0.1 U/L (0-1), negative anti-neutrophil cytoplasmic antibodies by immunofluorescence, proteinase 3 <0.1 U/mL (0-3), myeloperoxidase <0.1 U/mL (0-5), complement C3 1.4g/L (0.75-1.65), C4 0.27g/L (0.14-0.54), rheumatoid factor <20 U/mL (<30), negative cryoglobulins, and negative hepatitis B and C serology. She underwent percutaneous renal biopsy (Figure 5). This showed an interstitial lymphocytic infiltrate (CD20 and CD5 positive), consistent with CLL. Additionally, the glomeruli showed membranoproliferative change with thickening and double-contouring of the basement membrane and immunostaining positive for IgG and C3 but negative for IgA and IgM; staining for κ and λ light chains was not performed. Congo red and amyloid P stains were also negative. These changes were felt secondary to her CLL, and she was therefore commenced on treatment with six cycles of rituximab and bendamustine delivered every four weeks between June and November 2016. Clinical response was excellent, with her serum creatinine falling from a peak of 327 μmol/L to 120 μmol/L within six weeks of starting treatment. Computed tomography scan in December 2016 showed no evidence of lymphadenopathy, and in February 2017, three months after completing

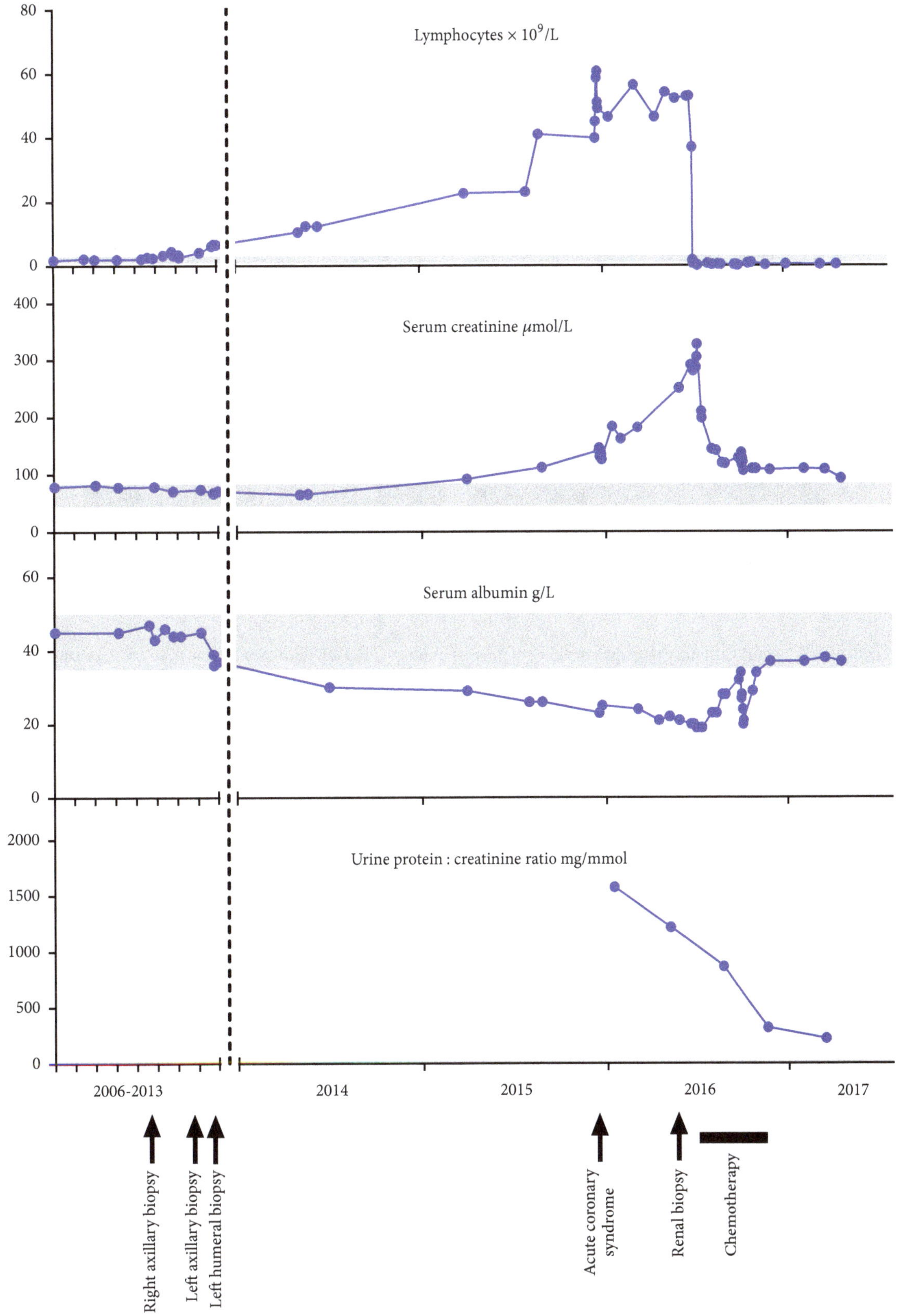

FIGURE 3: Patients laboratory investigations and clinical events. Shaded areas represent reference ranges.

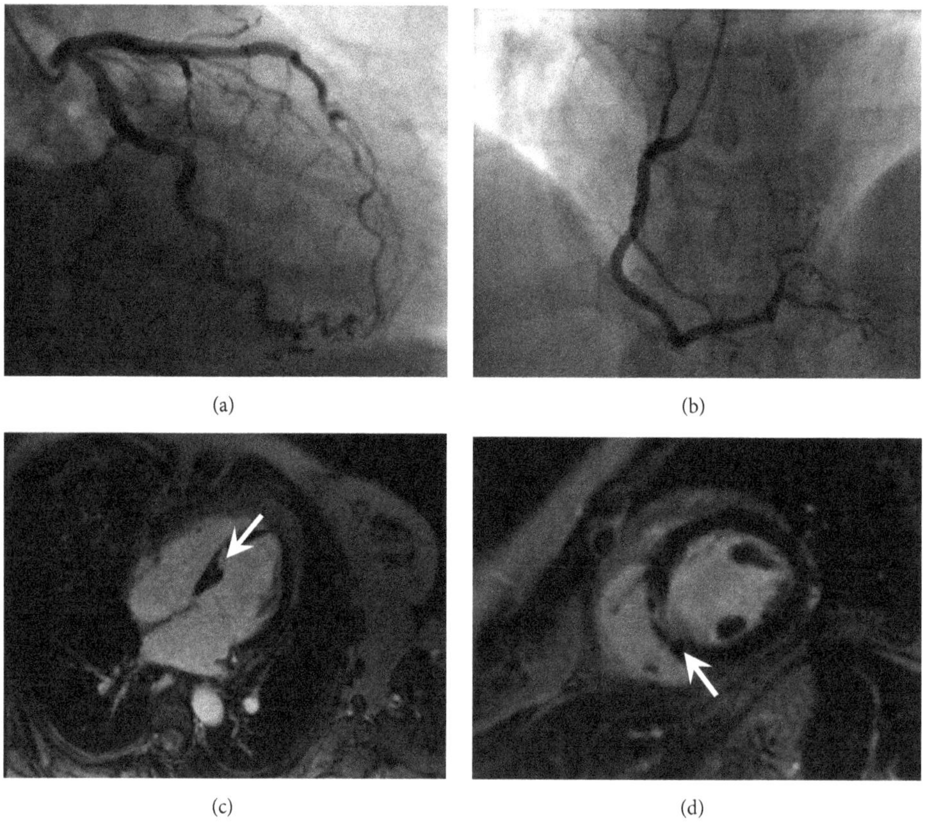

FIGURE 4: Cardiac imaging: (a) Coronary angiogram showing normal unobstructed left coronary artery. (b) Coronary angiogram showing normal unobstructed right coronary artery. (c) Left ventricle 4 chamber cardiac MRI late gadolinium enhancement image showing area of near transmural infarction in the mid septum. (d) Left ventricle short axis cardiac MRI late gadolinium enhancement image at the papillary muscle level showing area of near transmural infarction of the mid septum.

therapy, serum creatinine was 109 μmol/L, albumin 38 g/L, and lymphocyte count 0.4×10^9/L; however, she still had significant proteinuria with a urine protein:creatinine ratio of 226 mg/mmol. Serum electrophoresis revealed only a faint IgG λ paraprotein band which was too small to quantify. Echocardiogram showed a left ventricular ejection fraction of 63%, with no regional wall motion abnormality.

2. Discussion

CLL is one of the commonest haematological malignancies in adults, with an incidence of around 600 per million in the Western world [1]. Clinical presentation is variable and may include features such as asymptomatic peripheral lymphocytosis, lymphadenopathy, increased incidence of infection, autoimmune phenomena (e.g., haemolytic anaemia, thrombocytopaenia), and B symptoms (fever, unintentional weight loss, night sweats, and severe fatigue) [1].

The clinical course of CLL can vary greatly. Many patients remain asymptomatic for decades and require no specific intervention. However, factors that may mandate active treatment include disease stage, evidence of disease progression (e.g., cytopaenias, progressive lymphadenopathy, and/or splenomegaly), and the presence of constitutional B symptoms, or when transformation to high-grade lymphoma occurs (Richter's transformation) [1]. Our patient had CLL with deposits at multiple sites (including lymph nodes, breast, and bone) but initially required no treatment as she was otherwise asymptomatic. However, soon after her peripheral blood lymphocyte count began to rise, she developed an acute coronary syndrome followed by heavy proteinuria and worsening renal function.

Renal insufficiency is not uncommon in patients with CLL, present in one study in 7.5% of patients at diagnosis, rising to 16.1% during follow-up [2]. Lymphocytic infiltration of the kidneys (that can mimic an acute or chronic interstitial nephritis) is frequent, occurring in up to 90% of patients at autopsy, but does not have a significant impact on renal function in the majority of cases [3]. Other potential causes of renal dysfunction include volume depletion, sepsis, nephrotoxic drugs, hypercalcaemia, tumour lysis syndrome, thrombotic microangiopathy (TMA), and obstructive uropathy (e.g., ureteric compression by lymphadenopathy) [4]. More rarely, there can be an associated glomerulonephritis (GN) as in our patient.

In two large retrospective studies of renal biopsies in patients with CLL and small lymphocytic lymphoma (SLL), membranoproliferative glomerulonephritis (MPGN, also known as mesangiocapillary GN) was the commonest lesion; others included minimal change disease, membranous

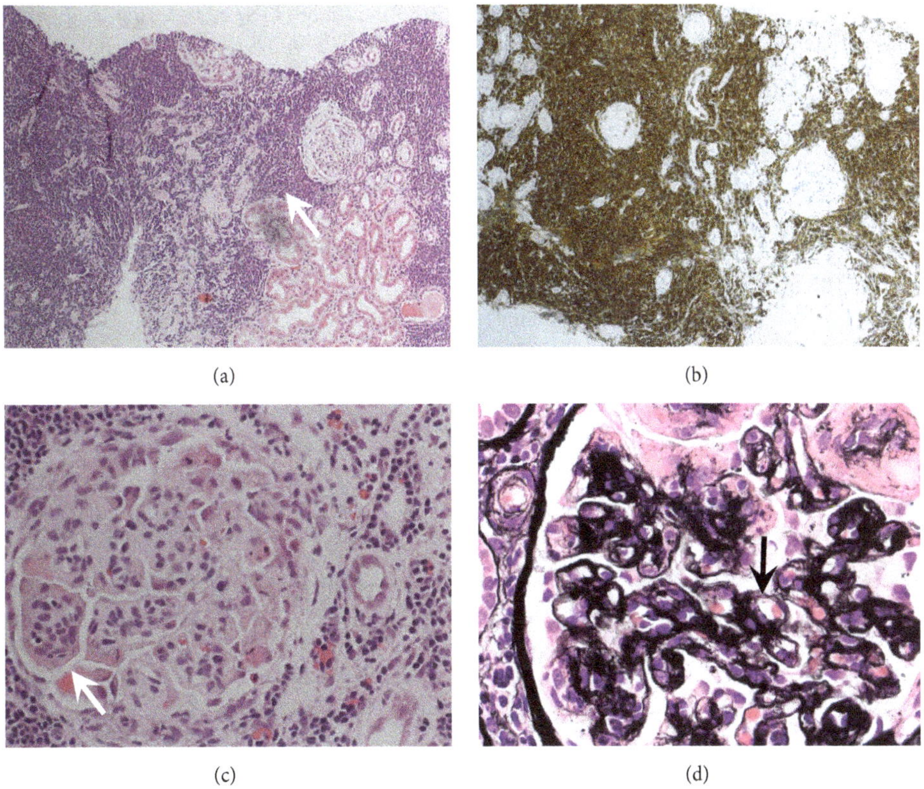

FIGURE 5: Percutaneous renal biopsy: (a) Haematoxylin and eosin stain showing dense lymphoid infiltrate. (b) Immunoperoxidase stain showing positive staining of lymphocytes for CD5. (c) Haematoxylin and eosin stain showing lobulation of glomeruli in keeping with MPGN. (d) Silver stain showing thickening and double contouring of basement membrane in keeping with MPGN.

GN, light chain cast nephropathy, TMA, and amyloidosis [4, 5]. The pathophysiology of MPGN in CLL is thought to involve deposition of paraprotein M components [6], for example, cryoglobulinaemia (most commonly type 2) with activation of the complement system, or noncryoprecipitating monoclonal IgG deposition without complement activation [7]. This has been termed "proliferative glomerulonephritis with monoclonal IgG deposits" (PGNMID) and can be mistaken as an immune-complex GN due to the fact that they both share similar histopathological findings (membranoproliferative or endocapillary proliferative GN with nonorganized granular deposits) [8]. More recently, it has been recognised that monoclonal IgM deposition may also lead to MPGN (although only two cases have been reported in association with CLL) [9, 10], described as "proliferative glomerulonephritis with monoclonal IgM deposits" (PGNMIMD) [9–11].

The clinical presentation of MPGN is most frequently a nephritic picture with features such as hypertension, haematuria, proteinuria (often nephrotic range), active urine sediment, and renal impairment. The next commonest indication for renal biopsy in CLL is nephrotic syndrome [4, 5, 12]. Since the signs and symptoms of renal involvement may be mild or subtle, even with fairly advanced disease, it is crucial to maintain a high index of suspicion and a low threshold for renal biopsy. Additionally, renal insufficiency has been shown to be an independent prognostic indicator in CLL and can influence therapeutic decisions [13]. Renal manifestations can regress following treatment of the underlying CLL [4, 5], and thus where renal involvement is identified, initiation of appropriate anti-CLL therapy should be considered. In some cases, the decision to initiate treatment may not be straightforward, and renal dysfunction can restrict the choice of chemotherapeutic agent(s). Our patient showed an excellent clinical improvement after six cycles of rituximab and bendamustine. To our knowledge, this is the third report of a case of CLL-associated proliferative GN managed successfully with a rituximab and bendamustine-based regimen leading to substantial renal improvement [14].

The other interesting aspect in this patient is her acute coronary syndrome. She had typical ischaemic symptoms and a troponin rise with MRI and echocardiogram showing full thickness infarction and hypokinesia, but in the absence of a prior cardiac history or traditional cardiovascular risk factors and with normal coronary angiography. As this happened at a time when her disease was progressing (demonstrated by a rising peripheral lymphocyte count and worsening renal function), we hypothesize that her CLL played a pathophysiological role.

Although cardiac infiltration by CLL and other lymphoproliferative disorders is well-described (occurring in 20% of patients in one postmortem series) [15], reports of consequent cardiac dysfunction are less common. A high peripheral leucocyte count itself has been demonstrated to increase the risk of (and mortality from) acute coronary artery thrombosis and to stimulate chronic atherosclerosis and microvascular occlusion. Multiple potential mechanisms have been suggested including leucocyte aggregation and adhesion with vessel plugging, activation of the coagulation system, interaction with platelets to promote thrombin generation, increased expression of monocyte and neutrophil tissue factors, and release of soluble mediators such as proteases, reactive oxygen species, growth factors, interleukins, and myeloperoxidase [16–18]. Patients with CLL may also develop amyloid infiltration of the heart, either paraprotein-related AL amyloid [19] or, less commonly, non-AL; the latter group appears to have a better prognosis [20]. Amyloid can also deposit within vessels causing occlusion [21]. CLL infiltration of the pericardium may lead to constrictive pericarditis [15, 22] and of the aortic valve to aortic stenosis [23].

In 1980, Applefield *et al.* reported a 47-year-old man with CLL who died from congestive cardiac failure. Postmortem examination showed endocardial fibroelastosis and leukaemic infiltration of the endocardium, myocardium, and coronary arteries [24]. More recently, Assiri *et al.* described an 83-year-old man with CLL who died following an acute myocardial infarct. Autopsy showed infiltration of the coronary artery walls by leukaemic cells but, unlike our patient, also significant atheromatous disease [25]. Finally, Xu *et al.* documented a 65-year-old woman with Richter's progression of CLL who presented with an acute myocardial infarct. She had a peripheral leucocyte count of 316×10^9/L and an IgM paraprotein of 0.3g/dL. She underwent plasmapheresis to reduce her leucocyte count but died despite this. Postmortem examination showed lymphomatous infiltrates in the myocardium, epicardium, and endocardium with occlusion of small vessels; immunohistochemistry showed IgM heavy chain and λ light chain deposition in a subintimal distribution [26]. It is thus plausible that our patient's acute cardiac event was related to her CLL.

In summary, new clinical signs or symptoms in patients with CLL should prompt consideration of whether these may represent disease complications and thus be an indication to commence treatment for CLL, even in the absence of more classical criteria. Close liaison between different medical specialties is vital in optimising outcome.

References

[1] T. J. Kipps, F. K. Stevenson, C. J. Wu et al., "Chronic lymphocytic leukaemia," *Nature Reviews Disease Primers*, vol. 3, p. 16096, 2017.

[2] T. D. Shanafelt, K. G. Rabe, C. A. Hanson, T. G. Call, S. Schwager, S. A. Parikh et al., "Renal disease in patients with chronic lymphocytic leukemia (CLL)," *Blood*, vol. 122, p. 5302, 2013.

[3] J. B. Schwartz and A. M. Shamsuddin, "The effects of leukemic infiltrates in various organs in chronic lymphocytic leukemia," *Human Pathology*, vol. 12, no. 5, pp. 432–440, 1981.

[4] P. Strati, S. H. Nasr, N. Leung et al., "Renal complications in chronic lymphocytic leukemia and monoclonal B-cell lymphocytosis: the mayo clinic experience," *Haematologica*, vol. 100, no. 9, pp. 1180–1188, 2015.

[5] A.-L. Poitou-Verkinder, A. Francois, F. Drieux et al., "The spectrum of kidney pathology in B-cell chronic lymphocytic leukemia / small lymphocytic lymphoma: a 25-year multicenter experience," *PLoS ONE*, vol. 10, no. 3, Article ID e0119156, 2015.

[6] B. Moulin, P. M. Ronco, B. Mougenot, A. Francois, J.-P. Fillastre, and F. Mignon, "Glomerulonephritis in chronic lymphocytic leukemia and related B-cell lymphomas," *Kidney International*, vol. 42, no. 1, pp. 127–135, 1992.

[7] G. Favre, C. Courtellemont, P. Callard et al., "Membranoproliferative glomerulonephritis, chronic lymphocytic leukemia, and cryoglobulinemia," *American Journal of Kidney Diseases*, vol. 55, no. 2, pp. 391–394, 2010.

[8] S. H. Nasr, A. Satoskar, G. S. Markowitz et al., "Proliferative glomerulonephritis with monoclonal IgG deposits," *Journal of the American Society of Nephrology*, vol. 20, no. 9, pp. 2055–2064, 2009.

[9] Y. Oe, K. Joh, M. Sato et al., "Proliferative glomerulonephritis with monoclonal IgM-κ deposits in chronic lymphocytic leukemia/small lymphocytic leukemia: case report and review of the literature," *CEN Case Reports*, vol. 2, no. 2, pp. 222–227, 2013.

[10] S. Sethi, L. Zand, N. Leung et al., "Membranoproliferative glomerulonephritis secondary to monoclonal gammopathy," *Clinical Journal of the American Society of Nephrology*, vol. 5, no. 5, pp. 770–782, 2010.

[11] M. Yahata, I. Nakaya, S. Takahashi, T. Sakuma, H. Sato, and J. Soma, "Proliferative glomerulonephritis with monoclonal IgM deposits without Waldenström's macroglobulinemia: case report and review of the literature," *Clinical Nephrology*, vol. 77, no. 03, pp. 254–260, 2012.

[12] W. Wung, S. Ananthakrishnan, and B. A. Jonas, "Proteinuria, hypoalbuminemia, and chronic lymphocytic leukemia: an unusual trio," *Journal of Investigative Medicine High Impact Case Reports*, vol. 6, Article ID 2324709618764207, 2018.

[13] P. Strati, K. G. Chaffee, S. J. Achenbach et al., "Renal insufficiency is an independent prognostic factor in patients with chronic lymphocytic leukemia," *Haematologica*, vol. 102, no. 1, pp. e22–e25, 2017.

[14] K. Fischer, P. Cramer, R. Busch et al., "Bendamustine in combination with rituximab for previously untreated patients with chronic lymphocytic leukemia: a multicenter phase II trial of the German Chronic Lymphocytic Leukemia Study Group," *Journal of Clinical Oncology*, vol. 30, no. 26, pp. 3209–3216, 2012.

[15] M. Barcos, W. Lane, G. A. Gomez et al., "An autopsy study of 1206 acute and chronic leukemias (1958 to 1982)," *Cancer*, vol. 60, no. 4, pp. 827–837, 1987.

[16] I. Benedek, E. Lázár, J. Sándor-Kéri, S. Bíró, S. Jakab, and I. Benedek, "Acute coronary syndromes in patients with hematological disorders," *Journal Of Cardiovascular Emergencies*, vol. 2, no. 4, pp. 159–168, 2016.

[17] M. Madjid, I. Awan, J. T. Willerson, and S. W. Casscells, "Leukocyte count and coronary heart disease: implications for risk assessment," *Journal of the American College of Cardiology*, vol. 44, no. 10, pp. 1945–1956, 2004.

[18] B. S. Coller, "Leukocytosis and ischemic vascular disease morbidity and mortality: is it time to intervene?" *Arteriosclerosis, Thrombosis, and Vascular Biology*, vol. 25, no. 4, pp. 658–670, 2005.

[19] D. Liu, H. T. Uqdah, and A. D. Gordy, "An unusual case of chronic lymphocytic leukemia, multiple myeloma and cardiac amyloidosis," *Journal of Community Hospital Internal Medicine Perspectives (JCHIMP)*, vol. 7, no. 4, pp. 230–233, 2017.

[20] T. V. Kourelis, M. Gertz, C. Zent et al., "Systemic amyloidosis associated with chronic lymphocytic leukemia/small lymphocytic lymphoma," *American Journal of Hematology*, vol. 88, no. 5, pp. 375–378, 2013.

[21] S. K. Peng, W. J. French, A. H. Cohen, and R. E. Fausel, "Light chain cardiomyopathy associated with small-vessel disease," *Archives of Pathology & Laboratory Medicine*, vol. 112, pp. 844–846, 1988.

[22] H. W. Habboush, J. Dhundee, D. Al Okati, and A. G. Davies, "Constrictive pericarditis in B cell chronic lymphatic leukaemia," *Clinical & Laboratory Haematology*, vol. 18, no. 2, pp. 117–119, 1996.

[23] M. Chisté, E. Vrotsos, C. Zamora, and A. Martinez, "Chronic lymphocytic leukemia/small lymphocytic lymphoma involving the aortic valve," *Annals of Diagnostic Pathology*, vol. 17, no. 3, pp. 295–297, 2013.

[24] M. M. Applefeld, S. D. Milner, R. D. Vigorito, and A. M. Shamsuddin, "Congestive heart failure and endocardial fibroelastosis caused by chronic lymphocytic leukemia," *Cancer*, vol. 46, no. 6, pp. 1479–1484, 1980.

[25] A. H. Assiri, M. Lamba, and J. P. Veinot, "Chronic lymphocytic leukemia involving the coronary arteries with accompanying acute myocardial infarction," *Cardiovascular Pathology*, vol. 14, no. 6, pp. 324–326, 2005.

[26] L. Xu, C. Drachenberg, and A. Burke, "Intimal IgM lambda paraprotein deposition in myocardial arteries resulting in acute myocardial infarction and sudden death," *Pathology*, vol. 43, no. 7, pp. 732–734, 2011.

8

Radiologically Guided Renal Artery Embolization with an Amplatzer Vascular Plug as a Rescue Therapy for Refractory Nephrotic Syndrome in AL-Amyloidosis

I. Spozio Züst,[1] H. R. Räz,[1] and F. Burkhalter[2]

[1] *Division of Nephology, Kantonsspital Baden, Switzerland*
[2] *Clinic for Transplant Immunology and Nephrology, University Hospital Basel, Switzerland*

Correspondence should be addressed to I. Spozio Züst; isabel.spoziozuest@ksb.ch

Academic Editor: Rumeyza Kazancioglu

Nephrotic syndrome is common in immunoglobulin light-chain (AL) amyloidosis and successful therapy may pose a challenge. We report the case of a 63-year-old patient with severe nephrotic syndrome due to primary renal AL-amyloidosis with well-preserved renal function at first presentation. Therapy with high dose steroids, loop diuretics, and ACE-inhibitors did not affect his proteinuria and he was seriously disabled because of symptomatic orthostatic hypotension and anasarca. With the patient's informed consent, medical nephrectomy was tried with nonsteroidal-anti-inflammatory drugs (NSAIDs), cyclosporine, and aminoglycosides, with significant deterioration of his renal function, but without relevant effect on his proteinuria. Despite adequate anticoagulation life threatening thrombotic and bleeding complications occurred. Total renal ablation was finally achieved using an Amplatzer vascular plug Typ IV (AVP 4) with a self-expanding Nitinol mesh design, which was placed in both main renal arteries in the same intervention. The patient became completely anuric, protein loss stopped, and serum albumin slowly rose to normal levels. The patient's clinical condition dramatically improved and he regained his full mobility at the price of a lifelong renal replacement therapy. To our knowledge, this is the first reported usage of such a vascular occluder in the setting of refractory nephrotic syndrome with normal kidney function at the time of first presentation.

1. Background

Nephrotic syndrome refractory to conventional therapy is a well-known complication of renal light chain (AL) amyloidosis. Beside the treatment of the underlying disease, therapy options are symptomatic and include low-salt diet, diuretics, ACE-inhibitors, and angiotensin-receptor blockers (ARB). In unaffected severe proteinuria medical nephrectomy with NSAIDs, calcineurin-inhibitors, aminoglycosides or radio-contrast-agents may be tried. As a treatment of last resort, surgical nephrectomy needs to be discussed or alternatively radiologically guided embolization of the renal arteries can be an option. Bilateral renal artery embolization was developed in the early nineteen-seventies as a treatment for renal cell carcinoma [1, 2] and was first described 1975 for the treatment of nephrotic syndrome [3]. For renal artery embolization, various materials are used with different success- and complication rates [4, 5]. A common side effect is postembolization syndrome with a reported frequency of 47-100% [6]. It is characterized by fever, flank pain, leukocytosis, and an elevated lactate dehydrogenase in the first few hours up to a few days after the embolization procedure.

2. Case

We report the case of a 63-year-old patient who presented to the nephrology department with an overt nephrotic syndrome and a normal kidney function. He had a history of arterial hypertension under medical treatment for several years. Our investigations revealed the presence of a light chain plasma cell dyscrasia IgG kappa and IgA kappa/lambda with a Bence Jones proteinuria type lambda, not fulfilling the criteria of a multiple myeloma on bone marrow biopsy (plasma cell infiltration < 10%). A kidney biopsy revealed a severe diffuse glomerular, vascular, and interstitial amyloidosis of the AL-lambda type with slight interstitial fibrosis (10%) and tubular atrophy. Immediately after the kidney biopsy, a self-limiting macrohematuria occurred and at the same time an isolated muscular vein thrombosis of the left lower leg was diagnosed. The next day the patient was admitted to the emergency unit with a subacute ST-elevation myocardial infarction. Coronary angiography showed a primary spiral dissection with occlusion of the left anterior descending artery (LAD). In the echocardiography the left ventricular function appeared moderately reduced with anterior dyskinesia, not suggestive of a cardiac amyloidosis. In addition to aspirin, an oral anticoagulation with dicoumarol was started. Meanwhile, the patient's urinary protein/creatinine ratio rose to 2175 mg/mmol, the serum albumin level dropped to 11 g/l, and he developed anasarca. Severe orthostatic hypotension with several falls made him completely bed-ridden. Medical nephrectomy to reduce proteinuria was started with initially Celecoxib (100 mg bid) due to unchanged proteinuria additionally with cyclosporine (200mg bid). A further rise of creatinine was observed up to 400 μmol/l, but urine volume and proteinuria did not decline, and the clinical condition of the patient worsened. To ameliorate overhydration and due to the reduced renal function, haemodialysis was started. The patient's condition improved slightly and his body weight could be stabilized but his urine volume remained between 0.5 and 1.5 litres per day. Still he remained severely orthostatic and was completely immobilized. Repeated echocardiography showed a severe reduced left ventricular function with a thrombus in the left ventricle despite oral anticoagulation and a pelvic deep venous thrombosis developed additionally. Dicoumarol and thalidomide were stopped and low molecular weight heparin (LMWH) was started. Two weeks later, the patient suffered an ischemic insult in the region of the posterior cerebral artery. LMWH was replaced by unfractionated heparin. He was in critical clinical condition and the decision for a renal ablation with radiologically guided embolization of both renal arteries was made in order to stop the proteinuria and save the patient's life. Two AVP 4 were placed by an interventional radiologist through a 5-F SOS catheter in both renal arteries using a standard femoral artery approach. The result was a complete occlusion of the left renal artery and an almost complete occlusion of the right renal artery. During the procedure, the patient received an epidural anaesthesia with bupivacaine and a prophylactic antibiotic treatment with piperacillin/tazobactam. Despite his severe illness, the patient tolerated the intervention well. A moderate postembolization syndrome developed with ischemic flank pain and fever up to 38.1°C, and LDH rose up to 786 U/l. The pain could be controlled by continuing the epidural anaesthesia for 48 h. Urinary output ceased completely, serum albumin levels normalized slowly during follow-up, and prophylactic antibiotic treatment was stopped after 5 days and normalization of the transient elevated C-reactive protein. The patient's general condition improved dramatically. He could be fully mobilized again, and over time he was able to go regularly for a walk and take a few laps in his swimming pool daily with an acceptable quality of life on maintenance hemodialysis. Without any further chemotherapy however, signs of systemic amyloidosis progressively developed 4 years after the intervention. Over time liver and spleen massively enlarged, ascites developed and recurrent pleural effusion was successfully treated by Talcum-Pleurodesis. As consequence of coronary heart disease and chronic renocardial syndrome, left ventricular ejection fracture worsened again. The patient complained of fading strength of his legs with difficulty to climb stairs and finally 8 years after the intervention he died from the consequences of systemic amyloidosis.

Table 1: Reported indications of renal embolization.

Reported indications
Palliative treatment of renal cell carcinoma
Refractory renal hypertension in ESRD or transplant patients
Transplant rejection
Nephrotic syndrome refractory to treatment
Chronic urinary fistulas
Traumatic renal hemorrhage

3. Discussion

Our patient suffered from life threatening nephrotic syndrome caused by renal amyloidosis of the AL-Lambda Type due to a plasma cell dyscrasia not fulfilling the diagnostic criteria of a multiple myeloma. Because of severe hypoalbuminemia, generalized oedema, and immobilizing orthostasis an unsuccessful medical nephrectomy was performed. After further several thrombotic and bleeding complications despite adequate anticoagulation, nephrectomy was considered as last resort. Regarding the desperate clinical condition of the patient, a surgical nephrectomy was considered inacceptable. To induce anuria, we consequently decided to embolize both renal arteries. This technique was developed in the early nineteen-seventies as a palliative therapy for surgically unresectable renal cell carcinoma. Soon after the first successful reports in cancer patients, the use of this technique was expanded to other indications (Table 1).

Data of total renal embolization are sparse and anecdotic and restricted to a few case reports and small case series [4, 7–13]. Controlled data are missing only reflecting the fact that such a radical procedure, with the consequence of lifetime dialysis, remains a rescue therapy after all other options have failed [10–13]. The technique is not standardized. There are descriptions of a great variety of materials used as emboli, depending on the desired arterial occlusion-level, i.e., the level of arteries at which occlusion should take place (main artery, segmental or subsegmental arteries, and capillaries). The complications of the technique depend on the embolization-material used. As a rule of thumb complication rate rises with the use of smaller particles occluding at a lower vascular level. Ethanol, cyanoacrylate ("superglue"), and maize starch occlude at the capillary level. Segmental blocks are achieved with gelatine or acrylate spheres. To occlude the main renal artery directly, balloons, metal coils, and self-expanding wire meshes are used. The most common side effect of the procedure is postembolization syndrome with a reported frequency of 47-100% [6]. In the literature,

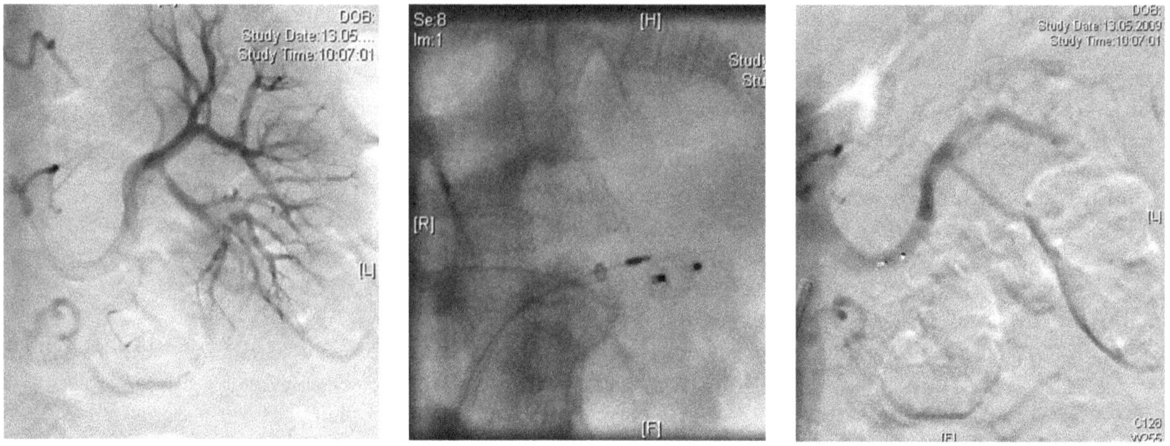

(a) Renal angiogram before embolization showing the entire arterial tree

(b) Placement of the Amplatzer vascular plug in the left renal artery

(c) Angiogramm after renal artery embolization without renal blood flow

FIGURE 1

the syndrome is characterized by fever, bilateral flank pain, leukocytosis, elevated blood sedimentation rate, rising levels of C-reactive protein, and lactate dehydrogenase. Subileus may occur. It is generally a benign condition of a few days duration and responds well to symptomatic treatment with nonsteroidal anti-inflammatory drugs or steroids. It is considered to be the consequence of kidney tissue necrosis. Sepsis and abscess formation due to super infection of a necrotic kidney have rarely been described [14]. In nephrotic syndrome technical success rates with renal embolization of 100% are reported [7, 8, 10–13, 15]. With embolization on the capillary level, anuria normally develops. Accidental embolization of the infrarenal vascular bed has been reported to occur in around ten percent of patients [6], especially when small embolization particles or fluids are used. This can be prevented by transient proximal occlusion of the main renal artery with a balloon prior to injection of the embolization material. For our patient we chose the technique that was available, easily feasible, and allowing the occlusion of both renal arteries in the same session. We used an AVP 4, a self-expanding wire mesh (Nitinol®), which is normally used for peripheral vascular embolization [16]. It is placed under radiological guidance by coaxial technique (Figure 1). The advantage of using an AVP 4 is that it can be delivered through a 0.038 inch guidewire-compatible diagnostic catheter and so eliminates the need for sheath or guiding catheter exchange. In contrast to coils, there is a higher success rate of complete occlusion, a low risk of distal embolization, and the possibility of repositioning if needed. In order to prevent ischemic pain, the patient received epidural anesthesia. After this proximal embolization with an Amplatzer device the patient continued to produce very low amounts of urine due to residual blood supply from renal capsular vessels. Postembolization syndrome was only mild with fever up to 38.1°C and a slightly elevated LDH. After the procedure, our patient recovered, was able to walk 4 km daily, and had the chance to live further 8 years with an acceptable quality of life.

In conclusion, proximal embolization of both kidneys with Amplatzer vascular plugs in a single intervention is feasible, safe, and successful and gave our patient the chance to continue his life with an acceptable quality of life for several years at the price of lifelong dialysis dependency. The percutaneous embolization of the kidneys is a valid and alternative procedure to the surgery with a lower risk for complications and high success rate using an AVP 4.

Authors' Contributions

All authors participated in writing of the paper and the performance of the research.

References

[1] S. Kadir, F. F. Marshall, R. I. White Jr., S. L. Kaufman, and K. H. Barth, "Therapeutic embolization of the kidney with detachable silicone balloons," *The Journal of Urology*, vol. 129, no. 1, pp. 11–13, 1983.

[2] D. Turini, G. Nicita, C. Fiorelli, C. Selli, and N. Villari, "Selective transcatheter arterial embolization of renal carcinoma: an original technique," *The Journal of Urology*, vol. 116, no. 4, pp. 419–421, 1976.

[3] C. T. Dotter, M. L. Goldman, and J. Rosch, "Instant selective arterial occlusion with isobutyl 2 cyanoacrylate," *Radiology*, vol. 114, no. 1, pp. 227–230, 1975.

[4] M. J. Schwartz, E. B. Smith, D. W. Trost, and E. D. Vaughan Jr., "Renal artery embolization: clinical indications and experience from over 100 cases," *BJU International*, vol. 99, no. 4, pp. 881–886, 2007.

[5] D. Hom, D. Eiley, J. H. Lumerman, D. N. Siegel, E. R. Goldfischer, and A. D. Smith, "Complete renal embolization as an alternative to nephrectomy," *The Journal of Urology*, vol. 161, no. 1, pp. 24–27, 1999.

[6] J.-M. Neuerburg and K. Lehrmann, "Transarterial embolization of the kidney: Review of the literature," *RöFo - Fortschritte Auf Dem Gebiet Der Röntgenstrahlen Und Der Bildgebenden Verfahren*, vol. 176, no. 6, pp. 809–816, 2004.

[7] S. H. Duda, A. Raible, T. Risler, P. E. Huppert, H.-J. Brambs, and M. Gregor, "Therapeutic bilateral renal artery embolization in the nephrotic syndrome," *Deutsche Medizinische Wochenschrift*, vol. 119, no. 3, pp. 58–62, 1994.

[8] D. H. Golwyn Jr., W. D. Routh, M. Y. M. Chen, W. B. Lorentz, and R. B. Dyer, "Percutaneous transcatheter renal ablation with absolute ethanol for uncontrolled hypertension or nephrotic syndrome: Results in 11 patients with end-stage renal disease," *Journal of Vascular and Interventional Radiology*, vol. 8, no. 4, pp. 527–533, 1997.

[9] F. S. Keller, M. Coyle, J. Rosch, and C. T. Dotter, "Percutaneous renal ablation in patients with end-stage renal disease: alternative to surgical nephrectomy," *Radiology*, vol. 159, no. 2, pp. 447–451, 1986.

[10] J. J. Olivero, J. P. Frommer, and J. M. Gonzalez, "Medical nephrectomy: the last resort for intractable complications of the nephrotic syndrome," *American Journal of Kidney Diseases*, vol. 21, no. 3, pp. 260–263, 1993.

[11] Y. Solak, I. Polat, H. Atalay, and S. Turk, "When urine is no longer beneficial: Renal artery embolisation in severe nephrotic syndrome secondary to amyloidosis," *Amyloid*, vol. 17, no. 1, pp. 24–26, 2010.

[12] A. Maeda, K. Takeda, H. Kondou et al., "Percutaneous renal artery embolization in a patient with severe nephrotic syndrome which continued after the introduction of hemodialysis," *Internal Medicine*, vol. 50, no. 23, pp. 2899–2904, 2011.

[13] Y. Solak, O. Koc, R. Ucar et al., "Renal artery embolization in severe nephrotic syndrome," *Hemodialysis International*, vol. 20, no. 3, pp. 407–413, 2016.

[14] C. González-Satué, L. Riera, E. Franco, E. Escalante, J. Dominguez, and N. Serrallach, "Percutaneous embolization of the failed renal allograft in patients with graft intolerance syndrome," *BJU International*, vol. 86, no. 6, pp. 610–612, 2000.

[15] T. Tikkakoski, M. Leppänen, J. Turunen, S. Anderson, and H. Södervik, "Percutaneous transcatheter renal embolization with absolute ethanol for uncontrolled nephrotic syndrome: case reports," *Acta Radiologica*, vol. 42, no. 1, pp. 80–83, 2001.

[16] C. Ferro, U. G. Rossi, G. Bovio, F. Petrocelli, and S. Seitun, "The AMPLATZER vascular plug 4: Preliminary experience," *CardioVascular and Interventional Radiology*, vol. 33, no. 4, pp. 844–848, 2010.

9

Successful Initiation of Dialysis with a 20-Year-Old Buried Peritoneal Dialysis Catheter: Case Report and Literature Review

**Ankur Gupta,[1,2] Susan Lavoie,[1,2] Brian Blew,[3]
Mohan Biyani,[1,2] and Brendan B. McCormick[1,2]**

[1]*Division of Nephrology, Department of Medicine, University of Ottawa and The Ottawa Hospital, Canada*
[2]*Kidney Research Centre, University of Ottawa, Canada*
[3]*Department of Surgery, University of Ottawa and the Ottawa Hospital, Canada*

Correspondence should be addressed to Brendan B. McCormick; bmccormick@toh.on.ca

Academic Editor: Phuong Chi Pham

Buried peritoneal dialysis (PD) catheters are typically inserted several weeks or months before the anticipated need for dialysis. Occasionally, renal function unexpectedly stabilizes after the surgery, and a patient may go years before the catheter is needed. We report a case of successful initiation of PD with a twenty-year-old buried catheter. We outline the steps needed to optimize the catheter function and review the benefits of the buried PD catheter.

1. Introduction

Since the late 1990s, our centre has inserted buried peritoneal dialysis (PD) catheters using a modified Moncrief-Popovitch technique [1, 2]. The technique was originally described in 1993 as a method for reducing the rate of PD peritonitis [3, 4]. It was postulated that allowing the catheter to heal in the sterile subcutaneous tissue would prevent the primary formation of bacterial biofilm. Delayed exteriorization of the catheter would allow for complete healing of the subcutaneous cuff which would then act as a physical barrier to biofilm formation. Studies did indeed show less biofilm formation with buried PD catheters [5], but this did not consistently translate into reduced rates of PD peritonitis [6–8]. Subsequently, buried PD catheters have been promoted as a way to increase PD utilization by allowing for insertion of a maintenance free access months before it is actually required, similar to early insertion of an arteriovenous fistula [9].

We have reported an ideal time window of exteriorization ranging from 6-weeks to 5-months as this seems to be associated with the lowest risk of primary failure and lowest need for intervention after exteriorization [10]. Furthermore, time to first peritonitis increases with increased length of time embedded suggesting that a well-healed and mature tunnel may lead to less early peritonitis [10]. However, it is postulated that the risk of fibrin plugging, omental wrapping, and catheter migration increases with time the catheter is not in use [10, 11].

2. Case

A now 76-year-old male underwent buried PD catheter insertion in 1998 at the Ottawa Hospital. He had membranous glomerulopathy and stage 5 chronic kidney disease (CKD) with an estimated glomerular filtration rate (eGFR) of 13 mL/min/1.73m2. Over the ensuing years, he continued to have subnephrotic proteinuria and was managed with perindopril. The renal function remained relatively stable and only began to decline in late 2017. He consented to initiation of PD in February 2018 after his eGFR dropped to 7 mL/min/1.73m2. A plain radiograph of the abdomen showed the PD catheter optimally positioned in the true pelvis (Figure 1(a)).

The exteriorization procedure was performed in the Home Dialysis Unit. A 0.5 cm skin incision was made 2 cm distal to the superficial cuff and a loop of the catheter was mobilized and the fibrin was cleared off the catheter. The distal catheter did not glide out easily. With the assistance of a surgeon, a second incision was made over the distal end of the catheter and it was separated from the subcutaneous

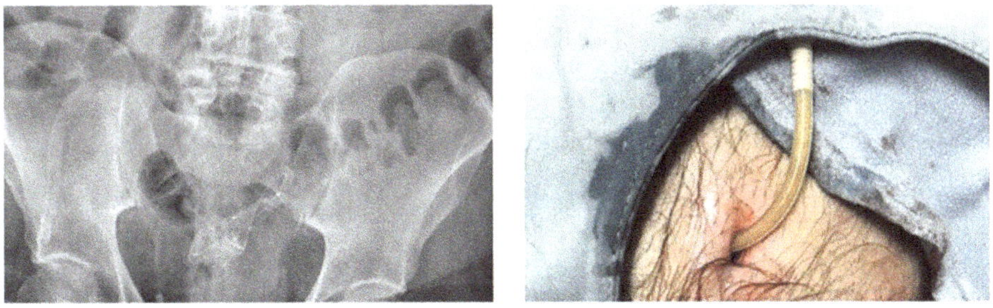

(a) (b)

FIGURE 1: (a) Plain radiograph of the abdomen showing position of catheter prior to exteriorization. (b) Catheter immediately after exteriorization.

tissue by dissection and the end of the catheter was cut off (Figure 1(b)). A large fibrin plug was removed from the lumen of the catheter with push and pull syringe aspiration. The flow remained very sluggish. Tissue plasminogen activator (tPA) was instilled into the catheter and by the following day the inflow significantly improved but outflow was still slow.

Two days later, a cathetergram and guide wire manipulation of the catheter was then arranged through interventional radiology. The initial contrast injection showed the PD catheter localized within a pocket of fibrous tissue communicating with the greater peritoneal cavity along the right pelvic wall. Two angled glide-wires were utilized to clear fibrin out of the lumen of the catheter and a torque cable was then used to flip the draining loop out of the fibrous pocket into the greater peritoneal cavity. Following this, outflow improved and the patient was able to successfully initiate continuous ambulatory PD (CAPD). We have documented a filling time of 6 minutes and drain time of 9 minutes. His clinical course has otherwise been uneventful.

3. Discussion

This case highlights a successful exteriorization and initiation of CAPD with a buried catheter that had lain dormant for almost 20 years. To our knowledge, this is the longest reported period of time between implantation of a buried PD catheter and successful initiation of PD. The exteriorization procedure was more challenging than usual as the free end of the catheter required surgical dissection whereas it normally glides out easily. We encountered the expected challenges with fibrin plugging of the catheter, but with a combination of syringe aspiration, tPA instillation, and guidewire manipulation, we were able to successfully initiation PD.

The early placement of a buried PD catheter has numerous advantages [2]. During the time that the catheter is buried, no maintenance is required and the exteriorization is an elective outpatient procedure. The completely healed catheter tunnel at the time of exteriorization allows for the use of full dwell volumes with lower leak risk. Other benefits include flexibility in PD initiation, reduced need for bridging hemodialysis in urgent starts, low rates of infectious complications, and cuff extrusion. While there are occasional reports of visceral perforation with a dormant PD catheter [12], similar reports of trauma have occurred with other methods of catheter insertion [13].

Our current report confirms that there is no upper limit of time after which a buried PD catheter should not be used due to presumed futility. Although we continue to recommend two to six months as the ideal time period for implantation of buried PD catheter prior to use, we strongly suggest that exteriorization of a long buried PD catheter should always be attempted before resorting to other dialysis accesses or modalities.

References

[1] D. E. Pagé and C. Turpin, "A simple and inexpensive method of subcutaneous implantation of catheter distal segment using a Tenckhoff curled catheter," *Peritoneal Dialysis International*, vol. 20, no. 1, pp. 85–87, 2000.

[2] B. B. McCormick, P. A. Brown, G. Knoll et al., "Use of the embedded peritoneal dialysis catheter: experience and results from a North American center," *Kidney International Suppl*, vol. 103, pp. S38–S43, 2006.

[3] J. W. Moncrief, R. P. Popovich, L. J. Broadrick, Z. Z. He, E. E. Simmons, and R. A. Tate, "The Moncrief-Popovich catheter: a new peritoneal access technique for patients on peritoneal dialysis," *ASAIO Journal*, vol. 39, no. 1, pp. 62–65, 1993.

[4] J. W. Moncrief, R. P. Popovich, M. Dasgupta, J. W. Costerton, E. Simmons, and B. Moncrief, "Reduction in peritonitis incidence in continuous ambulatory peritoneal dialysis with a new catheter and implantation technique," *Peritoneal Dialysis International*, vol. 13, Suppl 2, pp. S329–S331, 1993.

[5] M. K. Oasgupta, K. B. Bettcher, R. A. Ulan et al., "Relationship of adherent bacterial biofilms to peritonitis in chronic ambulatory peritoneal dial ysis," *Peritoneal Dialysis International*, vol. 7, no. 3, pp. 168–173, 1987.

[6] M. S. Park, A. S. Yim, S. H. Chung et al., "Effect of prolonged subcutaneous implantation of peritoneal catheter on peritonitis rate during CAPD: a prospective randomized study," *Blood Purification*, vol. 16, no. 3, pp. 171–178, 1998.

[7] A. Danielsson, L. Blohmé, A. Tranæus, and B. Hylander, "A prospective randomized study of the effect of a subcutaneously

"buried" peritoneal dialysis catheter technique versus standard technique on the incidence of peritonitis and exit-site infection," *Peritoneal Dialysis International*, vol. 22, no. 2, pp. 211–219, 2002.

[8] C.-C. Wu, P.-F. Su, and S.-S. Chiang, "A prospective study to compare subcutaneously buried peritoneal dialysis catheter technique with conventional technique," *Blood Purification*, vol. 25, no. 3, pp. 229–232, 2007.

[9] M. K. Dasgupta, "Moncrief-Popovich catheter and implantation technique: the AV fistula of peritoneal dialysis," *Advances in Chronic Kidney Disease*, vol. 9, no. 2, pp. 116–124, 2002.

[10] P. A. Brown, B. B. McCormick, G. Knoll et al., "Complications and catheter survival with prolonged embedding of peritoneal dialysis catheters," *Nephrology Dialysis Transplantation* , vol. 23, no. 7, pp. 2299–2303, 2008.

[11] J. H. Crabtree and R. J. Burchette, "Peritoneal dialysis catheter embedment: surgical considerations, expectations, and complications," *The American Journal of Surgery*, vol. 206, no. 4, pp. 464–471, 2013.

[12] J. Yao, L. Witherspoon, B. B. McCormick, E. Belanger, and J. E. Warren, "Abdominal visceral perforation by buried peritoneal dialysis catheters: cause or coincidence?" *Seminars in Dialysis*, vol. 31, no. 3, pp. 305–308, 2018.

[13] K. Abreo and A. Sequeira, "Bowel perforation during peritoneal dialysis catheter placement," *American Journal of Kidney Diseases*, vol. 68, no. 2, pp. 312–315, 2016.

10

Treating TNF Receptor Associated Periodic Fever Syndrome in End-Stage Renal Failure

J. Coutinho,[1] R. S. Chorão,[1] M. Oliveira,[2] and C. R. Santos[1]

[1]*Hospital Amato Lusitano, Castelo Branco, Portugal*
[2]*Centro Hospitalar Cova da Beira, Covilhã, Portugal*

Correspondence should be addressed to J. Coutinho; joanacoutinho_@hotmail.com

Academic Editor: Raoul Bergner

Tumor necrosis factor receptor associated periodic syndrome (TRAPS) is a rare monogenic autoinflammatory disease. Its most severe manifestation is secondary amyloidosis. A 44-year-old male presented with nephrotic syndrome. Kidney biopsy was conclusive for secondary amyloidosis. The patient and his children had a history of recurrent febrile periods since infancy. All subjects were positive for a heterozygous variant of the TNFRSF1A gene, confirming TRAPS diagnosis. The patient progressed to end-stage renal failure and developed recurrent pericarditis episodes. He was started on anakinra while on hemodialysis with marked reduction of his serum amyloid A protein (SAA) levels. Meanwhile he received a cadaveric renal transplant and maintains anakinra treatment. Despite renal failure being the most feared complication of AA amyloidosis caused by TRAPS, little data is available about safety of anti-IL-1 treatment in patients with severe kidney failure. The authors report this case of a patient on dialysis treated with anakinra in which no complications were registered. Though amyloidosis is established, the authors believe containing its progression and reducing inflammatory activity can improve patient prognosis and reduce recurrence of amyloidosis in kidney transplant, as has been demonstrated in transplanted patients due to familial Mediterranean fever amyloidosis.

1. Introduction

Periodic fever associated syndromes are monogenic autoinflammatory diseases with autosomal patterns of genetic transmission. These hereditary febrile syndromes lack features of adaptive immune dysregulation and have been proposed to be caused by innate immune defects. Innate immune system dysregulation causes a pathogenic proinflammatory state driven by inflammasome activation and consequently excessive production of inflammatory cytokines, namely, interleukin-1-beta [1–3].

Tumor necrosis factor receptor associated periodic syndrome (TRAPS) caused by mutation of the TNF receptor superfamily 1A gene was first characterized in 1999, though the disease had been previously described as familial Hibernian fever in 1982 [4]. Though the disease has no cure, in the last decade IL-1 receptor antagonists have emerged as the first-line treatment option for TRAPS patients [5, 6], being effective in both acute clinical symptom control and postponing of the appearance of amyloidotic complications [1, 6, 7]. Though in the past anti-IL-1 drugs were thought to be reductant when amyloid deposition had already caused significant damage to vital organs, more recent evidence points out that these agents are effective in controlling inflammation, containing amyloidosis, and improving quality of life and possibly some regression of amyloidosis could occur [7–9]. Also a great benefit in cardiovascular protection could derive from controlling inflammation itself [10, 11].

Late diagnosis of TRAPS can entail serious complications in terms of prognosis and pose difficulties for treatment. Despite renal failure being the most feared complication of TRAPS, little data is available about safety of anti-IL-1 treatment in patients with severe kidney failure.

2. Case Presentation

We report the case of a 44-year-old male referred by the family doctor to our nephrology clinic due to the uncontrolled hypertension and renal failure. The patient had a 3-year history of hypertension and hypercholesterolemia and he was taking the following medications: propranolol 40 mg, simvastatin 20 mg, losartan 50 mg, and nifedipine 60 mg.

This patient presented to our outpatient clinic with uncontrolled hypertension (195/110 mmHg), leg edemas that extended to the lower thighs, and complaints of fatigue and headaches. On this first consultation, the patient provided blood and urine workup from 3 months earlier that documented normocytic, normochromic anemia (Hb 12 g/dL), an elevation of creatinine and BUN to 1.9 mg/dL and 66 mg/dL, respectively, and proteinuria of 4.0 g/24 hours. He also had a renal ultrasound reporting normal sized, normal contoured, hyperechogenic kidneys bilaterally with slight corticomedullary dedifferentiation.

The patient was hospitalized with the diagnosis of nephrotic syndrome. The initial workup included a 24-hour urine collection with total proteinuria of 7.36 g, a urinary sediment with many hyaline casts, and a complete blood workup that revealed serum creatinine 2.5 mg/dL, a PTH level of 82 pg/mL, and a slight prolongation of prothrombin time. Subsequent full laboratory and imaging screening tests ruled out infectious and neoplastic or autoimmune disorders. The only positive finding was a left ventricular and auricular hypertrophy with a normal systolic function and ejection fraction, seen on echocardiogram.

From his personal medical history, he had been hospitalized on three occasions, twice in a surgical department for an appendectomy and a cholecystectomy and once in a cardiology department due to suspicion of rheumatic fever that was never confirmed. Apart from the family doctor he denied any other regular medical follow-up. He denied smoking, drugs, or excessive alcohol intake. He also denied contact with animals, except for his dog, and had never travelled abroad. From his family history, there was a history of hypertension from his father and breast cancer from his mother and one younger sister that is healthy. He had no knowledge of consanguinity or congenital diseases within his family.

During the 2-week period the patient was hospitalized, a rapidly progressive worsening of kidney function was observed with creatinine levels reaching 6.3 mg/dL accompanied by serious anemia and an altered coagulation function test needing transfusional support. The prothrombin time was not corrected with fresh frozen plasma and in need of performing a kidney biopsy, we opted for starting the patient on corticosteroids with oral prednisolone 1 mg/kg.

On the 15th day of hospitalization, the hematologic disturbances stabilized, hypertension was controlled, and a kidney biopsy was performed. Over the next days, under corticosteroids the patient's clinical status improved, with concurrent stabilization of kidney function and the anemia, to creatinine level 2.80 mg/dL and hemoglobin 11.8 g/dL. Diet modifications, antihypertensive medication, and chelators of potassium and phosphorus as well as iron therapy had been introduced, with good response, and the patient was discharged on this medication. He waited for the kidney biopsy results as an outpatient and was summoned up for consultation and reevaluation at our nephrology clinic as soon as we had the results.

The kidney biopsy revealed complete sclerosis of the glomeruli with invasion of mesangium and capillaries by an amorphous substance, with 2 glomeruli presenting hyaline mesangial proliferation. Tubules were completely atrophic and there was diffuse interstitial fibrosis with a moderate lymphocitary infiltrate. There was arteriolar hyalinosis at the vascular poles staining positive with Congo red, with normal appearance of the remnant vessels. Immunohistochemistry was negative for complement, free light chains or immunoglobulins. Evaluation for the presence of serum amyloid A (SAA) protein was positive in both the vessels and glomeruli.

Considering the biopsy results we asked the patient to come in for a clinical interview with his wife. On this interview, the patient recalled a long-time history of febrile periods since he was 9 years old that had faded with age and therefore he did not consider relevant. He had been investigated as a child but no conclusion had been made. According to the wife, their two male children suffered from a similar kind of recurrent fevers since they were about 3 years old which had been investigated by their pediatrician but so far no diagnosis had been made. Our patient reported his febrile periods lasted approximately 1 week to 10 days, with no cyclic clockwork recurrence, sometimes attributed to stressful events but mostly unpredictable, and did not respond to classic antipyretics such as ibuprofen or paracetamol. These febrile periods were often accompanied by headaches or myalgia that was focal and migratory, but he denied pharyngitis, skin rashes or urticaria, aphthous ulcers, abdominal pain, arthritis, or vomiting. His children had febrile periods with somewhat different characteristics, as they lasted longer, usually 2 weeks, had a cyclic recurrence 6 months apart, and were mostly accompanied by abdominal pain and migratory arthritis. Neither the patient nor his children had any dysmorphology. His children had normal psychomotor development for their ages, 6 and 8 years old, respectively. The whole family was tested for serum amyloid A protein (SAA). The father was positive (90.3 mg/L, normal <6.4) and the children were negative.

Considering such family history and the fever recurrence in the absence of any suspected infection, the diagnostic algorithm of periodic fever syndrome was considered and corticosteroid therapy was gradually tapered. The fact that both children were affected made us focus on disorders with an autosomal dominant pattern of transmission. Though the father and children had some phenotypic variability, the febrile periods were > 1 week long in all of them, they had consistently 2 to 3 episodes a year, and they all lacked lymphadenopathies and cutaneous or ophthalmologic manifestations, which made us think of TRAPS as the most probable diagnosis.

The family was referred to a geneticist and was tested for TNF receptor mutations. All subjects were positive in heterozygosity for a missense variant mutation (c.242G>T p.Cys81Phe) of the TNFRSF1A gene on chromosome 12, and the diagnosis of TRAPS was confirmed. When these results were known, the family was referred to the rheumatology department to be considered for treatment with IL-1 receptor antagonists. The children were started on anakinra and up until the moment of submission of this article, the children have had no complications of treatment and they have not had any febrile episode for 2 years.

In the meanwhile, the patient continued follow-up in our nephrology clinic and had the need for hospitalization twice, 11 and 13 months after the first hospitalization, due to recurrent pericarditis that did not respond to NSAIDs nor corticosteroid therapy but did respond partially to colchicine. Approval for the use of anakinra in our patient took longer, as anakinra is not approved for use in patients with severe renal failure. Despite control of hypertension and dyslipidemia and partial remission of proteinuria, the patient had a protracted course into end-stage renal failure starting hemodialysis 15 months after the first hospitalization. While on hemodialysis the patient was started on anakinra (100 mg every two days, subcutaneously). Throughout treatment the patient had no serious complication and remained symptom-free, with marked reduction of his serum amyloid A protein levels (3.3 mg/L).

The patient received a successful cadaveric renal transplant in December 2017, 15 months after starting dialysis, and maintains treatment with anakinra until today, which was adjusted after kidney transplantation to 100 mg daily, subcutaneously.

3. Discussion

Periodic fever associated syndromes are monogenic autoinflammatory diseases with autosomal patterns of genetic transmission. Among the classic periodic fever syndromes TRAPS is generally distinguished by being characterized by longer febrile periods, with an average of 7 days to 3 weeks; however there is great interindividual variability in clinical features [2, 12]. Most typical clinical features associated with TRAPS, apart from fever, are abdominal pain (75%), headaches (68%), and focal migratory myalgia (64%) [2], though many others have been described [12–14]. There seems to be a difference on clinical manifestations between patients with pediatric and adult disease onset, with older patients tending to have longer attacks duration and presenting more frequently with chest pain and headache, while abdominal pain, vomiting, cervical adenitis, and pharyngitis predominate in pediatric patients [14]. Recurrent pericarditis is common, especially when disease onset is in adulthood and is more frequently associated with low penetrance mutations, though it was not this patient's case [15, 16].

To date there are more than 170 sequence variant mutations of the TNFRSF1A gene listed on ClinVar [17], though the exact clinical significance of some mutations is unknown. Mutations affecting certain cysteine residues of the TNF receptor seem to be associated with more serious disease and higher risk of systemic amyloidosis, though there is not an exact correlation between genetic mutation and clinical phenotype. Missense mutations, like the mutation our family has, are nonconservative amino acid substitutions, which is likely to impact secondary protein structure and consequently its function [5, 18, 19]. Missense variants in the cysteine residues (C81G/R/Y) and in nearby residues (T79M/K, C84R/Y/S, E85D) have been reported in the Human Gene Mutation Database in association with periodic fever [20]. The largest series of patients with TNFRSF1A gene mutations, EUROFEVER/EUROTRAPS, reported that pathogenic mutations affecting cysteine residues occurred in about 27% of TRAPS patients [2]. Notably, patients with such mutations had a 25% risk of developing secondary amyloidosis, in contrast to patients with low penetrance mutations (R92Q, P46L) which have a 2% risk of developing systemic amyloidosis [1, 2, 7]. The exact mechanism by which a mutation of the TNF receptor leads to activation of inflammatory response is not completely understood, probably because not all mutations share the same mechanism of disease. Some variants of the TNF receptor mutation course with decreased levels of the soluble TNF receptor which lead to insufficient neutralization of excess TNFα. These variants often respond to etanercept, an anti-TNFα monoclonal antibody [8]. However, some genetic variants seem to produce misfolded TNF receptors which are retained in the endoplasmic reticulum and act as sensitizers to small stimuli from the innate immune system, causing the cells to have an exaggerated inflammatory response from trivial stimuli [9]. Consistent with this last theory, called the "misfolding hypothesis," is the demonstration that cysteine residues are involved in formation of intramolecular disulfide bonds, essential to maintain the three-dimensional structure of TNFR1 [10].

Primary treatment of TRAPS targets symptom control and secondary treatment focuses on prevention of long-term complications, namely, AA amyloidosis. Acute symptom control was classically treated with colchicine and oral corticosteroids, with variable results. In the last decade IL-1 receptor antagonists have emerged as the first-line treatment option for TRAPS patients [20–26], being effective in both acute and long-term treatment. Currently 3 anti-IL-1 drugs are available; all of them are renally excreted and caution is advised for use in patients with renal failure. Anakinra, a recombinant homolog of the human IL-1 receptor that competitively inhibits binding of IL-1-alpha and IL-1-beta to its receptor, was the first of its class and has the handicap of needing daily subcutaneous administration with frequent skin reactions. Long-lasting drugs targeting IL-1-beta, such as canakinumab and rilonacept, have better tolerability [11, 27] and are administered subcutaneously every 4 to 6 weeks; however trials evaluating their safety profile in renal failure are lacking. Data regarding the use of IL-1 receptor antagonists in patients with end-stage renal failure is limited to case reports of single patients [28–30], both using anakinra.

Current evidence points to anti-IL-1 drugs being effective, even when significant organ damage has occurred, by controlling inflammation and containing further amyloid deposition. Apart from symptomatic control with anakinra our patient was offered a cadaveric renal transplantation, both of which greatly improved his quality of life. The patient should maintain anakinra throughout his life to prevent long-term complications of this autoinflammatory disorder. Whether this drug will be absolutely effective in containing amyloid deposition in the renal allograft should be a matter for future studies.

Abbreviations

IL-1: Interleukin-1-beta
SAA: Serum amyloid A protein
TNF: Tumor necrosis factor
TNFR1: Tumor necrosis factor receptor 1
TRAPS: Tumor necrosis factor receptor associated periodic fever syndrome.

Consent

Written consent from the patient was obtained for all procedures during investigation and for publication of the article. A copy of the consent form can be made available for review by the editor of this journal.

Disclosure

R. S. Chorão, M. Oliveira, and C. R. Santos are coauthors. All the authors have read and approved of the manuscript to be submitted.

References

[1] L. Cantarini, O. M. Lucherini, I. Muscari et al., "Tumour necrosis factor receptor-associated periodic syndrome (TRAPS): State of the art and future perspectives," *Autoimmunity Reviews*, vol. 12, no. 1, pp. 38–43, 2012.

[2] H. J. Lachmann, R. Papa, and K. Gerhold, "The phenotype of TNF receptor-associated autoinflammatory syndrome (TRAPS) at presentation: a series of 158 cases from the Eurofever/EUROTRAPS international registry," *Annals of the Rheumatic Diseases*, vol. 73, no. 12, pp. 2160–2167, 2014.

[3] D. Rigante, G. Lopalco, A. Vitale et al., "Key facts and hot spots on tumor necrosis factor receptor-associated periodic syndrome," *Clinical Rheumatology*, vol. 33, no. 9, pp. 1197–1207, 2014.

[4] M. F. McDermott, B. W. Ogunkolade, E. M. McDermott et al., "Linkage of familial hibernian fever to chromosome 12p13," *American Journal of Human Genetics*, vol. 62, no. 6, pp. 1446–1451, 1998.

[5] S. L. Rebelo, S. E. Bainbridge, M. R. Amel-Kashipaz et al., "Modeling of tumor necrosis factor receptor superfamily 1A mutants associated with tumor necrosis factor receptor-associated periodic syndrome indicates misfolding consistent with abnormal function," *Arthritis & Rheumatology*, vol. 54, no. 8, pp. 2674–2687, 2006.

[6] http://www.hgmd.org.

[7] N. Ravet, S. Rouaghe, C. Dodé et al., "Clinical significance of P46L and R92Q substitutions in the tumour necrosis factor superfamily 1A gene," *Annals of the Rheumatic Diseases*, vol. 65, no. 9, pp. 1158–1162, 2006.

[8] S. Stojanov, C. Dejaco, P. Lohse et al., "Clinical and functional characterisation of a novel TNFRSF1A c.605T>A/V173D cleavage site mutation associated with tumour necrosis factor receptor-associated periodic fever syndrome (TRAPS), cardiovascular complications and excellent response to etanercept treatment," *Annals of the Rheumatic Diseases*, vol. 67, no. 9, pp. 1292–1298, 2008.

[9] A. Simon, H. Park, R. Maddipati et al., "Concerted action of wild-type and mutant TNF receptors enhances inflammation in TNF receptor 1-associated periodic fever syndrome," *Proceedings of the National Acadamy of Sciences of the United States of America*, vol. 107, no. 21, pp. 9801–9806, 2010.

[10] A. A. Lobito, F. C. Kimberley, J. R. Muppidi et al., "Abnormal disulfide-linked oligomerization results in ER retention and altered signaling by TNFR1 mutants in TNFR1-associated periodic fever syndrome (TRAPS)," *Blood*, vol. 108, no. 4, pp. 1320–1327, 2006.

[11] F. De Benedetti, M. Gattorno, J. Anton et al., "Canakinumab for the treatment of autoinflammatory recurrent fever syndromes," *The New England Journal of Medicine*, vol. 378, no. 20, pp. 1908–1919, 2018.

[12] I. Aksentijevich, J. Galon, M. Soares et al., "The tumor-necrosis-factor receptor-associated periodic syndrome: new mutations in *TNFRSF1A*, ancestral origins, genotype-phenotype studies, and evidence for further genetic heterogeneity of periodic fevers," *American Journal of Human Genetics*, vol. 69, no. 2, pp. 301–314, 2001.

[13] E. Aganna, I. Aksentijevich, G. A. Hitman et al., "Tumor necrosis factor receptor-associated periodic syndrome (TRAPS) in a Dutch family: evidence for a TNFRSF1A mutation with reduced penetrance," *European Journal of Human Genetics*, vol. 9, no. 1, pp. 63–66, 2001.

[14] E. Ruiz-Ortiz, E. Iglesias, A. Soriano et al., "Disease phenotype and outcome depending on the age at disease onset in patients carrying the R92Q low-penetrance variant in TNFRSF1A gene," *Frontiers in Immunology*, vol. 8, p. 299, 2017.

[15] L. Cantarini, O. M. Lucherini, R. Cimaz et al., "Idiopathic recurrent pericarditis refractory to colchicine treatment can reveal tumor necrosis factor receptor-associated periodic syndrome," *International Journal of Immunopathology and Pharmacology*, vol. 22, no. 4, pp. 1051–1058, 2009.

[16] L. Cantarini, O. M. Lucherini, A. Brucato et al., "Clues to detect tumor necrosis factor receptor-associated periodic syndrome (TRAPS) among patients with idiopathic recurrent acute pericarditis: results of a multicentre study," *Clinical Research in Cardiology*, vol. 101, no. 7, pp. 525–531, 2012.

[17] https://clinvarminer.genetics.utah.edu/submissions-by-variant/NM_001065.3%28TNFRSF1A%29%3Ac.242G%3ET%20%28p.Cys81Phe%29.

[18] I. Todd, P. M. Radford, K. Draper-Morgan et al., "Mutant forms of tumour necrosis factor receptor I that occur in TNF-receptor-associated periodic syndrome retain signalling functions but show abnormal behaviour," *The Journal of Immunology*, vol. 113, no. 1, pp. 65–79, 2004.

[19] A. A. Lobito, T. L. Gabriel, J. P. Medema, and F. C. Kimberley, "Disease causing mutations in the TNF and TNFR superfamilies: Focus on molecular mechanisms driving disease," *Trends in Molecular Medicine*, vol. 17, no. 9, pp. 494–505, 2011.

[20] N. Ter Haar, H. Lachmann, S. Özen et al., "Treatment of autoinflammatory diseases: results from the Eurofever registry

and a literature review," *Annals of the Rheumatic Diseases*, vol. 72, no. 5, pp. 678–685, 2013.

[21] N. M. Ter Haar, M. Oswald, J. Jeyaratnam et al., "Recommendations for the management of autoinflammatory diseases," *Annals of the Rheumatic Diseases*, vol. 74, no. 9, pp. 1636–1644, 2015.

[22] A. Vitale, D. Rigante, O. M. Lucherini et al., "Biological treatments: new weapons in the management of monogenic autoinflammatory disorders," *Mediators of Inflammation*, vol. 2013, Article ID 939847, 16 pages, 2013.

[23] M. Gattorno, M. A. Pelagatti, A. Meini et al., "Persistent efficacy of anakinra in patients with tumor necrosis factor receptor-associated periodic syndrome," *Arthritis & Rheumatism*, vol. 58, no. 5, pp. 1516–1520, 2008.

[24] Z. B. Özçakar, S. Özdel, S. Yılmaz, E. D. Kurt-Şükür, M. Ekim, and F. Yalçınkaya, "Anti-IL-1 treatment in familial Mediterranean fever and related amyloidosis," *Clinical Rheumatology*, vol. 35, no. 2, pp. 441–446, 2016.

[25] L. Obici, A. Meini, M. Cattalini et al., "Favourable and sustained response to anakinra in tumour necrosis factor receptor-associated periodic syndrome (TRAPS) with or without AA amyloidosis," *Annals of the Rheumatic Diseases*, vol. 70, no. 8, pp. 1511-1512, 2011.

[26] C. A. Dinarello and J. W. M. van der Meer, "Treating inflammation by blocking interleukin-1 in humans," *Seminars in Immunology*, vol. 25, no. 6, pp. 469–484, 2013.

[27] F. La Torre, M. Caparello, and R. Cimaz, "Canakinumab for the treatment of TNF-receptor associated periodic syndrome," *Expert Review of Clinical Immunology*, vol. 13, no. 6, pp. 513–523, 2017.

[28] C. Moser, G. Pohl, I. Haslinger et al., "Successful treatment of familial Mediterranean fever with anakinra and outcome after renal transplantation," *Nephrology Dialysis Transplantation*, vol. 24, no. 2, pp. 676–678, 2009.

[29] S. Gentileschi, D. Rigante, A. Vitale et al., "Efficacy and safety of anakinra in tumor necrosis factor receptor-associated periodic syndrome (TRAPS) complicated by severe renal failure: a report after long-term follow-up and review of the literature," *Clinical Rheumatology*, vol. 36, no. 7, pp. 1687–1690, 2017.

[30] K. S. Stojanovic, Y. Delmas, P. U. Torres et al., "Dramatic beneficial effect of interleukin-1 inhibitor treatment in patients with familial Mediterranean fever complicated with amyloidosis and renal failure," *Nephrology Dialysis Transplantation*, vol. 27, no. 5, pp. 1898–1901, 2012.

11

Apheresis Therapy for Steroid-Resistant Idiopathic Nephrotic Syndrome: Report on a Case Series

Hamza Naciri Bennani,[1] Thomas Jouve,[1,2] Johan Noble,[1,2] Lionel Rostaing,[1,2] Paolo Malvezzi,[1] and Rachel Tetaz[1]

[1]*Service de Néphrologie, Hémodialyse, Aphérèses et Transplantation Rénale, CHU Grenoble-Alpes, Grenoble, France*
[2]*Université Grenoble Alpes, Grenoble, France*

Correspondence should be addressed to Lionel Rostaing; lrostaing@chu-grenoble.fr

Academic Editor: Yoshihide Fujigaki

Idiopathic nephrotic syndrome (INS) represents 15%–30% of adulthood glomerulopathies. Corticosteroids have been the main treatment for decades and are effective in 70% of minimal-change disease patients and ~30% of focal segmental glomerulosclerosis patients. Multidrug-resistant (steroids, calcineurin-inhibitors, cyclophosphamide, mycophenolate-mofetil, rituximab) idiopathic nephrotic syndrome is a major therapeutic challenge in nephrology. Apheresis (double-filtration plasmapheresis or semi specific immunoadsorption) could act by eliminating the circulating factor (apolipoproteinA1b, solubleCD40L, suPAR) increasing glomerular permeability seen in INS. The aim of the study was to report the outcome of three patients with multidrug-resistant INS treated successfully with apheresis.

1. Introduction

Idiopathic nephrotic syndrome (INS) causes ~90% of childhood glomerulopathies and between 15%–30% of adulthood glomerulopathies [1]. INS is the result of either minimal-change disease (MCD) or focal-segmental glomerulosclerosis (FSGS). In adult patients, first-line treatment relies on steroids, leading to full-remission in 70% of MCD patients [2] and ~30% of FSGS patients [3]. Complete remission of proteinuria with prednisone is a major prognostic factor. In cases of steroid-dependence or steroid-resistant INS, second-line therapy relies on calcineurin-inhibitors, cyclophosphamide, mycophenolate-mofetil (MMF), or rituximab [4]. In ~50% of cases, steroid-resistant INS evolves to end-stage kidney disease within 6–8 years. When INS does not respond to immunosuppressive drugs, apheresis can be considered (e.g., double-filtration plasmapheresis (DFPP) or semi specific immunoadsorption (IA)).

DFPP (plasma separator Plasmaflo™ OP-056 W; Cascadeflo™ EC20; Asahi Kasei Medical, Tokyo, Japan) is an apheresis technique that removes high molecular-weight proteins (alpha2-macroglobulin, LDL, fibrinogen, and immunoglobulins mainly IgM). The blood passes through the first filter, which is used to separate cellular components consisting of white blood cells, red blood cells, and platelets from the plasma. The plasma without the cellular components will pass through the second filter where the macromolecules are selectively removed. Semi-specific immunoadsorption (Immunosorba® or Globaffin® columns; Fresenius Medical Care, Bad-Homburg, Germany) initially involves a centrifugation separating the plasma and cellular components. The plasma is then treated with an adsorptive membrane to selectively remove immunoglobulins (IgA, IgM, and IgG).

Several reports of the literature involve antibodies or circulating factor with regard to the mechanism of proteinuria in INS that triggers podocytes causing the increased glomerular permeability (e.g., apolipoproteinA1b, solubleCD40L, suPAR) [5]. These antibodies and/or this circulating factor would also be the cause of recurrence INS on the kidney allograft [5]. Apheresis could act by eliminating the antibodies and the circulating factor.

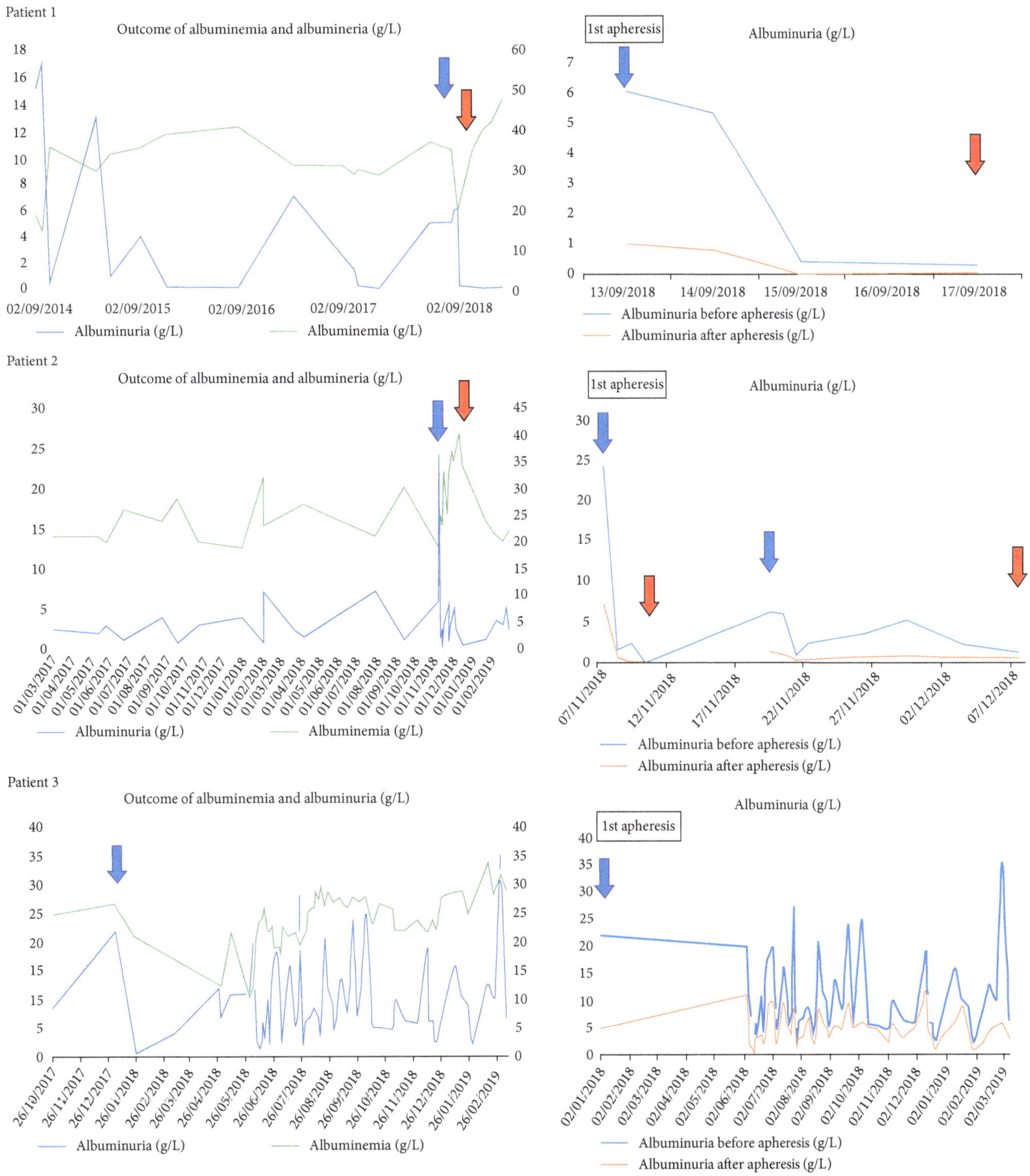

FIGURE 1: Outcome of albuminemia and albuminuria (g/L) for three patients. The blue arrow corresponds to the beginning of apheresis therapy and the red arrow corresponds to the stop of apheresis therapy. On the x axis are dates of the sessions and y axis on the left side albuminuria (g/L) and on the right side albuminemia (g/L).

Full remission is defined as having proteinuria <0.5 g/day and albuminemia >30 g/L; partial remission is defined as proteinuria >0.5 g/day, and albuminemia >30 g/L, or a 50% reduction in the initial proteinuria [6].

Herein, we report on three adult patients with immunosuppressive-resistant INS and that they were successfully treated with apheresis (Figure 1).

2. Case Series

2.1. Patient 1. A 66-year-old male was diagnosed in 2014 with MCD (proteinuria 15 g/L/ albuminemia 19 g/L). He was initially treated with steroids, which gave a good response, but he became steroid-dependent (20 mg/d). When corticosteroid therapy was decreased (<20 mg/d), proteinuria increased to

13 g/L. He, thereafter, received four infusions of rituximab (1 gr each) over a 3-year period, with low steroid doses. The first 3 infusions of rituximab allowed a complete remission during, respectively, 3, 1, and 8 months: at the time of each relapse proteinuria was found to be at 4, 7, and 5 g/L, respectively. At the time of the fourth relapse he received an infusion of rituximab (the 4th one); this induced partial remission; however, one month later proteinuria reincreased to 6 g/L.

In September 2018, he had a fifth relapse (proteinuria 6 g/L/ albuminemia 28 g/L). At that point, he received DFPP (one daily session for 4 consecutive days) followed by one infusion of rituximab (1 gr), and subsequently, remission (>10 months) (>6 months) with proteinuria at 0.09 g/L and albuminemia at 46 g/L. He was weaned-off steroids at the end of DFPP sessions. His renal function remained normal (i.e., estimated glomerular-filtration rate (eGFR) at 89 mL/min/1.73 m^2 according to CKD-EPI formula).

2.2. Patient 2. A 44-year-old woman was diagnosed with MCD when aged 13. She achieved remission with steroids. During her second pregnancy in 2016, she had a relapse of MCD (proteinuria 2.5 g/L/albuminemia 21 g/L) and was placed on steroid therapy without success. Therefore, from early 2017 to November 2018, she was successively treated with MMF, rituximab, and tacrolimus without success. A second kidney biopsy confirmed MCD.

In November 2018, proteinuria was 6 g/L and albuminemia 19 g/L under tacrolimus. She was started on IA therapy, i.e., one daily session for 4 days, which induced remission (proteinuria 0.26 g/L albuminemia 23 g/L). After one week without IA, proteinuria reappeared (proteinuria 5 g/L, and albuminemia 25 g/L); thus, IA therapy was resumed (i.e., one session/day 4 days, then two sessions per week for two weeks). This resulted in partial remission (proteinuria 1.6 g/L albuminemia 40 g/L). However, she refused to continue IA therapy, corticoids, and tacrolimus. Currently, proteinuria fluctuates between 2 and 5 g/L, and albuminemia is between 20 and 25 g/L. Renal function is normal (i.e., eGFR is 106 mL/min/1.73 m^2).

2.3. Patient 3. A 39-year-old male was diagnosed in October 2017 with MCD; proteinuria was 8.8 g/L and albuminemia was 25 g/L. Partial remission was achieved with steroids. Tacrolimus was then added, but was stopped after 3 months because of no improvement in proteinuria (proteinuria 12 g/L albuminemia 13 g/L). In June 2018, apheresis was started, alternating DFPP (up to 18) and IA (up to 36 sessions). In addition, he received an infusion of rituximab (1 gr) every 3 months, and MMF was added. We were unable to stop apheresis because of a relapse within 8–10 days. At present, he receives one apheresis session/week and is no longer taking immunosuppressive therapy; proteinuria fluctuates between 3 and 10 g/L, and albuminemia between 25 and 35 g/L. His eGFR is 79 mL/min/1.73m^2.

To summarize, these three cases of immunosuppressive-resistant INS that received apheresis allowed (i) full remission in one case (with steroid withdrawal), (ii) partial remission in one case with apheresis dependency (one session/ week); and (iii) partial remission with IA dependency in the third case, but the patient refused long-term therapy.

3. Discussion

The physiopathology of FSGS is still unknown and relies on the existence of a permeability circulating factor (suPAR) or antibodies (anti-CD40 antibody, protein tyrosine-phosphatase receptor type O antibody, apoliprotein, ...) [5]. A recent study identified anti-ubiquitin carboxyl-terminal hydrolase 1 autoantibody (UCHL-1) as a cause of proteinuria in INS. This antibody induces proteinuria and podocyte foot effacement in mice [7]. If autoantibody (ies) is/are involved in the pathophysiology of INS, rituximab and apheresis may be the best therapy for corticosteroid-resistant INS. Rituximab is a B-lymphocyte depleting monoclonal antibody that targets CD20. It can influence the production of the circulating factor that results in INS and it inhibits actin-cytoskeleton breakdown in podocytes to reduce proteinuria [8]. On the other hand, apheresis could act by directly eliminating the antibodies and the circulating factor.

In a review paper, Muso et al. reported that apheresis resulted in 54%–86% remission in adults with steroid-resistant INS [9]. In a prospective multicenter study that included 44 steroid/cyclosporine-resistant adults with INS (12 MCD and 28 FSGS) apheresis achieved partial remission in 23% after 9.6+/−2.7 sessions [10] and was 84% more efficacious when started earlier (i.e. at <8 weeks vs. later [43% success]).

Raina et al. reported on 11 steroid/cyclosporine-resistant children with INS where apheresis induced remission in 64%, i.e., proteinuria decreased from 9.7+/−2.5 to 1 +/0.5 g/d [11]. Similarly, Nattes et al. [12] gave IA (10 sessions over a 2-week period) to 14 steroid/calcineurin-inhibitor-resistant children with INS (58% were FSGS); this resulted in full or partial remission in 50% and 15% of cases, respectively.

4. Conclusion

Until now, there has been no consensus on when to implement apheresis in immunosuppressive-resistant INS (in both children and adults). However, the literature and our experience suggest that DFPP or IA can be added in INS when conventional therapies have failed.

References

[1] V. Audard, P. Lang, and D. Sahali, "Pathogénie du syndrome néphrotique à lesions glomérulaires minimes," *Médecine/ Sciences*, vol. 24, pp. 853–858, 2008.

[2] J. Hogan and J. Radhakrishnan, "The treatment of minimal change disease in adults," *Journal of the American Society of Nephrology*, vol. 24, no. 5, pp. 702–711, 2013.

[3] S. M. Korbet, "Treatment of primary FSGS in adults," *Journal of the American Society of Nephrology*, vol. 23, no. 11, pp. 1769–1776, 2012.

[4] S. M. Korbet and W. L. Whittier, "Management of adult minimal change disease," *Clinical Journal of American Society of Nephrology*, vol. 14, no. 6, pp. 911–913, 2019.

[5] M. Delville, T. K. Sugdel, C. Wei et al., "A circulating antibody panel for pretransplant prediction of FSGS recurrence after kidney transplantation," *Science Translational Medicine*, vol. 6, no. 256, p. 256ra136, 2014.

[6] Haute Autorité de Santé, "Syndrome néphrotique idiopathique de l'adulte," https://www.has-sante.fr/portail/upload/docs/application/pdf/2014-12/pnds_-_syndrome_nephrotique_idiopathique_de_ladulte.pdf.

[7] A. Jamin, L. Berthelot, A. Couderc et al., "Autoantibodies against podocytic UCHL1 are associated with idiopathic nephrotic syndrome relapses and induce proteinuria in mice," *Journal of Autoimmunity*, vol. 89, pp. 149–161, 2018.

[8] V. Audard, N. Kamar, D. Sahali et al., "Rituximab therapy prevents focal and segmental glomerulosclerosis recurrence after a second renal transplantation," *Transplant International*, vol. 25, no. 5, pp. e62–e66, 2012.

[9] E. Muso, "Beneficial effect of LDL-apheresis in refractory nephrotic syndrome," *Clinical and Experimental Nephrology*, vol. 18, no. 2, pp. 286–290, 2014.

[10] E. Muso, M. Mune, T. Hirano et al., "A prospective observational survey on the long-term effect of LDL apheresis on drug-resistant nephrotic syndrome," *Nephro Extra*, vol. 5, no. 2, pp. 58–66, 2015.

[11] R. Raina and V. Krishnappa, "An update on LDL apheresis for nephrotic syndrome," *Pediatric Nephrology*, 2018.

[12] E. Nattes, D. Karra, L. Dehoux, M. Peuchmaur, T. Kwon, and G. Deschênes, "Remission of proteinuria in multidrug-resistant idiopathic nephrotic syndrome following immunoglobulin immunoadsorption," *Acta Pediatrica*, vol. 108, no. 4, pp. 757–762, 2019.

12

Propofol Infusion Syndrome in the Postoperative Period of a Kidney Transplant

Edgar Dehesa-López,[1,2,3] **Sergio Saul Irizar-Santana**,[1,2] **Rolando Claure-Del Granado**,[4] **and Rafael Valdez-Ortiz**[5]

[1]*Department of Internal Medicine and Nephrology, Hospital Civil de Culiacán, Culiacán, Mexico*
[2]*Centro de Investigación y Docencia en Ciencias de la Salud, Universidad Autónoma de Sinaloa, Culiacán, Mexico*
[3]*Instituto Mexicano del Seguro Social (IMSS), Mexico*
[4]*Division of Nephrology, Hospital Obrero #2 – C.N.S., Cochabamba, Bolivia*
[5]*Department of Nephrology, Hospital General de México, Mexico City, Mexico*

Correspondence should be addressed to Edgar Dehesa-López; edgar.dehesa@gmail.com

Academic Editor: Anja Haase-Fielitz

Sedation during medical procedures poses a risk to any patient, and the use of specific anesthetic agents should be carefully considered to avoid adverse outcomes. We report on a patient with propofol infusion syndrome diagnosed during the post-operative period of a renal transplant. A 58-year-old female on chronic hemodialysis due to end stage kidney disease secondary to microscopic polyangiitis underwent kidney transplant from a deceased donor. Anesthetic induction was performed with fentanyl, propofol, and cisatracurium, and maintained with continuous propofol infusion. In the recovery room, the patient developed somnolence, tachypnea, and thoracoabdominal dissociation secondary to residual neuromuscular block. An arterial-blood gas test indicated acidemia, high pCO_2, low HCO_3, and mildly increased serum lactate. The patient remained hemodynamically stable, on volume-controlled ventilation, with sedation by continuous propofol infusion. Blood gas tests revealed persistent acidemia without tissue hypoperfusion. Doppler ultrasound of the renal graft reported adequate blood flow and serum triglycerides were elevated. A diagnosis of propofol infusion syndrome was made, and infusion ceased. A decrease in serum lactate levels was observed, with normalization 4 h later. This case highlights the importance of considering adverse effects of anesthetic agents as the cause of post-operative complications when prolonged sedation is required.

1. Introduction

Renal transplantation is currently the best therapeutic option for treating end-stage kidney disease (ESKD) [1, 2]. Current pre-transplant evaluation of the anesthetic, medical, surgical, and immunological risks of the renal recipient makes this a safe procedure, with a low complication rate [3–5]. Propofol is a powerful general anesthetic agent with a short half-life, and characterized by its immediate action and rapidly reversible sedation, which make it popular for sedation during medical or surgical procedures and for maintained sedation in ICUs [6, 7]. Propofol infusion syndrome (PRIS) is a rare, potentially fatal condition first described in children in the 1990s, and later reported in adults. It is generally associated with high doses or prolonged use of propofol infusion, and characterized by metabolic acidosis, rhabdomyolysis of skeletal and cardiac muscle, arrhythmias (bradycardia, atrial fibrillation, ventricular and supraventricular tachycardia, bundle branch block, and asystole), myocardial failure, renal failure, and hepatomegaly [8]. We present a case of severe lactic acidosis, secondary to PRIS, in the post-operative period of a kidney transplant.

2. Case Presentation

A 58-year-old female was diagnosed with ESKD secondary to microscopic polyangiitis, refractory to initial treatment with methylprednisolone, intravenous cyclophosphamide, and

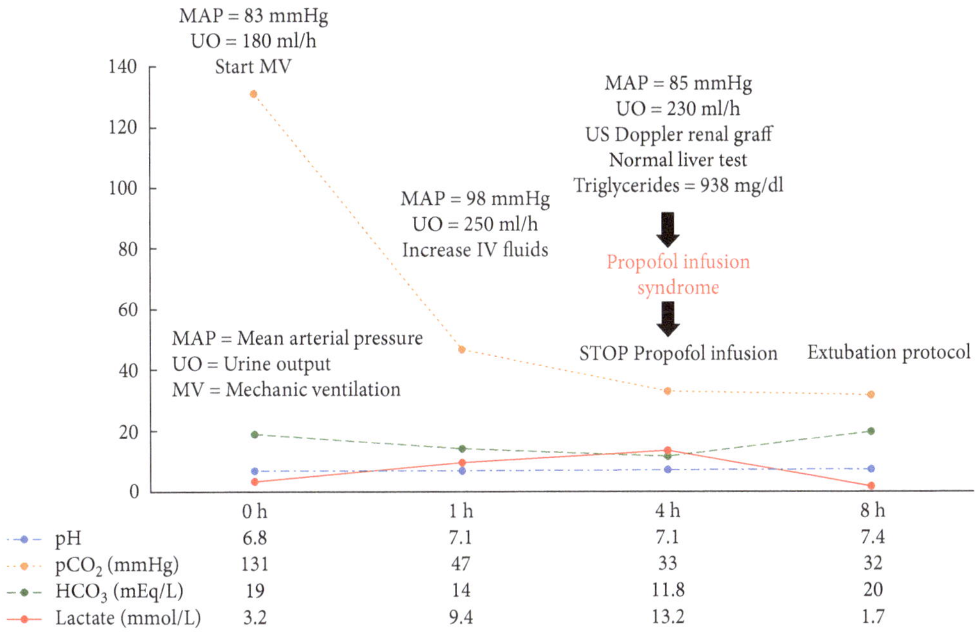

Figure 1: Evolution of gasometric parameters during treatment of patient.

plasmapheresis. She remained on chronic, intermittent hemodialysis 3 times a week for 16 months and had diuresis (800 ml/24 h), without any clinical or biochemical activity of microscopic polyangiitis in the past 6 months. She successfully completed the protocol for a kidney transplant from a deceased donor, which was performed in August of 2018. Crossmatch test was negative, blood type was A+ (donor 26-year-old female, blood type O+), and the induction immunosuppression regimen used was methylprednisolone (1000 mg, IV) and basiliximab (20 mg, IV). The surgical procedure was performed under total general intravenous anesthesia, induced with fentanyl (3 μ/kg), propofol (1.5 mg/kg), and cisatracurium (100 μ/kg). Anesthesia was maintained with continuous infusion of propofol (100–200 μ/Kg/min). Two arterial anastomoses, one venous and one ureterovesical, were made without complications. Adequate perfusion of the graft was corroborated, and 200 ml of spontaneous diuresis was observed by the end of the surgical procedure. The patient remained hemodynamically stable during surgery, which lasted 3 h, with a cold ischemia time of 10 h and surgical bleeding less than 500 ml. In the recovery room, the patient developed somnolence, tachypnea, and thoracoabdominal dissociation secondary to residual neuromuscular block. An arterial-blood gas test revealed a pH of 6.8, pCO_2 131 mmHg, pO_2 212 mmHg, HCO_3 19 mmol/L, and lactate 3.2 mmol/L. The patient was intubated and transferred to the intensive care unit (ICU) for mechanical ventilation support. In the ICU, the patient remained on volume-controlled ventilation, was hemodynamically stable, and remained sedated with continuous propofol infusion at 0.5 mg/kg/h. A venous-blood gas test performed 1 h later showed that pH increased to 7.10, pCO_2 47 mmHg, pO_2 59 mmHg, HCO_3 14 mmol/L, and increased lactate levels (9.4 mmol/L) (Figure 1). Common causes of type A and B lactic acidosis were ruled out due to a lack of arterial hypotension and tissue hypoperfusion, presence of spontaneous renal graft diuresis, normal oxygen saturation, and normal liver tests. Three hours after increasing intravenous fluids, a new venous-blood gas test showed persistent acidemia with a pH of 7.16, pCO_2 33 mmHg, pO_2 60 mmHg, HCO 11.8 mmol/L, and increased lactate levels (13.2 mmol/L), despite maintaining hemodynamic stability, with MAP >65 mmHg without vasopressor treatment, urinary output 200–300 ml/h, and being afebrile without any clinical data demonstrating tissue hypoperfusion (Figure 1). No auricular or ventricular arrhythmia was documented, and her serum level of creatine phosphokinase was normal (143 U/L). Doppler ultrasound of the renal graft reported adequate blood flow at the principal and polar renal arteries. Once the main causes of lactic acidosis were ruled out, we reviewed less frequent causes of unexplained lactic acidosis and found that propofol infusion syndrome (PRIS) could be the cause in our patient. We proceeded to measure serum triglyceride levels, which were 964 mg/dl (Figure 2), and the patient was diagnosed with PRIS. Propofol infusion was stopped, and correction of metabolic acidosis and a progressive decrease in serum lactate levels were observed, with normalization 4 h later (pH 7.4, pCO_2 32 mmHg, HCO_3 20 mmol/L, and lactate 1.7 mmol/L) (Figure 1). The patient was extubated without complications and transferred to the hospital ward. Progressive decrease and normalization of serum triglyceride and creatinine levels were documented, and she was discharged on postoperative day 4 with no other complications.

3. Discussion

The first cases of a rare, but potentially lethal complication associated with the use of propofol infusion were reported in pediatric patients in 1990 [9]. This complication was

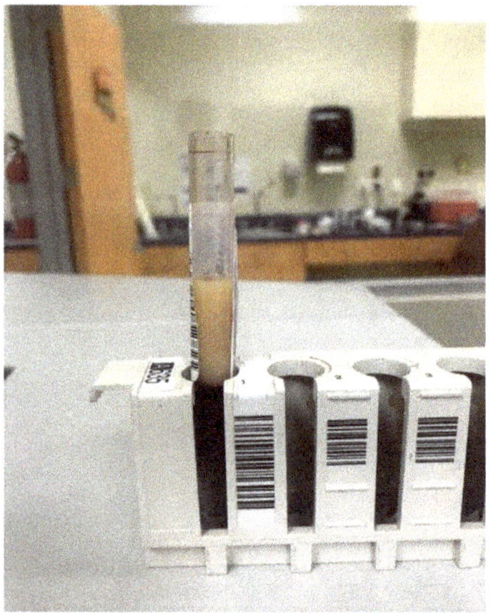

FIGURE 2: Image shows the patient's lipemic serum.

characterized by severe lactic acidosis, rhabdomyolysis, and increased lipemia, with cardiac, hepatic, and renal dysfunction. These pediatric cases were then followed by an increasing number of reported cases in adults, especially in those treated with high doses (>5 mg/kg/h) or prolonged infusions (>48 h) of propofol [10].

The incidence rate of PRIS is difficult to assess due to the use of different diagnostic criteria. Roberts et al. prospectively studied 1,017 ICU patients at 11 academic medical centers treated with propofol infusion for at least 24 h, reporting an incidence of 1.1% [10]. Hemphill et al. recently conducted a narrative review of all cases of PRIS published between 1989 and 2018, documenting a total of 168 cases, of which 44 were in the pediatric population and 124 in the adult population [11]. Since there is variability in the diagnostic criteria used, the authors proposed a definition for PRIS, which is a syndrome that occurs in critically ill patients receiving either high doses (>5 mg/kg/h) or long duration (>48 h) propofol infusions, with one or more of otherwise unexplained symptoms including metabolic acidosis, rhabdomyolysis, electrocardiographic changes with or without acute kidney injury, hyperkalemia, lipidemia, cardiac failure, fever, elevated liver enzymes, or increased lactate levels.

Hemphill et al. also proposed to classify clinical features of PRIS into primary and secondary. Primary features include metabolic acidosis, electrocardiographic changes, and rhabdomyolysis, and secondary features include acute kidney injury, hyperkalemia, lipidemia, cardiac failure, fever, elevated liver enzymes, and increased lactate levels [11]. According to this classification, the diagnosis of PRIS in our patient was based on the presence of 1 primary clinical feature (metabolic acidosis) and 2 secondary features (raised serum lactate levels, and lipidemia).

The primary features most frequently reported by the authors were metabolic acidosis (77%), electrocardiographic changes (62.8%), and rhabdomyolysis (62%). Secondary features most frequently observed were acute kidney injury (50.4%), hyperkalemia (33.6%), raised lactate serum levels (31%), arterial hypotension (31%), cardiac failure (25%), and lipidemia (22.1%) [11]. Multisystem involvement was a frequent finding, with involvement of 3 organs in 29.2%, 4 organs in 23.9%, 2 organs in 20.4%, and 6 organs in 5.3% of cases, with only 15.9% of cases presenting with the involvement of a single organ [11].

From the first reported cases, a wide variety of risk factors for developing PRIS have been identified, including cumulative propofol dose [12, 13], infusion duration [13], sepsis [14], steroids [15], vasopressors [16], fasting [15], critical illness [10], rich fat and low carbohydrate diet [14], inborn errors in mitochondrial fatty-acid oxidation [17], and cranioencephalic trauma [12]. The main risk factors consistently associated with PRIS are accumulated dose and duration of propofol infusion [11, 13]. However, it is important to emphasize that cases of PRIS with multisystem compromise have been reported with low doses of propofol [18]. Krajcova et al. reviewed 153 cases of PRIS and were able to differentiate features dependent on dosage from those related to infusion duration [13]. Features of PRIS dependent on dosage were heart failure, metabolic acidosis, fever, and hypotension. Features dependent on infusion duration were arrhythmias and electrocardiographic changes. Features dependent on high dosage and prolonged duration were rhabdomyolysis and hypertriglyceridemia [13]. Finally, the idiosyncratic features of PRIS (independent of dose and infusion duration) most frequently observed were hepatomegaly and acute kidney injury [13]. In our case, the patient presented a mild form of PRIS due to early diagnosis and immediate discontinuation of propofol infusion.

In our case, the risk factors that likely contributed to the development of PRIS were severe respiratory acidosis during post-anesthetic recovery, use of high doses of methylprednisolone during the induction of immunosuppression, and ESKD. The latter may have caused accumulation of propofol, despite using the recommended doses and a short infusion time. Ickx et al. documented that the pharmacokinetics and pharmacodynamics of propofol are not affected during the induction and maintenance of general anesthesia in patients with ESKD, and that the kidneys do not contribute significantly to extra-hepatic clearance [19]. However, Fodale et al. more recently showed that kidneys have an important role in intrinsic clearance of propofol, contributing up to 27% of total body clearance [8]. An explanation for these contradictory results is use of different pharmacokinetic models to determine total body clearance of propofol [20].

The pathophysiology of PRIS is complex and multifactorial. It is characterized by injury and cell death secondary to imbalance between energy supply and demand within the cells. Propofol interferes with mitochondrial fatty-acid oxidation by inhibiting the enzymatic activity of palmitoyl-transferase I, which causes an energy deficit within cells, and accumulation of free fatty acids in the serum and various organs [21, 22]. This energy deficit mainly affects skeletal and cardiac muscle cells, causing rhabdomyolysis and myocardial dysfunction, respectively [15]. Rhabdomyolysis leads to the release and elevation of intracellular products such as myoglobin, creatinine phosphokinase, potassium, and lactic acid, which can trigger or aggravate kidney damage and acidosis.

At the cardiovascular level, accumulation of free fatty acids has been associated with cardiac arrhythmias [15]. Propofol inhibits β-adrenergic receptors and blocks cardiac calcium channels, which results in a shock state that can evolve to refractory cardiogenic shock, requiring intravenous catecholamines, which can also trigger or aggravate kidney damage and acidosis [15, 23, 24]. It is important to emphasize that these features can often be explained by the patient's critical illness (sepsis, septic shock, traumatic brain injury, etc.), which can mask PRIS and delay its diagnosis.

The prognosis of PRIS is variable and depends of severity and degree of systemic involvement. Hemphill et al. documented a mortality rate of 48% in adult patients and 52% in pediatric patients with the main factors related to mortality being propofol infusion rate, accumulated dose, and infusion duration [11]. Clinical features associated with mortality in adult patients were electrocardiographic changes, arterial hypotension, hyperkalemia, and cranioencephalic trauma. Systemic involvement of multiple organs was also associated with higher mortality in adult patients [11]. Our patient did not present any of the clinical features or dose/duration criteria associated with propofol-induced mortality.

Treatment of PRIS includes immediate suspension of propofol infusion, general support measures, and cardiopulmonary and renal support, if necessary [25]. There is no specific treatment, so early diagnosis is crucial for successful treatment. Awareness of clinical profiles and increased monitoring of patients receiving propofol infusion constitutes the best measures for an early diagnosis. Specific recommendations to reduce the incidence of PRIS are: avoid infusions >5 mg/kg/h and for >48 h. In addition, carbohydrates should be provided to prevent lipemia. It is important to monitor blood pH, lactate levels, and creatine phosphokinase in patients receiving high doses or prolonged infusions of propofol, which cannot be avoided [11, 15, 26].

4. Conclusions

PRIS is a rare but potentially lethal complication that usually occurs in patients receiving propofol infusions at either high doses (>5 mg/kg/h) or for long durations (>48 h). Clinical features and systemic involvement are variable; therefore, awareness of the clinical entity and high level of suspicion are the best measures for early diagnosis. PRIS should be considered as a differential diagnosis in patients on propofol infusion who develop unexplained severe lactic acidosis.

References

[1] R. A. Wolfe, V. B. Ashby, E. L. Milford et al., "Comparison of mortality in all patients on dialysis, patients on dialysis awaiting transplantation, and recipients of a first cadaveric transplant," *New England Journal of Medicine*, vol. 341, no. 23, pp. 1725–1730, 1999.

[2] G. C. Oniscu, H. Brown, and J. L. R. Forsythe, "Impact of cadaveric renal transplantation on survival in patients listed for transplantation," *Journal of the American Society of Nephrology*, vol. 16, no. 6, pp. 1859–1865, 2005.

[3] F. Hovaguimian, M. Schläpfer, and B. Beck-Schimmer, "Organ protection in allograft recipients: anesthetic strategies to reduce postoperative morbidity and mortality," *Current Opinion in Organ Transplantation*, vol. 19, no. 2, pp. 121–130, 2014.

[4] A. Humar and A. J. Matas, "Surgical complications after kidney transplantation," *Seminars in Dialysis*, vol. 18, no. 6, pp. 505–510, 2005.

[5] H.-U. Meier-Kriesche, S. Li, R. W. G. Gruessner et al., "Immunosuppression: evolution in practice and trends, 1994–2004," *American Journal of Transplantation*, vol. 6, no. 5p2, pp. 1111–1131, 2006.

[6] G. Trapani, C. Altomare, G. Liso, E. Sanna, and G. Biggio, "Propofol in anesthesia. Mechanism of action, structure-activity relationships, and drug delivery," *Current Medicinal Chemistry*, vol. 7, no. 2, pp. 249–271, 2000.

[7] K. M. Ho and J. Y. Ng, "The use of propofol for medium and long-term sedation in critically ill adult patients: a meta-analysis," *Intensive Care Medicine*, vol. 34, no. 11, pp. 1969–1979, 2008.

[8] V. Fodale and E. La Monaca, "Propofol infusion syndrome: an overview of a perplexing disease," *Drug Safety*, vol. 31, no. 4, pp. 293–303, 2008.

[9] T. J. Parke, J. E. Stevens, A. S. Rice et al., "Metabolic acidosis and fatal myocardial failure after propofol infusion in children: five case reports," *British Medical Journal*, vol. 305, no. 6854, pp. 613–616, 1992.

[10] R. J. Roberts, J. F. Barletta, J. J. Fong et al., "Incidence of propofol-related infusion syndrome in critically ill adults: a prospective, multicenter study," *Critical Care*, vol. 13, no. 5, R169 pages, 2009.

[11] S. Hemphill, L. McMenamin, M. C. Bellamy, and P. M. Hopkins, "Propofol infusion syndrome: a structured literature review and analysis of published case reports," *British Journal of Anaesthesia*, vol. 122, no. 4, pp. 448–459, 2019.

[12] O. L. Cremer, K. G. Moons, E. A. Bouman, J. E. Kruijswijk, A. M. G. A. de Smet, and C. J. Kalkman, "Long-term propofol infusion and cardiac failure in adult head-injured patients," *The Lancet*, vol. 357, no. 9250, pp. 117–118, 2001.

[13] A. Krajčová, P. Waldauf, M. Anděl, and F. Duška, "Propofol infusion syndrome: a structured review of experimental studies and 153 published case reports," *Critical Care*, vol. 19, no. 1, article no. 398, 2015.

[14] K. Ahlen, C. J. Buckley, D. B. Goodale, and A. H. Pulsford, "The 'propofol infusion syndrome': the facts, their interpretation and implications for patient care," *European Journal of Anaesthesiology*, vol. 23, no. 12, pp. 990–998, 2006.

[15] B. Vasile, F. Rasulo, and A. Candiani, N. Latronico, "The pathophysiology of propofol infusion syndrome: a simple name for a complex syndrome," *Intensive Care Medicine*, vol. 29, no. 9, pp. 1417–1425, 2003.

[16] H. Smith, G. Sinson, and P. Varelas, "Vasopressors and propofol infusion syndrome in severe head trauma," *Neurocritical Care*, vol. 10, no. 2, pp. 166–172, 2009.

[17] J. Parness, M. Savard, and A. F. Turgeon, "Propofol-related infusion syndrome heralding a mitochondrial disease: case report," *Neurology*, vol. 82, no. 5, pp. 461–462, 2014.

[18] T. M. Merz, B. Regli, H.-U. Rothen, and P. Felleiter, "Propofol infusion syndrome—a fatal case at a low infusion rate," *Anesthesia & Analgesia*, vol. 103, no. 4, p.1050, 2006.

[19] B. Ickx, I. D. Cockshott, L. Barvais et al., "Propofol infusion for induction and maintenance of anaesthesia in patients with end-stage renal disease," *British Journal of Anaesthesia*, vol. 81, no. 6, pp. 854–860, 1998.

[20] D. Takizawa, H. Hiraoka, F. Goto, K. Yamamoto, and R. Horiuchi, "Human kidneys play an important role in the elimination of propofol," *Anesthesiology*, vol. 102, no. 2, pp. 327–330, 2005.

[21] J.-P. Vollmer, S. Haen, H. Wolburg et al., "Propofol related infusion syndrome: ultrastructural evidence for a mitochondrial disorder," *Critical Care Medicine*, vol. 46, no. 1, pp. e91–e94, 2018.

[22] A. Wolf, P. Weir, P. Segar, J. Stone, and J. Shield, "Impaired fatty acid oxidation in propofol infusion syndrome," *The Lancet*, vol. 357, no. 9256, pp. 606–607, 2001.

[23] W. Zhou, H. J. Fontenot, S.-N. Wang, and R. H. Kennedy, "Propofol-induced alterations in myocardial β-adrenoceptor binding and responsiveness," *Anesthesia & Analgesia*, vol. 89, no. 3, pp. 604–608, 1999.

[24] W. Zhou, H. J. Fontenot, S. Liu, and R. H. Kennedy, "Modulation of cardiac calcium channels by propofol," *Anesthesiology*, vol. 86, no. 3, pp. 670–675, 1997.

[25] D. A. Diedrich and D. R. Brown, "Analytic reviews: propofol infusion syndrome in the ICU," *Journal of Intensive Care Medicine*, vol. 26, no. 2, pp. 59–72, 2011.

[26] V. Papaioannou, C. Dragoumanis, V. Theodorou, and I. Pneumatikos, "The propofol infusion 'syndrome' in intensive care unit: from pathophysiology to prophylaxis and treatment," *Acta Anaesthesiologica Belgica*, vol. 59, no. 2, pp. 79–86, 2008.

13

Relapsed Acute Lymphoblastic Leukemia Presenting as Acute Renal Failure

Ashley Rose,[1] **Samuel Slone,**[1] **and Eric Padron**[2]

[1]*Internal Medicine, University of South Florida, Tampa, FL 33602, USA*
[2]*Malignant Hematology, H. Lee Moffitt Cancer Center and Research Institute, Tampa, FL 33602, USA*

Correspondence should be addressed to Ashley Rose; ashleyrose2@health.usf.edu

Academic Editor: Yoshihide Fujigaki

Acute lymphoblastic leukemia (ALL) is the second most common acute leukemia in adults. It is an aggressive hematologic neoplasm, with a bimodal age distribution typically presenting in childhood and the 6th decade of life (Terwilliger and Abdul-Hay, 2017). Renal injury in ALL is common and can occur through many different mechanisms, such as prerenal acute kidney injury, acute tubular necrosis, renovascular disease, obstruction, glomerulonephritis, and parenchymal infiltration of tumor cells (Luciano and Brewster, 2014). Infiltration of kidneys by leukemia cells is common; however a resultant injury only occurs in about 1% of patients, and renal failure is even more rare (Luciano and Brewster, 2014). Renal failure due to bilateral infiltration of tumor cells has been reported in only a few cases and is thought to be a poor prognostic indicator (Luciano and Brewster, 2014; Sherief et al., 2015). Biopsy is essential to the diagnosis of renal infiltration of leukemia. We present a case of acute renal failure secondary to bilateral renal infiltration of ALL presenting as the first sign of relapse in a young man.

1. Introduction

Acute lymphoblastic leukemia (ALL) is the second most common acute leukemia in adults with 75% of cases developing from hematopoietic precursors of B-cell lineage [1]. Kidney involvement and injury in leukemia can occur in a variety of different ways such as prerenal acute kidney injury (AKI), acute tubular necrosis (ATN), parenchymal infiltration by the tumor cells, renovascular diseases, obstruction, glomerulonephritis, and electrolyte/acid-base disturbances [2]. AKI secondary to infiltration of ALL is rare, with renal failure being even more rare [2]. The following is a case of acute renal failure secondary to diffuse renal involvement by B-cell ALL as the first sign of relapse, successfully treated with immunotherapy and steroids.

2. Case Presentation

A 37-year-old Hispanic male with a history of B-cell acute lymphocytic leukemia (ALL) presented to the emergency department with left sided flank pain and hematuria. He was previously treated with multiple lines of therapy including several chemotherapy regimens with relapsed/refractory disease. He underwent CAR-T cell therapy in April 2017 and achieved complete remission. He went on to have a mismatched allogeneic hematopoietic stem cell transplant in August 2017 which was complicated by *E. coli* bacteremia and BK cystitis induced hematuria. Soon after, he presented to clinic with acute renal failure and had a ureteral stent placed for left hydronephrosis. Imaging at that time showed symmetric enlargement and decreased density of the kidneys. Serum BK/adenovirus studies were negative. Urine cytology showed benign urothelial cells. Repeat bone marrow biopsy at that time showed 80% cellularity with 80% lymphoblasts. The patient was started on Inotuzumab in March 2018. Repeat bone marrow biopsy following cycle 1 showed no evidence of residual B-cell ALL.

The patient then presented to the emergency department in May 2018 with left sided flank pain and hematuria. Laboratory analysis demonstrated creatinine of 3.9 mg/dL compared to a baseline of 0.6-0.9 mg/dL just 2 weeks earlier. Urinalysis showed negative nitrites, negative leukocyte esterase, >500 protein, 6-10 WBC, 3-5 RBC, and few granular and hyaline casts. Imaging at that time was unchanged from prior

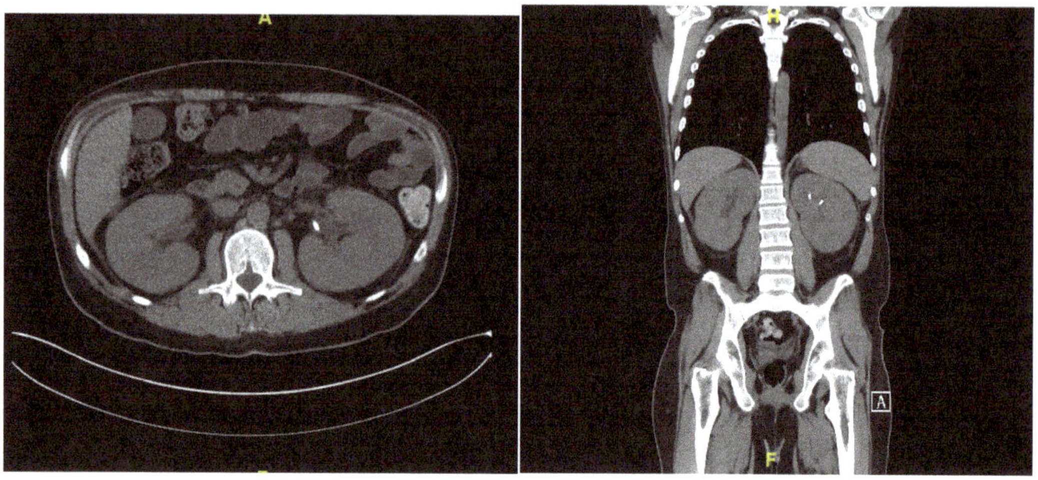

FIGURE 1: (a), (b) Computed tomography scan showing symmetric enlargement and hypoattenuation of bilateral kidneys with associated fat stranding involving the renal sinuses and perinephric fat. Left sided urinary stent in in place. No hydronephrosis or nephrolithiasis.

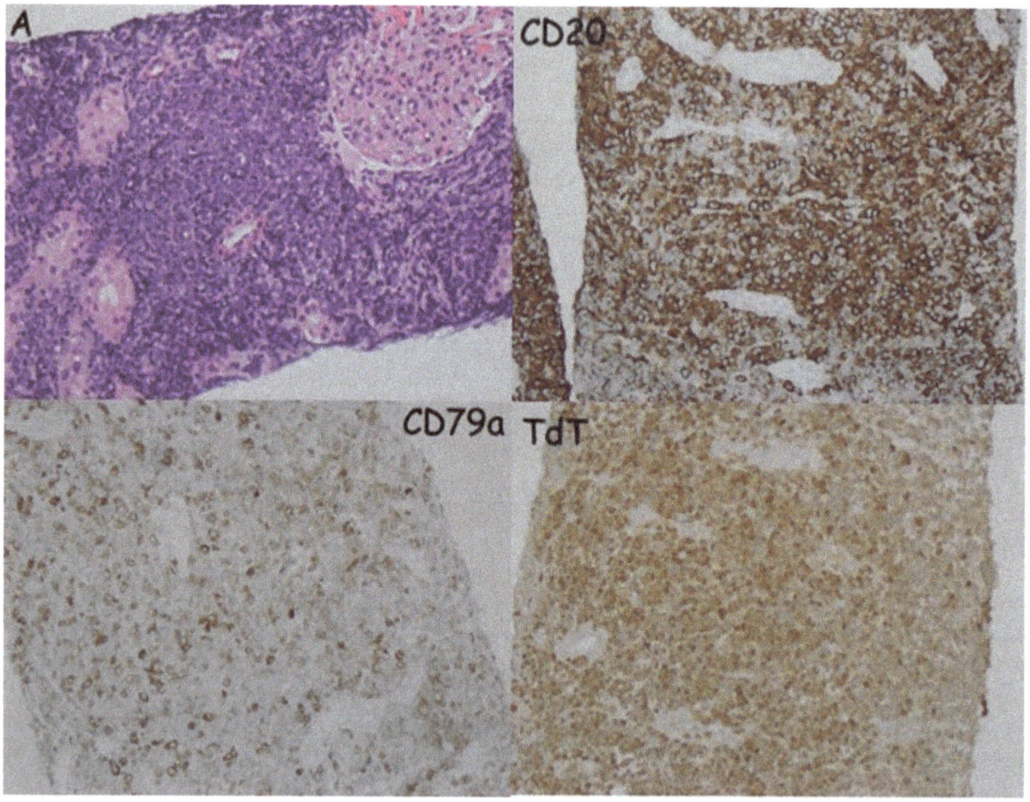

FIGURE 2: Fine needle aspiration of the kidney. *Top left:* H&E stain shows blue tumor cells infiltrating the kidney, pushing the tubules and glomeruli apart. *Top right:* CD20 marker positivity, which is associated with B-cells. *Bottom left:* CD79 marker positivity, which is associated with B-cells. *Bottom right:* Terminal deoxynucleotidyl transferase (TdT) positivity, often seen in acute lymphoblastic leukemia.

imaging, showing symmetric kidney enlargement (Figure 1). Negative work-up included BK viral load, ANCA, anti-GBM antibody, and complement levels. Urine eosinophils were positive. Repeat bone marrow biopsy showed diffuse involvement of B-cell ALL, consistent with relapse. Blood chemistries and uric acid were not consistent with tumor lysis syndrome. Fine needle aspiration of the kidney was performed and demonstrated diffuse invasion of the renal parenchyma by lymphoblasts with positive CD20, CD79, and TdT stains consistent with renal invasion by ALL (Figure 2). The patient had significant oliguria during the first week of hospitalization, with a low daily output of 600mL on day 4. The patient was started on cycle 2 of Inotuzumab as well as Solumedrol 125mg daily for two days, then Prednisone 80mg daily for 5 days followed by a prolonged taper. The patient had significant improvement in hematuria, oliguria, and flank pain following initiation of treatment. His creatinine trended down to 1.5 mg/dL prior to discharge. The patient never required hemodialysis. Unfortunately, several weeks after discharge, the patient presented to the hospital with sepsis secondary to pneumonia and ultimately passed away.

3. Discussion

The reported incidence of ALL is estimated to be 1.6/100,000 with a bimodal distribution with the first peak occurring in childhood and the second peak occurring around age 50 [1]. ALL is an aggressive form of cancer with only 30-40% of patient's achieving remission [1]. Malignant lymphoid cells can accumulate in the bone marrow, peripheral blood, or extramedullary sites with the most common locations being lymph nodes, the spleen, and the liver [1].

Acute kidney injury and renal failure are well recognized complications of leukemia. The most common form of kidney injury in leukemia is related to prerenal AKI in the setting of volume depletion (poor PO intake, diarrhea, anorexia, early satiety) [2]. ATN is also common as either an extension of the disease itself (lysozyme-induced tubular necrosis and tumor lysis syndrome) or secondary to a complication commonly seen in the disease process such as sepsis [2]. Glomerular disease can also be seen with hematologic malignancies. In ALL, the most common types of glomerular lesions are minimal change disease (secondary to lysozymuria induced tubular damage) and focal segmental glomerular sclerosis (more common in children) [2]. Kidney infiltration is common in hematologic malignancies and can be seen in 60-90% of patients, with one study of 1200 autopsy cases showing the prevalence of ALL infiltration of the kidney in ~54% of patients at time of death [3].

AKI secondary to infiltration is seen in ~1% of acute leukemia with renal failure secondary to leukemic infiltration being even more rare [2]. In patients with a hematologic malignancy and unexplained renal failure, infiltration should be suspected especially in the setting of widespread disease [4]. Renal failure in these patients is thought to be secondary to acute tubular compression and disruption of the microvasculature leading to ATN [2]. Typical symptoms associated with kidney infiltration secondary to leukemia include hematuria, flank pain, frothy urine [2]. When infiltration is suspected, kidney biopsy is typically pursued as the extent of infiltration can give prognostic information regarding the malignancy as the rate of infiltration parallels the stage and grade of the disease [2]. Leukemic infiltration of the kidneys tends to occur in the late stages of ALL [5]. Renal infiltration has been associated with a poor prognosis [5].

This case represents a rare occurrence of renal failure secondary to leukemic infiltration of bilateral kidneys presenting as a first sign of relapse in this young patient. The patient had already received multiple lines of therapy for relapsed/refractory ALL. Biopsy was obtained proving the etiology of renal failure, and treatment was initiated promptly. The patient had significant improvement in renal function within a few days of therapy, further proving the cause of his renal dysfunction. It is critical to consider leukemic infiltration in a leukemia patient presenting with renal dysfunction. Once common causes are ruled out, biopsy should be obtained and treatment should be initiated. Unfortunately, this patient ultimately passed away due to sepsis.

References

[1] T. Terwilliger and M. Abdul-Hay, "Acute lymphoblastic leukemia: a comprehensive review and 2017 update," *Blood Cancer Journal*, vol. 7, no. 6, p. e577, 2017.

[2] R. L. Luciano and U. C. Brewster, "Kidney involvement in leukemia and lymphoma," *Advances in Chronic Kidney Disease*, vol. 21, no. 1, pp. 27–35, 2014.

[3] M. Barcos, W. Lane, and G. A. Gomez, "An atuopsy study of 1206 acute and chronic leukemias (1958 to 1982)," *Cancer*, vol. 60, no. 4, pp. 827–837, 1987.

[4] G. T. Obrador, B. Price, Y. O'Meara et al., "Acute renal failure due to lymphomatous infiltration of the kidneys," *Journal of the American Society of Nephrology*, vol. 8, no. 8, pp. 1348–1354, 1997.

[5] L. M. Sherief, S. F. Azab, M. M. Zakaria et al., "Renal presentation in pediatric acute leukemia: report of 2 cases," *Medicine*, vol. 94, no. 37, p. e1461, 2015.

14

Lymphoma-Associated Monoclonal Cryoglobulinemic Glomerulonephritis and Relationship with Hepatitis C Virus Infection: A Case Report

Sangeeta Mutnuri,[1] Hania Kassem,[1] John Badalamenti,[1] You-Wen Qian,[2] Christopher Marquez,[2] and Marjan Afrouzian[1,2]

[1]*Department of Internal Medicine, University of Texas Medical Branch, Galveston, TX, USA*
[2]*Department of Pathology, University of Texas Medical Branch, Galveston, TX, USA*

Correspondence should be addressed to Marjan Afrouzian; maafrouz@utmb.edu

Academic Editor: David Mudge

We report a case of type I cryoglobulinemic glomerulonephritis in a patient with chronic hepatitis C who presented with acute renal failure. The renal biopsy revealed membranoproliferative GN (MPGN) due to cryoglobulinemia with unexpected monoclonal Kappa restriction on immunofluorescence microscopy, suggesting an underlying hematopoietic malignancy. The bone marrow biopsy revealed presence of marginal zone lymphoma. Our case raises awareness regarding possibility of monoclonality in the renal biopsy of HCV-infected patients and exemplifies the crucial role the renal biopsy plays in detecting lymphoid malignancies where clinical features are ambiguous.

1. Introduction

Monoclonal (type I) cryoglobulinemic glomerulonephritis (mCGN) is an uncommon diagnosis, usually reported in association with lymphoproliferative malignancies [1]. Hepatitis C virus (HCV) infection-associated cryoglobulinemia, on the other hand, is a much more common disease, expected to affect the kidney by causing polyclonal (type II) cryoglobulinemic glomerulonephritis (pCGN) [2]. Herein, we introduce an HCV-infected patient who presented with renal failure and in whom the renal biopsy revealed cryoglobulinemic glomerulonephritis (CGN) with monoclonal light chain restriction. The incidences of pCGN and mCGN are compared and the importance of detecting monoclonality in the renal biopsies obtained from HCV-infected patients is entertained.

2. Case Report

2.1. Clinical History and Initial Laboratory Data. A 47-year-old Caucasian male with a history of HCV infection (genotype 3A) and hypertension was admitted with complaints of shortness of breath, dyspnea on exertion, lower extremity edema, abdominal distention, and decreased urine output for the past two months. Physical examination revealed an elevated jugular venous pulse to 8-10 cm of water, bibasilar crackles, an S3 gallop, bilateral lower extremity edema, and hepatosplenomegaly. He was hypertensive with a blood pressure of 183/111 mmHg. Laboratory tests revealed pancytopenia, hypoalbuminemia, hypocomplementemia, cryoglobulinemia, elevated HCV PCR levels, an elevated creatinine level, and an elevated rheumatoid factor level (Table 1). Urine microscopy revealed dysmorphic red blood cells (RBC) in addition to white blood cell (WBC) and RBC casts. He was also found to have nephrotic range proteinuria (9.5 g in 24 hours).

Retroperitoneal ultrasound only showed a small volume of ascites, 14 cm and 12 cm sized kidneys with no hydronephrosis. HCV-induced cryoglobulinemia was suspected and a kidney biopsy was performed.

TABLE 1: Patient's lab results on presentation.

Analyte	Reference Interval	Result
WBC	4.2-10.7 x $10^3/\mu L$	1.8
RBC	4.26-5.52 x $10^6/\mu L$	3.1
Hemoglobin	12.2-16.4 g/dL	9.1
Hematocrit	38.4-49.3 %	27.6
Platelets	150-328 x$10^3/\mu L$	86
Blood Urea Nitrogen (BUN)	7-23 mg/dL	42
Creatinine (Cr)	0.60-1.25 mg/dL	2.87
Albumin	3.5-5.0 g/dL	2.8
C3 complement	86-184 mg/dL	55
C4 complement	20.0-59.0 mg/dL	2.8
RF	<20 IU/mL	10700
HCV PCR -1st	IU/ml	890,318 (diluted 1:13)
HCV PCR (1 week later)	IU/ml	2,485,307
HCV PCR (2 weeks later)	IU/ml	6,790,390

Conversion factors for units: BUN in mg/dL to mmol/L, x0.357; Cr in mg/dL to μmol/L, x88.4; C4 complement in mg/dL to μmol/L, x0.05.
HCV PCR result interpretation.
Not detected: target not detected (not the same as negative).
<12 /ml: detected (but not quantifiable).
12-100,000,000 IU/ml.
>100,000,000 IU/ml: >upper limit of quantification.

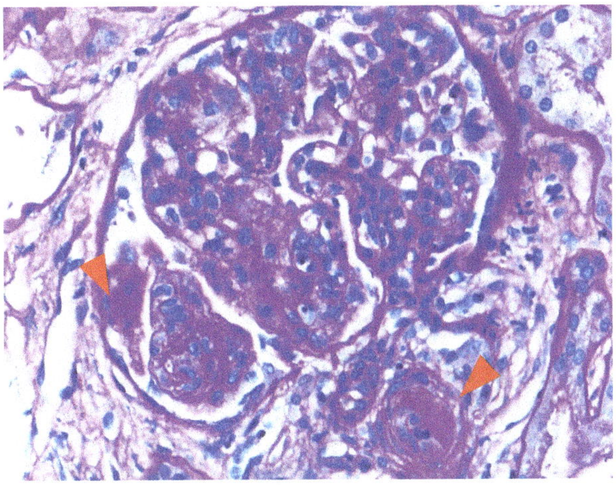

FIGURE 1: Light microscopy: presence of PAS-positive coagula of cryoglobulin in the glomerular capillaries and arterioles (arrowheads).

2.2. Pathology. Light microscopy (LM): of the twenty-six glomeruli present, one glomerulus showed segmental sclerosis with capsular adhesion. The remaining glomeruli revealed diffuse endocapillary proliferation with lobular simplification and glomerular influx of monocytes, neutrophils, and even eosinophils (one glomerulus). Many glomeruli contained PAS-positive intracapillary coagula of cryoglobulin (Figure 1), and small double contours were observed on silver stain. The interstitium contained sheets of lymphocytes in two foci and a lymphoid follicle with clear germinal center in another focus. Interstitial fibrosis, tubular atrophy, and arterial changes were minimal. One arteriole contained intraluminal cryoglobulin.

Immunofluorescence microscopy (IF): eleven glomeruli were present in the specimen processed for IF and revealed the following findings: IgM, Kappa, and C3 (3+) granular staining along peripheral capillary loops (Figure 2); IgG and Lambda (negative to trace) staining in the glomeruli. IgA, Clq, and Albumin were negative. Fibrinogen showed (1+) staining in some glomerular capillaries. Positive controls were satisfactory. As there was more than 2+ difference in intensity between Kappa and Lambda light chains, IgG, IgM, Kappa, and Lambda were repeated and the results of the second run were identical to the first run: presence of IgM with Kappa restriction was confirmed in the deposits.

Electron microscopy (EM): endocapillary proliferation, mesangial interposition, and presence of subendothelial and subepithelial electron dense deposits were observed in the single glomerulus present for electron microscopy (Figure 3). On high magnification, characteristic paired and curved

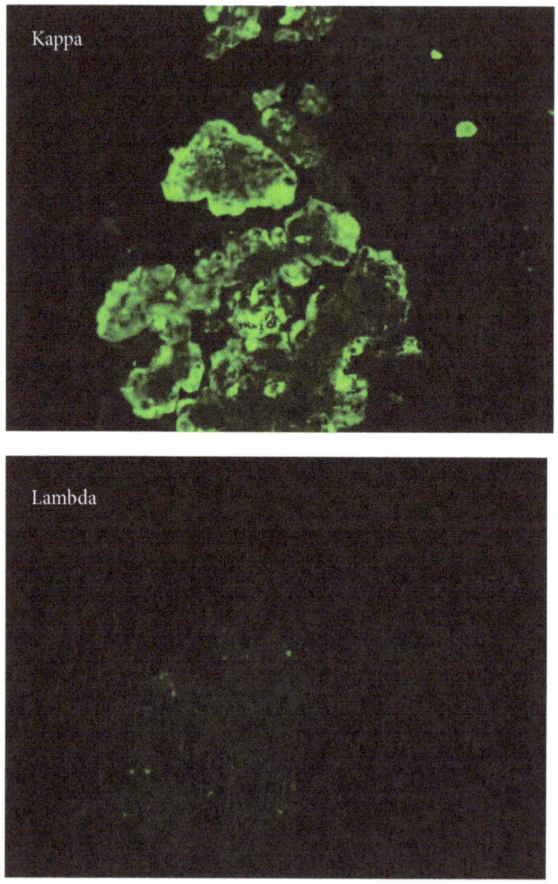

FIGURE 2: Immunofluorescence microscopy: Kappa light chain deposits within the glomerulus. Lambda light chain is negative.

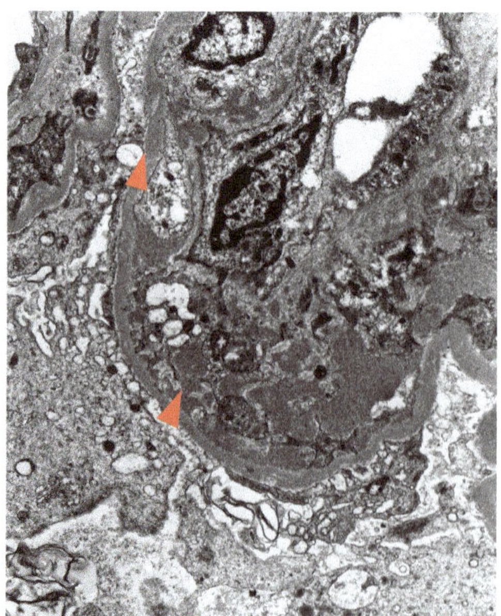

FIGURE 3: Electron microscopy: subendothelial and subepithelial electron dense deposits of cryoglobulins (arrowheads).

organized deposits of cryoglobulin were identified. Occasionally, the deposits revealed a microtubular pattern. Foot processes were focally effaced.

2.3. Summary of Findings and Follow-Up. The diagnosis of mCGN (with type III MPGN pattern) was rendered based on the presence of the following findings: features of MPGN (type III), intracapillary coagula of cryoglobulin (by LM), glomerular deposits of IgM with Kappa restriction (by IF), and organized deposits of cryoglobulins (by EM). The pathologist's suggestion regarding the possibility of an underlying B cell malignancy triggered further workup. Serum viscosity was within normal limits, but serum and urine protein electrophoresis revealed IgM monoclonal gammopathy. Computed tomography (CT) detected hepatosplenomegaly associated with retroperitoneal paraaortic lymph node enlargement. Bone survey did not reveal any lytic or blastic lesions; however, bone marrow biopsy results were consistent with bone marrow involvement by low-grade lymphoma, favoring Marginal Zone Lymphoma (MZL). Marrow biopsy showed multiple lymphoid aggregates in the background of trilineage maturing hematopoiesis. The lymphoid aggregates are composed of small-sized lymphoid cells without increased plasma cells or large atypical lymphoid cells. By immunohistochemistry studies, the lymphoid cells in the lymphoid aggregates are mostly PAX-5 and CD20 positive B cells. Plasma cells scattered in the marrow spaces are polyclonal and express both Kappa and Lambda. Flow cytometry detected about 3% of Kappa monoclonal B-cells expressing CD19, CD20, and CD22, but do not express CD5, CD10, or CD103. These findings support a diagnosis of marginal zone lymphoma rather than a lymphoplasmacytic lymphoma or hairy cell leukemia. The patient was initiated on a rituximab/dexamethasone-based regimen, which he tolerated well, with improvement of his renal function, urinary sediment, and proteinuria.

During the course of his hospitalization, hematology and infectious disease were consulted and they favored treating with the above regimen and planned a trial of direct acting antivirals at a later stage. At the most recent follow-up, patient is being continued on the abovementioned therapy and is being monitored by oncology closely.

3. Discussion

Our case report represents a combination of rarities and has multiple facets that need to be addressed separately.

3.1. Polyclonal and Monoclonal Cryoglobulins. The pathogenesis of HCV infection is closely related to chronic antigenic stimulation. Basically, in response to HCV infection, the virus core particle is captured by the dendritic cells, leading to B cell activation in the marginal zone of the lymphoid follicle, leading to B cell activation. [3] Subsequently, the activated dendritic cells release B lymphocyte activating factor (BAFF), which plays a key role in sustaining the clonal expansion of B cells. In about 20-56% of cases of HCV infection, this process leads to cryoglobulinemia, usually of mixed type (type II cryoglobulinemia) [1]. The mechanism of this polyclonal lymphoid activation is well known: once activated by the HCV antigens, the B cells synthesize large amounts of IgM with rheumatoid factor (RF) activity. These IgM-RF molecules bind HCV viral particles and lead to the formation of immune complexes capable of precipitation when exposed to cold temperatures, called cryoglobulins. These cryoglobulins bind specifically to the endothelial cells via C1q receptors and generate vasoactive peptides from the complement system. This in turn favors recruitment of inflammatory cells and mediates leukocytoclastic vasculitis [3]. While the polyclonal pathway is the most common pathway involved with HCV infection, rarely the infection presents itself with monoclonal cryoglobulinemia. In this case, our patient with chronic HCV antigenemia developed MZL and monoclonal cryoglobulinemia. The cryoglobulins subsequently affected the kidneys causing the uncommon type of MPGN type III.

3.2. Cryoglobulinemia and MPGN Type I versus MPGN Type III. About one-third of the patients who have mixed cryoglobulinemia develop renal involvement, which may present itself early on, in the form of an acute nephritic syndrome. More advanced cases typically have nephrotic range proteinuria. The most common renal manifestation and histologic feature of cryoglobulinemia is MPGN, specifically a common subtype of MPGN with subendothelial deposits, known as MPGN type I (not to be confused with type I cryoglobulinemia). Needless to mention that MPGN type I accounts for about 80% of renal biopsies with MPGN [2]. Less often, cryoglobulinemia presents itself in the kidney in the form of MPGN type III, which is the type encountered in our patient's biopsy and is the type that contains both subendothelial and subepithelial deposits. Therefore, our case not only deviates from the usual polyclonal pathway of B cell activation, it also presents itself with the least common histologic patter of MPGN. It is known that immune complex deposits that reach the subepithelial aspect of the glomerulus have less electron negativity (are more cationic) than those that remain in the subendothelial region. Therefore, it is conceivable that at least some of the immune complexes produced by the monoclonal B cell activation in our case have reached the subepithelial region due to their more cationic charge, while others with less cationic charge have been stopped by the electron negativity of the filtration barrier and retained in the subendothelial region. This dual property seen in outpatient can be explained by the viral envelope's dual B cell activation pathways explained above.

3.3. The role of Renal Biopsy and The Lesson Learned. Due to complex clinical presentations, there are very few reported cases of mCGN associated with gammopathies and Non-Hodgkin Lymphomas (NHL). [4] In those rare reported cases, it has always been the renal biopsy, specifically the IF findings that have unveiled the ambiguity and dictated the subsequent search for a gammopathy [4]. In a few recent large studies, notably the NCI-SEER, VA health system, and EPILYMPH consortium, a positive, modest increased risk of NHL has been documented in some HCV patients and MZL has been recognized as the most frequent type of lymphoid malignancy encountered [1, 5–7]. This association is further reinforced by several small clinical studies demonstrating regression of lymphomas in response to anti-HCV therapy [8, 9]. Conservative as well as immunosuppressive therapies have been used in a small number of patients with variable outcomes [4]. Multiple therapies have been used for malignancies in the setting of an underlying lymphoproliferative disease including interferon and rituximab therapy. However, mixed results have been obtained on therapies targeting lymphoma. More recently, newer agents, especially direct acting antivirals, have been shown to elicit good lymphoproliferative disease response in HCV associated lymphoproliferative disorders. This trial of interferon-free antiviral therapy is a huge step in establishing a casual relationship between HCV and lymphoproliferative disorders, as well as a guide to assist in treatment decisions [10]. At the present time, treatment decisions are being made based on clinical experience.

4. Conclusion

Our case represents a composite of multiple rarities:

(1) Monoclonal (type I) cryoglobulinemia which accounts for about 10-15% of total cases of cryoglobulinemias [2].

(2) mCGN which is a very rare diagnosis, with fewer than 50 cases reported so far in the literature [11].

(3) MPGN type III which is the least common histologic type of MPGN associated with cryoglobulinemia.

While HCV infection and monoclonal B cell proliferation is a notion that is well explored and understood, there are only a few case reports describing the concurrence of mCGN in HCV patients with malignancy [12]. Our case raises awareness mainly among nephropathologists regarding the possibility of monoclonality in the biopsy of HCV-infected patients, especially because polyclonality is the routine finding in these patients. Moreover, it is possible that the actual incidence of mCGN among HCV patients is higher than currently thought as monoclonality can be overlooked in the biopsies: a vigilant diagnosis of mCGN on renal biopsy could be of great assistance in early diagnosis and more effective management approaches, with better patient outcomes. Larger studies will be necessary in order to establish the true prevalence of type I cryoglobulinemic glomerulonephritis in HCV-infected patients.

Disclosure

Drs. Mutnuri, Kassem, Badalamenti, Qian, Marquez, and Afrouzian declare that they have no relevant financial interest.

References

[1] A. Tedeschi, C. Baratè, E. Minola, and E. Morra, "Cryoglobulinemia," *Blood Reviews*, vol. 21, no. 4, pp. 183–200, 2007.

[2] D. S. Viswanatha and A. Dogan, "Hepatitis C virus and lymphoma," *Journal of Clinical Pathology*, vol. 60, no. 12, pp. 1378–1383, 2007.

[3] F. Dammacco and D. Sansonno, "Therapy for hepatitis C virus-related cryoglobulinemic vasculitis," *The New England Journal of Medicine*, vol. 369, no. 11, pp. 1035–1045, 2013.

[4] S. Sethi, L. Zand, N. Leung et al., "Membranoproliferative glomerulonephritis secondary to monoclonal gammopathy," *Clinical Journal of the American Society of Nephrology*, vol. 5, no. 5, pp. 770–782, 2010.

[5] E. A. Engels, N. Chatterjee, J. R. Cerhan et al., "Hepatitis C virus infection and non-hodgkin lymphoma: Results of the NCI-seer multi-center case-control study," *International Journal of Cancer*, vol. 111, no. 1, pp. 76–80, 2004.

[6] T. P. Giordano, L. Henderson, O. Langdren et al., "Risk of non-Hodgkin lymphoma and lymphoproliferative precursor diseased in US veterans with hepatitis C virus," *JAMA*, vol. 297, pp. 2010–2017, 2007.

[7] A. Nieters, B. Kallinowski, P. Brennan et al., "Hepatitis C and risk of lymphoma: results of the european multicenter case-control study epilymph," *Gastroenterology*, vol. 131, no. 6, pp. 1879–1886, 2006.

[8] D. Saadoun, F. Suarez, F. Lefrere et al., "Splenic lymphoma with villous lymphocytes, associated with type II cryoglobulinemia and HCV infection: A new entity?" *Blood*, vol. 105, no. 1, pp. 74–76, 2005.

[9] O. Hermine, F. Lefrère, J. Bronowicki et al., "Regression of splenic lymphoma with villous lymphocytes after treatment of hepatitis C virus infection," *The New England Journal of Medicine*, vol. 347, no. 2, pp. 89–94, 2002.

[10] L. Arcaini, C. Besson, M. Frigeni et al., "Interferon-free antiviral treatment in B-cell lymphoproliferative disorders associated with hepatitis C virus infection," *Blood*, vol. 128, no. 21, pp. 2527–2532, 2016.

[11] A. Karras, L. H. Noël et al., "Renal involvement in monoclonal (type I) cryoglobuline- mia: two cases associated with IgG3 kappa cryoglobulin," *American Journal of Kidney Diseases*, vol. 40, no. 5, pp. 1091–1096, 2002.

[12] E. Chelioti, E. Efthimiou, M. Sotiraki, A. Papalexandrou, and M. Tsilivigkou, "Splenic marginal zone lymphoma and concurrent membranoproliferative glomerulonephritis with IgMKappa deposits in a HCV-seropositive patient," *Nephro-Urology Monthly*, vol. 6, no. 4, p. e18391, 2014.

15

Crescentic Glomerulonephritis and Membranous Nephropathy: A Rare Overlap

Mohamedanwar Ghandour,[1] **Heba Osman**,[2] **Samer Alkassis**,[3] **Alix Charles**,[3] **Kristina Zalewski**,[3] **Jarrett Weinberger**,[3] **Yahya Malik-Osman**,[1] **and Zeenat Y. Bhat**[1]

[1]*Department of Internal Medicine WSU SOM, Division of Nephrology Wayne State University, Detroit, MI, USA*
[2]*Department of Internal Medicine/Pediatrics, Wayne State University/Detroit Medical Center, Detroit, MI, USA*
[3]*Department of Internal Medicine WSU SOM, Wayne State University, Detroit, MI, USA*

Correspondence should be addressed to Mohamedanwar Ghandour; ha4202@wayne.edu

Academic Editor: Hernán Trimarchi

Background. Membranous nephropathy (MN) is a disease that affects the basement membrane of the glomeruli of the kidney resulting in proteinuria. The concurrent incidence of vasculitic glomerulonephritis and MN in the same patient is unusual. Herein, we report a case with this unusual combination. *Case.* Our patient is a 53-year-old Hispanic male with a medical history of tobacco use, type 2 diabetes mellitus, and hypertension who presented with hematuria and was found to have nephrotic range proteinuria and renal impairment. Blood workup revealed positive ANCA serology, which led to a renal biopsy that showed crescentic vasculitis in addition to membranous nephropathy. The patient was started on intermittent hemodialysis (HD) and treated initially with intravenous (IV) pulse steroids; subsequently, oral prednisolone and IV cyclophosphamide were initiated. The patient remained HD dependent at the time of discharge with the resolution of hematuria. A follow-up with an outpatient nephrology clinic was arranged. *Conclusion.* Membranous nephropathy complicated by crescentic glomerulonephritis has a more aggressive clinical course and decline in renal function compared to MN alone which can lead to initiating renal replacement therapy. However, immunosuppressive drugs can result in significant improvement of renal function if started early enough.

1. Introduction

Membranous nephropathy (MN) is a common etiology of nephrotic syndrome, especially in on-diabetic adults. Histologically, it is characterized by a light microscopy pattern of basement membrane thickening with deposition of immunoglobulins and complement proteins [1]. MN can be either idiopathic or associated with an underlying disease such as systemic lupus nephritis, other autoimmune disorders, malignancies, or drugs such as nonsteroidal anti-inflammatory drugs (NSAIDs) [2–4]. On the other hand, antineutrophil cytoplasmic autoantibody (ANCA)-associated vasculitis (AAV) is a group of chronic inflammatory diseases affecting small and medium-sized vessels. Literature reports rare cases of vasculitic or crescentic glomerulonephritis in membranous nephropathy, except in those cases associated with systemic lupus erythematosus [5, 6]. Herein, we report a rare case of crescentic glomerulonephritis with membranous nephropathy. To our knowledge, the immunopathogenesis of this uncommon overlap of membranous nephropathy and crescentic glomerulonephritis is limited.

1.1. Case Presentation. Our patient is a 53-year-old Hispanic male with a medical history of tobacco use, type 2 diabetes mellitus, and HTN who presented to the emergency department with hematuria and diarrhea for 4 days. He additionally complained of symptoms of chronic sinusitis and epistaxis that occurred all year round. His medications at home included tramadol, celecoxib, glipizide, metformin, lisinopril, and metoprolol. Physical examination was only remarkable for 1+ pitting edema in his lower extremities bilaterally and dental caries. There were no signs of

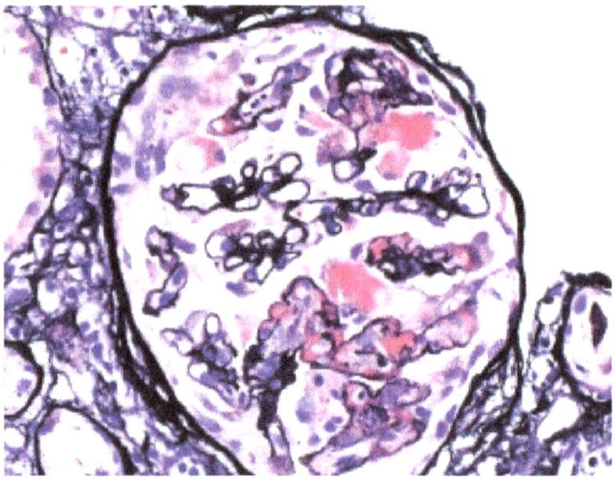

Figure 1: Light microscopy showing a glomerulus with focal segmental fibrinoid necrosis.

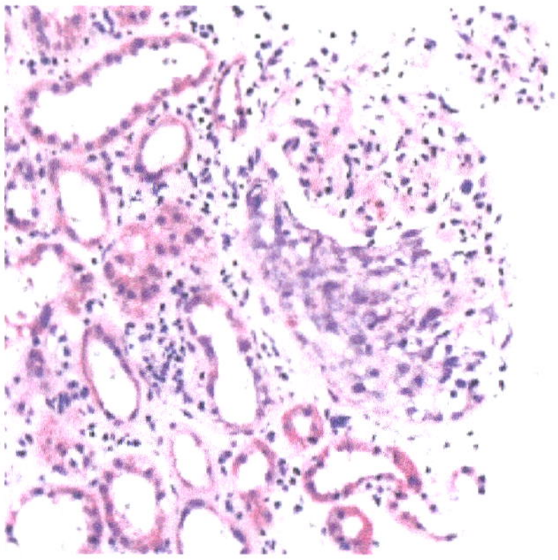

Figure 2: Light microscopy showing diffuse cellular crescent formation.

photosensitivity, malar rash, oral ulcers, lymphadenopathy, pericarditis, or sinus involvement. On admission, the patient was found to have a creatinine of 8.04 mg/dL (reference range 0.70–1.3 mg/dL). His baseline creatinine was 0.9 mg/dL less than eight months ago. His urinalysis revealed gross and microscopic hematuria, with RBC >100/HPF, 3+ protein, and no casts. A CT abdomen/pelvis was performed on admission which was unremarkable for any signs of obstruction; however, it revealed fibrotic changes in the lower lung bases. The urine protein creatinine ratio (UPCR) was 19.2 g/mg and low serum albumin was 2.7 gm/dL (reference range 3.5–5.7 gm/dL). ANCA antibody was positive; however, all viral markers (hepatitis B, C, syphilis EIA, and HIV), complement C3 and C4 levels, and autoimmune antibody profiles (ANA, rheumatoid factor, anti-ds DNA antibody, and antiglomerular basement membrane antibody) were all negative or within normal limits. The patient had high titers of myeloperoxidase (MPO) antibody. All other infectious workups such as urine culture and blood cultures were negative. CT of the lungs revealed interval worsening of fibrotic changes with honeycombing predominantly in the lung bases, suggesting usual interstitial pneumonia. Pulmonology was consulted and reported this was consistent with ANCA-associated lung involvement. Renal ultrasound showed normal kidney size with no hydronephrosis.

Renal biopsy was then performed which revealed membranous pattern glomerulonephritis with diffuse cellular crescents. There was moderate interstitial fibrosis, tubular atrophy with focal segmental fibrinoid necrosis (Figure 1). Light microscopy revealed 50% of sampled glomeruli had active cellular crescents (Figure 2). Immunohistochemical staining for phospholipase A2 receptor (PLA2R), thrombospondin type 1 domain-containing 7A (THSD7A), and neural epidermal growth factor-like 1 were negative. Immunofluorescence revealed granular capillary wall and mesangial staining for IgA (3+) and IgG (3+) (Figures 3 and 4). All the other stains were negative. Electron microscopy revealed extracapillary hypercellularity and segmental thickening in the glomerular capillary basement membranes with severe effacement of podocyte foot processes. There was no significant mesangial hypercellularity. Global subepithelial immune-type electron-dense deposits

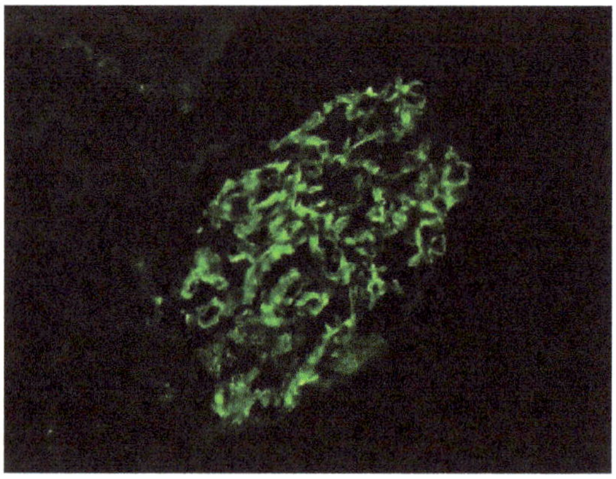

Figure 3: Immunofluorescence stained for IgA.

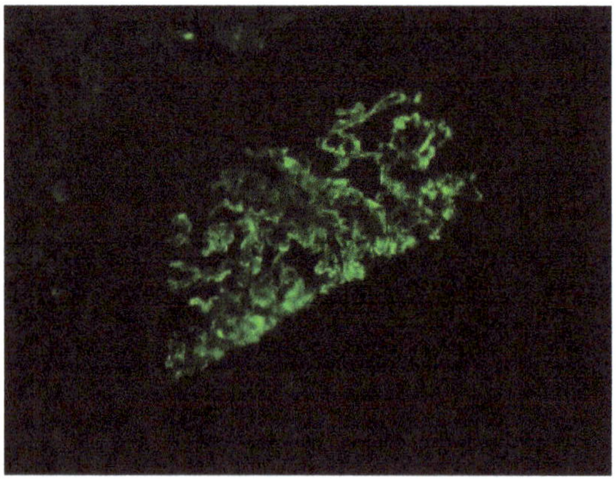

Figure 4: Immunofluorescence stained for IgG.

were identified, consistent with a membranous pattern with occasional intramembranous deposits.

Throughout his stay, the patient's creatinine continued to rise for which intermittent hemodialysis was initiated. The patient was also started on pulse dose steroids followed by maintenance steroids and intravenous cyclophosphamide. The patient reported a resolution of hematuria after the

Table 1: Clinical details of patients with membranous nephropathy and concomitant vasculitic glomerulonephritis.

Title/authors	Patient (age/sex)	PLA2R	ANCA by IF	ANCA specificity by ELISA	Treatment	Prognosis
Membranous nephropathy with proteinase 3-ANCA-associated vasculitis successfully treated with rituximab; Shun Yoshida, Shunichiro Hanai, Daiki Nakagomi, Kei Kobayashi, Kazuya Takahashi, Fumihiko Furuya [7]	73/F			PR3	Oral prednisolone and IV rituximab	Renal function immediately improved, along with symptoms and urinalysis abnormalities
Association of vasculitis glomerulonephritis with membranous nephropathy: A report of 10 cases; Tse WY, Howie AJ, Adu D, Savage CO, Richards NT, Wheeler DC, Michael J [1]	10 patients: 9 males/1 female, 30–70 years					Renal function improved in 3 patients; 2 patients required RRT; 3 patients died: one of systemic vasculitis and 2 of sepsis
	30/M		C-ANCA		Oral prednisolone and cyclophosphamide	Stable renal function. Complication: squamous lung CA 10 years after presentation
	39/M		Negative		Oral prednisolone and cyclophosphamide	Recovery. Complication: steroid-induced DM. Duration of follow-up: 7 months
	41/M		Negative		Oral prednisolone and cyclophosphamide	Stable renal function, duration of follow-up: 3 years
	58/F		Negative		Oral prednisolone and cyclophosphamide	Dialysis, duration of follow-up: 7 years
	63/M		NA		Oral prednisolone and azathioprine for 3 years, followed by prednisolone and cyclophosphamide	Death, duration of follow-up: 6 years
	64/M		P-ANCA		Oral prednisolone and azathioprine	Dialysis, duration of follow-up: 2 years
	65/M		P-ANCA		Oral prednisolone and cyclophosphamide	Recovery, duration of follow-up: 5 years
	65/M		Negative		Oral prednisolone and cyclophosphamide	Death (after 4 months)
	68/M		Negative		Oral prednisolone and cyclophosphamide	Death (after 2 months)
	70/M		C-ANCA		Oral prednisolone, cyclophosphamide, and plasma exchange	Recovery (duration of follow-up:4 years)
Membranous glomerulonephritis with ANCA-associated necrotizing and crescentic glomerulonephritis; Samih H. Nasr, Samar M. Said, Anthony M. Valeri, Michael B. Stokes, Naveed N. Masani, Vivette D. D'Agati, and Glen S. Markowitz [4]	64/M		C-ANCA	NA	Prednisone and cyclophosphamide	Resolution of pulmonary lesions, normalization of Cr, diminution of proteinuria
	68/F		NA	MPO	Prednisone	Normalization of Cr
	47/F		P-ANCA	MPO	Methylprednisolone and then prednisone and cyclophosphamide	Diminution of proteinuria and disappearance of crescents (on repeat bx)
	67/M		P-ANCA	MPO	Prednisone and azathioprine	Dialysis
	69/M		P-ANCA	MPO	Prednisone and cyclophosphamide	Normalization of Cr
	68/F		N/A	MPO	Prednisone and cyclophosphamide	Partial recovery
Co-occurrence of PLA2R-positive membranous nephropathy without crescents, and PR3-positive eosinophilic granulomatosis with polyangiitis; Yuexin Zhu, Qing Chang, Xiangyan Cao, Song Zheng, Peiling Li, Junjun Luan, Hua Zhou [8]	??	PLA2R positive	ANCA positive	PR3	Prednisone and cyclophosphamide	Recovery
Anti-neutrophil cytoplasmic antibody-positive eosinophilic granulomatosis with polyangiitis: can it cause membranous nephropathy? S B Mahmood, H Ahmad, J Wu, D Haselby, M M LeClaire, R Nasr [9]	63/F		P-ANCA	MPO	Rituximab	Recovery

Table 1: Continued.

Title/authors	Patient (age/sex)	PLA2R	ANCA by IF	ANCA specificity by ELISA	Treatment	Prognosis
Primary membranous nephropathy presenting with crescentic glomerulonephritis 25 years after initial presentation: A case report; David Massicotte-Azarniouch, Sean Barbour, Paula Blanco, Edward G Clark [10]	63/M	PLA2R positive	Negative ANCA	Negative	Prednisone and cyclophosphamide and then azathioprine for maintenance	Dialysis and then partial recovery
Anti-neutrophil cytoplasmic antibody-associated glomerulonephritis with detection of myeloperoxidase and phospholipase A2 receptor in membranous nephropathy lesions: report of two patients with microscopic polyangiitis; Tominaga K, Uchida T, Imakiire T et al. [11]	52/M	PLA2R positive	Not reported	MPO	Not reported	Not reported
	63/F	PLA2R positive	Not reported	MPO	Not reported	Not reported
Crescentic glomerulonephritis and membranous nephropathy: A rare coexistence; Olga Balafa, Rigas Kalaitzidis, Georgios Liapis, Sofia Xiromeriti, Fotios Zarzoulas, Georgios Baltatzis and Moses Elisaf [5]	58/M		p-ANCA		Prednisolone, cyclophosphamide, and plasmapheresis	Recovery, duration of follow-up: 3 months
	27 patients with ANCA-GN and characteristics of MN on renal biopsy	17 M and 10 F, with an age of 52.4 ± 17.7 years	25 p-ANCA positive; 2 c-ANCA positive	25 MPO positive and 2 PR3 positive	Prednisone and cyclophosphamide	11 of 27 (40.7%) died; 13 of 27 (48.1%) progressed to ESRD
Clinical and immunologic characteristics of patients with ANCA-associated glomerulonephritis combined with membranous nephropathy a retrospective cohort study in a single Chinese center; Zou, Rong; Liu, Gang; Cui, Zhao; Chen, Min; Zhao, Ming-Hui [12]	17 M and 10 F, with an age of 52.4 ± 17.7 years					ANCA-GN patients with MN had significantly poorer renal outcome ($P = 0.021$) and patients' survivals ($P = 0.036$) compared with the patients without MN No significant difference in causes of death between ANCA-GN patients with and without MN. Infection is the first cause of death in ANCA-GN patients with and without MN

Table 1: Continued.

Title/authors	Patient (age/sex)	PLA2R	ANCA by IF	ANCA specificity by ELISA	Treatment	Prognosis
Membranous nephropathy with crescents: A series of 19 cases; Erika F. Rodriguez, Samih H. Nasr, Christopher P. Larsen, Sanjeev Sethi, Mary E. Fidler, Lynn D. Cornell [13]	19 patients with ANCA and crescentic MN No patient had positive anti-dsDNA, hep B and C, or HIV	38% PLA2R positive	All negative	All negative		
	22/M		Negative	Negative	Prednisone and cyclophosphamide and then cyclosporine	Recovery, duration of follow-up: 138 months
	76/F		Negative	Negative	Prednisone and cyclophosphamide	Partial recovery, duration of follow-up: 26 months
	80/F		Negative	Negative	Mycophenolate mofetil and prednisone	Recovery, duration of follow-up:6 months
	69/F		Negative	Negative	Prednisone	ESRD, duration of follow-up: 1.5 months
	57/M		Negative	Negative	Prednisone and cyclophosphamide orally with remission; then azathioprine; then prednisone and cyclophosphamide	Duration of follow-up: 56 months
	41/M		Negative	Negative	Prednisone and cyclophosphamide	Worsening renal function, duration of follow-up:5 months
	20/F		Negative	Negative	None	ESRD, duration of follow-up: 35 months
	17/F		Negative	Negative	Enalapril	Recovery, duration of follow-up: 3 months
	50/M		Negative	Negative	Prednisone, cyclophosphamide, and mycophenolate	Partial recovery, duration of follow-up: 16 months
	5/F		Negative	Negative	Prednisone and mycophenolate (no response at 6 m); then, prednisone and cyclosporine; then, prednisone and tacrolimus	Recovery, duration of follow-up: 32 months
	86/M		Negative	Negative	Prednisone	Partial recovery, duration of follow-up: 11 months
	64/M		Negative	Negative	Prednisone and cyclosporine	Worsening renal function, duration of follow-up: 2 months
	72/F		Negative	Negative	Prednisone and cyclophosphamide	Partial recovery, duration of follow-up: 27 months
	62/M		Negative	Negative	Unknown	Partial recovery, duration of follow-up: 19 months
	64/M		Negative	Negative	Prednisone and cyclosporine (no response at 2 m); then 4 doses rituximab; then mycophenolate and prednisone (no response)	ESRD, duration of follow-up: 11 months
	72/M		Negative	Negative	Losartan	Partial recovery, duration of follow-up: 9 months
	58/M		Negative	Negative	Prednisone and cyclophosphamide orally for 2 m; then azathioprine for 1 y	Partial recovery, duration of follow-up: 11 months
	70/F		Negative	Negative	Unknown	Dialysis within 1 month
	56/M		Negative	Negative	Prednisone and cyclophosphamide	Partial recovery, duration of follow-up: 3 months

Table 1: Continued.

Title/authors	Patient (age/sex)	PLA2R	ANCA by IF	ANCA specificity by ELISA	Treatment	Prognosis
A case of membranous glomerulonephritis with superimposed anti-neutrophil cytoplasmic antibody-associated rapidly progressive crescentic glomerulonephritis; Yoo Hyung Kim, Hae Ri Kim, Young Rok Ham, Jae Woong Jeon, Sarah Chung, Dae Eun Choi, Kang Wook Lee and Ki Ryang Na [14]	65/M	Not reported	p-ANCA	MPO	Methylprednisolone and cyclophosphamide	ESRD
Membranous glomerulonephritis with superimposed ANCA-associated vasculitis: Another case report; Antonio Granata, Fulvio Floccari [15]	67/M	Not reported	p-ANCA	Not reported	Methylprednisolone and cyclophosphamide	Partial recovery

initiation of steroids; however, patient remained dialysis-dependent. The patient was discharged in a stable condition and scheduled for follow-up with the outpatient nephrology clinic.

2. Discussion

The primary antibodies identified in AAV are proteinase 3 (PR3) and myeloperoxidase (MPO)-ANCA antibodies. These autoantibodies are hallmarks of AAV, with PR3-ANCA being the most common in GPA, while MPO-ANCA is the most common in MPA. However, the association of vasculitic glomerulonephritis with membranous nephropathy is rare, estimated to be <5% of all membranous glomerulonephritis (MGN) cases, and is reported only in a handful of times in the literature [1]. Many concomitant MGN and AAV cases are also diagnosed together at presentation (Table 1). Our case had positive myeloperoxidase (MPO)-ANCA antibodies. The histological pattern of MGN is characterized by the formation of subepithelial immune complex deposits with changes to the glomerular basement membrane. Primary MGN occurs in approximately 75% of MGN cases and is caused by circulating anti-PLA2R antibodies against the podocyte antigens. In 25% of cases, secondary MGN occurs and is associated with hepatitis B, autoimmune diseases, thyroiditis, malignancies, and certain drug use such as nonsteroidal anti-inflammatory drugs (NSAIDs) [2].

Microscopic hematuria, proteinuria, and acute kidney failure are all common presentations of MGN associated with ANCA vasculitis [3, 4]. In a case series of 15 patients reported by Nikolopoulou et al., microscopic hematuria was detected in all of them except for one who was anuric. Moreover, proteinuria was also noticed with a median UPCR of 819.5 mg/mmol (reference range 88–5600) [3]. The reported case presented with UPCR was 19.2 g/day. Extra-renal symptoms are also common including fatigue, arthralgias, and malaise. A literature review done by Balafa et al., which included 38 patients with ANCA-positive MGN and 30 patients with ANCA-negative MGN, revealed that vasculitis symptoms predominated in the first group, but were absent in the second one [5].

The renal function at presentation along with the presence of antibodies may predict the clinical outcome. However, prognosis is variable with 40% of patients progressing to end-stage renal disease [3]. Patients with MGN and ANCA-associated NCGN are likely to have heavier proteinuria and a worse prognosis than patients with ANCA-associated NCGN alone [4]. In addition to higher levels of urinary protein excretion and decreased eGFR at the time of renal biopsy being risk factors for poor prognosis in MGN, crescent formation was reported to be another risk factor for worse renal outcome [6].

Prompt aggressive treatment can lead to stabilization of renal function and a significant decline in proteinuria. Treatment typically involves a combination of immunosuppressive agents such as steroids and cyclophosphamide and/or rituximab. Nasr et al.'s case series of 14 patients revealed that 5 out of 14 patients progressed to ESRD despite treatment; however, ANCA testing was repeated after treatment in 7 patients and revealed that 5 patients were seronegative [3]. In Nikolopolou et al.'s case series, 9 patients had stabilization or improvement of renal function, 6 had progressed to ESRD, and 4 died in the median 72-month follow-up period [4]. All the patients were treated with steroids, 10 with cyclophosphamide and 6 with rituximab [4]. There is currently not enough evidence to guide treatment when deciding between the addition of cyclophosphamide versus rituximab.

3. Conclusion

Our case of a 53-year-old man who was found to have both ANCA-associated GN and MGN with crescents on kidney biopsy represents a rare dual glomerulopathy. An overlap between MN and ANCA is rare and might require a histological diagnosis. Presentation with proteinuria, microscopic hematuria, and acute kidney injury should prompt treatment for rapidly progressive glomerulonephritis to prevent poor clinical outcomes and progression to end-stage renal disease.

Disclosure

The abstract was presented at the American Society of Nephrology.

References

[1] W. Tse, A. Howie, D. Adu et al., "Association of vasculitic glomerulonephritis with membranous nephropathy: a report of 10 cases," *Nephrology Dialysis Transplantation*, vol. 12, no. 5, pp. 1017–1027, 1997.

[2] A. B. Fogo, M. A. Lusco, B. Najafian, and C. E. Alpers, "AJKD atlas of renal pathology: membranous nephropathy," *American Journal of Kidney Diseases*, vol. 66, no. 3, pp. e15–e17, 2015.

[3] A. Nikolopoulou, I. Huang-Doran, S. P. McAdoo, M. E. Griffith, H. T. Cook, and C. D. Pusey, "Membranous glomerulonephritis with crescents," *Kidney International Reports*, vol. 4, no. 11, pp. 1577–1584, 2019.

[4] S. H. Nasr, S. M. Said, A. M. Valeri et al., "Membranous glomerulonephritis with ANCA-associated necrotizing and crescentic glomerulonephritis," *Clinical Journal of the American Society of Nephrology*, vol. 4, no. 2, pp. 299–308, 2009.

[5] O. Balafa, R. Kalaitzidis, G. Liapis et al., "Crescentic glomerulonephritis and membranous nephropathy: a rare coexistence," *International Urology and Nephrology*, vol. 47, no. 8, pp. 1373–1377, 2015.

[6] J. Wang, P. Zhu, Z. Cui et al., "Clinical features and outcomes in patients with membranous nephropathy and crescent formation," *Medicine (Baltimore)*, vol. 94, no. 50, Article ID e2294, 2015.

[7] S. Yoshida, S. Hanai, D. Nakagomi, K. Kobayashi, K. Takahashi, and F. Furuya, "Membranous nephropathy with proteinase 3-ANCA-associated vasculitis successfully treated

with rituximab," *Internal Medicine*, vol. 60, no. 1, pp. 145–150, 2021.

[8] Y. Zhu, Q. Chang, X. Cao et al., "Co-occurrence of PLA2R-positive membranous nephropathy without crescents, and PR3-positive eosinophilic granulomatosis with polyangiitis," *Clinical Nephrology*, vol. 92, no. 4, pp. 208–215, 2019.

[9] S. Mahmood, H. Ahmad, J. Wu, D. Haselby, M. LeClaire, and R. Nasr, "Anti-neutrophil cytoplasmic antibody-positive eosinophilic granulomatosis with polyangiitis: can it cause membranous nephropathy?" *Scandinavian Journal of Rheumatology*, vol. 48, no. 3, pp. 256-257, 2019.

[10] D. Massicotte-Azarniouch, S. Barbour, P. Blanco, and E. G. Clark, "Primary membranous nephropathy presenting with crescentic glomerulonephritis 25 years after initial presentation: a case report," *Clinical Nephrology*, vol. 90, no. 4, pp. 291–295, 2018.

[11] K. Tominaga, T. Uchida, T. Imakiire et al., "Anti-neutrophil cytoplasmic antibody-associated glomerulonephritis with detection of myeloperoxidase and phospholipase A2 receptor in membranous nephropathy-lesions: report of two patients with microscopic polyangiitis," *BMC Nephrology*, vol. 19, pp. 120–125, 2018.

[12] R. Zou, G. Liu, Z. Cui, M. Chen, and M. H. Zhao, "Clinical and immunologic characteristics of patients with ANCA-associated glomerulonephritis combined with membranous nephropathy: a retrospective cohort study in a single Chinese center," *Medicine (Baltimore)*, vol. 94, no. 37, Article ID e1472, 2015.

[13] E. F. Rodriguez, S. H. Nasr, C. P. Larsen, S. Sethi, M. E. Fidler, and L. D. Cornell, "Membranous nephropathy with crescents: a series of 19 cases," *American Journal of Kidney Diseases*, vol. 64, no. 1, pp. 66–73, 2014.

[14] Y. H. Kim, H. R. Kim, Y. R. Ham et al., "A case of membranous glomerulonephritis with superimposed anti-neutrophil cytoplasmic antibody-associated rapidly progressive crescentic glomerulonephritis," *Chonnam Medical Journal*, vol. 51, no. 2, pp. 102–105, 2015.

[15] A. Granata and F. Floccari, "Membranous glomerulonephritis with superimposed ANCA-associated vasculitis: another case report," *Clinical Kidney Journal*, vol. 4, no. 1, pp. 80-81, 2011.

16

Rapidly Progressive Glomerulonephritis Secondary to IgA Nephropathy in a Patient with Systemic Lupus Erythematosus

Amol M. Patel,[1] Lily Anne Romero Karam,[1] Stephanie C. Fuentes Rojas,[1] Warren E. Redfearn,[1] Luan D. Truong,[2] and Juan M. Gonzalez[3]

[1]*Department of Internal Medicine, Houston Methodist Hospital, Houston, TX, USA*
[2]*Department of Pathology and Genomic Medicine, Houston Methodist Hospital, Houston, TX, USA*
[3]*Department of Internal Medicine, Division of Nephrology, Houston, TX, USA*

Correspondence should be addressed to Amol M. Patel; ampatel@houstonmethodist.org

Academic Editor: Yoshihide Fujigaki

Lupus nephritis is a common manifestation of systemic lupus erythematosus (SLE). IgA nephropathy is a common type of primary glomerulonephritis. Renal manifestations in SLE patients are often due to lupus nephritis; however, renal diseases unrelated to lupus nephritis are rarely reported. While crescentic IgA nephropathy with rapid clinical progression is rare, its development in patients with SLE in the absence of lupus nephritis is even more unusual. A 74-year-old woman with a history of SLE without known renal involvement, chronic kidney disease stage IIIa, congestive heart failure, hypertension, and type 2 diabetes mellitus presented with acute kidney injury. Her creatinine continued to rise rapidly. Renal biopsy revealed mesangial proliferative glomerulonephritis with crescent formation. Immunofluorescent staining showed IgA and C3 mesangial deposition and absence of C4 and C1q, consistent with IgA nephropathy. She received a course of methylprednisolone and plasmapheresis. Unfortunately, her renal function continued to deteriorate, and she was started on hemodialysis which was continued after hospital discharge. This case illustrates crescentic IgA nephropathy without lupus nephritis as the cause of acute kidney injury in a patient with SLE. It highlights the observation that renal diseases other than lupus nephritis can develop in SLE patients.

1. Introduction

Renal disease is common among patients with systemic lupus erythematosus (SLE); however, renal diseases unrelated to lupus nephritis (LN) in these patients are rarely reported.

LN affects about 50% of patients with SLE [1]. Clinically, LN is divided into six subtypes: minimal mesangial LN (class I), mesangial proliferative LN (class II), focal proliferative LN (class III), diffuse proliferative LN (class IV), membranous LN (class V), and advanced sclerosing LN (class VI) [2]. On histology, LN is classically characterized by the so-called "full house" pattern under immunofluorescent microscopy, staining positively for IgG, IgA, IgM, C3, and C1q [3].

Globally, the most commonly observed glomerulopathy is IgA nephropathy (IgAN) [4]. It is characterized by circulating IgA immune complexes which contribute to glomerular inflammation, glomerular capillary damage, and mesangial proliferation. The range of clinical manifestations of IgAN is broad, from asymptomatic microscopic hematuria to rapidly progressive glomerulonephritis (RPGN). Although the two most common clinical presentations are asymptomatic hematuria and progressive kidney disease, IgAN can be fatal with the largest case series of 113 patients showing a rate of progression to ESRD of 42.5% at 1 year despite immunotherapy [5].

We report a case of acute renal injury secondary to RPGN of IgAN in a patient with SLE in the absence of LN. RPGN of IgAN is rare, and more unusual is this presentation in a patient with SLE without LN.

2. Case Presentation

A 74-year-old woman with a history of SLE on hydroxychloroquine without known renal involvement, chronic kidney disease stage (CKD) IIIa, heart failure with reduced

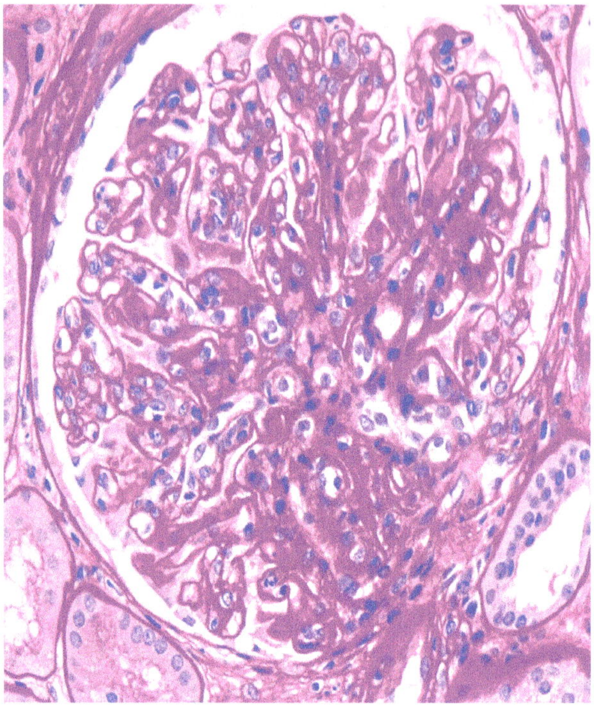

FIGURE 1: There is global moderate mesangial siderosis and hypercellularity (periodic acid-Schiff, x400).

ejection fraction, hypertension, and type 2 diabetes mellitus (T2DM) presented to the emergency department with progressive chest "heaviness" which had started several days prior to admission. In addition, she complained of swelling in both feet and at least three-pound weight gain.

Upon admission she was afebrile, blood pressure ranged 150-180/70-80 mm Hg, heart rate was about 50 bpm, and oxygen saturation was above 95% on room air. She was a well-developed, nonobese woman in no significant distress and nontachypneic. Pertinent physical exam findings included no jugular venous distention, no crackles audible at base of lungs, heart with regular rate and rhythm with no extra sounds or murmurs, nondistended abdomen, trace peripheral leg edema, and no visible rashes. Laboratory tests were significant for sodium 129 mEq/L, potassium 4.2 mEq/L, chloride 98 mEq/L, CO2 20 mEq/L, BUN 46 mg/dL, and creatinine 3.4 mg/dL. Her baseline creatinine based on the most recent reading one month prior to admission was 1.1 mg/dL. Urinalysis was significant for a specific gravity of 1.006, RBC 142, and WBC 8 per HPF. No casts of dysmorphic cells were seen. Proteinuria was 2+, and a random urine protein-to-creatinine ratio was 1.48.

Her creatinine continued to rise rapidly, and by day 6 of hospitalization it was 6.4 mg/dL. Due to these findings, a renal biopsy was performed. Up to 21 glomeruli were present per tissue section, and two of them showed global sclerosis. Two other glomeruli showed segmental sclerosis and the remaining glomeruli were open. There was global diffuse marked mesangial sclerosis and hypercellularity, and there was no obvious endocapillary cell proliferation or inflammatory cell infiltrate. Three of the open glomeruli also displayed segmental or circumferential predominantly cellular crescent. There was multifocal chronic tubulointerstitial injury characterized by atrophic tubules, interstitial fibrosis, and mild mononuclear inflammatory cell infiltrate, all which accounted for about 20-40% of the cortical tissue area. Figures 1 and 2 are biopsies seen in light microscopy with the former showing mesangial proliferation and the latter demonstrating a crescent on silver stain. Immunofluorescent staining showed marked IgA and C3 mesangial deposition, weak linear IgG staining of the glomerular basement membrane, and absence of C4 and C1q which was consistent with IgA nephropathy. There are also changes suggestive of diabetic nephropathy, in keeping with the clinical history of diabetes. These changes include thickened lamina densa and linear IgG of the glomerular basement membrane and mesangial sclerosis. Immunofluorescent staining positive for IgA and C3 is seen in Figures 3 and 4, respectively. Staining for C4 and C1q was both negative with the latter seen on Figure 5. In addition, electron microscopy showed uniform thickening of lamina densa of glomerular basement membrane, marked mesangial sclerosis, and hypercellularity, and some electron dense deposits were identified in the mesangial areas and subepithelial location which can be seen in Figures 6 and 7. Ultimately, given the histological findings, the biopsy was diagnosed as mesangial proliferative glomerulonephritis with crescent formation. Findings were not comparable with lupus nephritis, especially the immunofluorescent findings. The significant mesangial IgA staining raised the likelihood of IgA nephropathy.

Her serologic work-up included anti-dsDNA antibody (1:80), ANA (1:320), and normal serum complement levels.

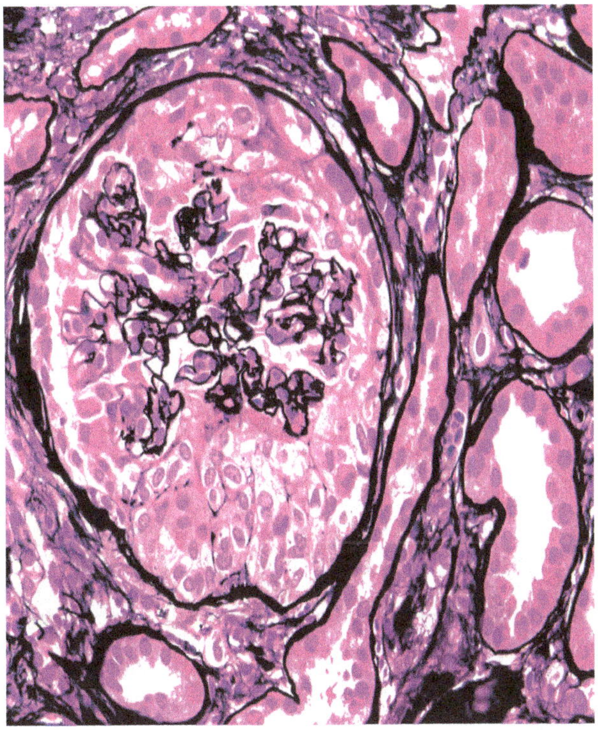

FIGURE 2: Circumferential cellular crescent is present, associated with collapse of the underlying glomerular capillaries (methenamine silver, x400).

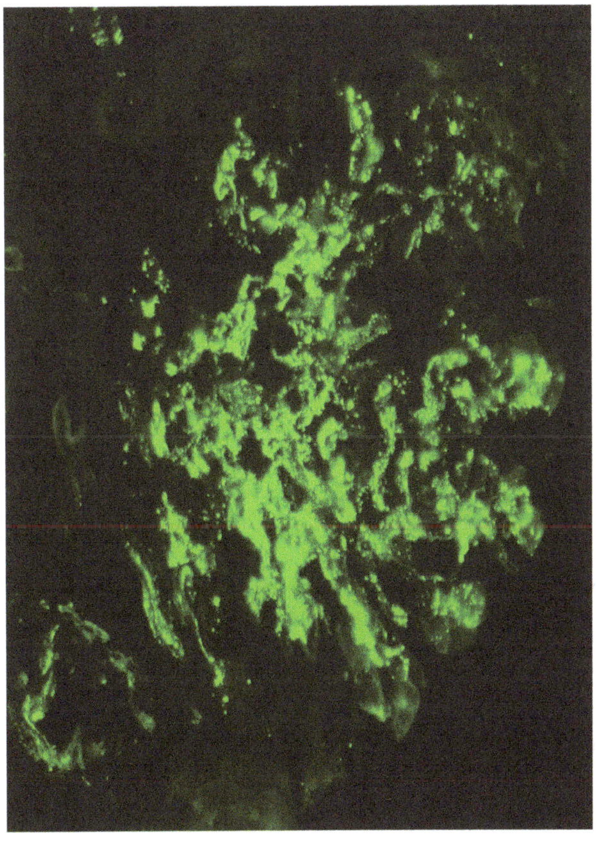

FIGURE 3: Global 3+ mesangial deposit of immunoglobulin A is present (immunofluorescent, x 400).

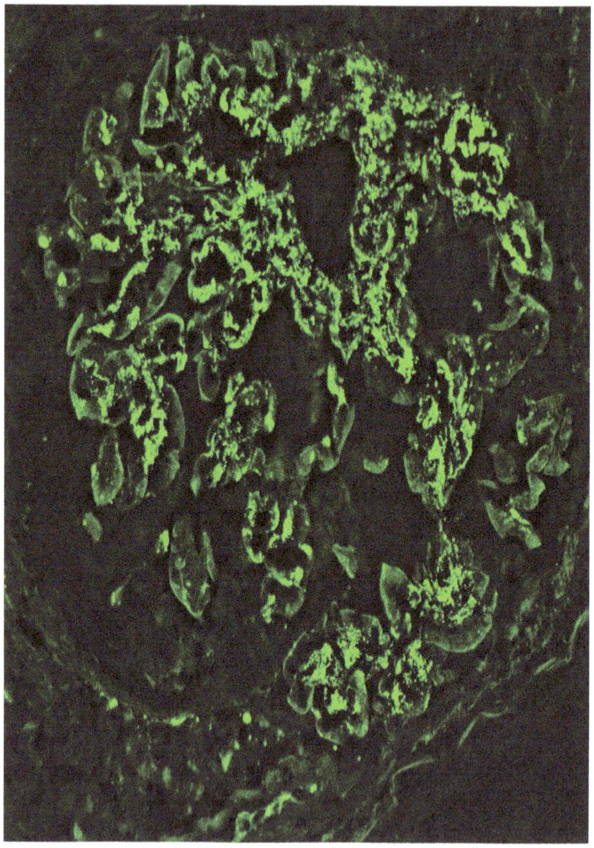

FIGURE 4: Global 3+ mesangial deposit of complement component C3 is present (immunofluorescent, x 400).

FIGURE 5: There is no glomerular deposition of complement component C1q present (immunofluorescent, x 400).

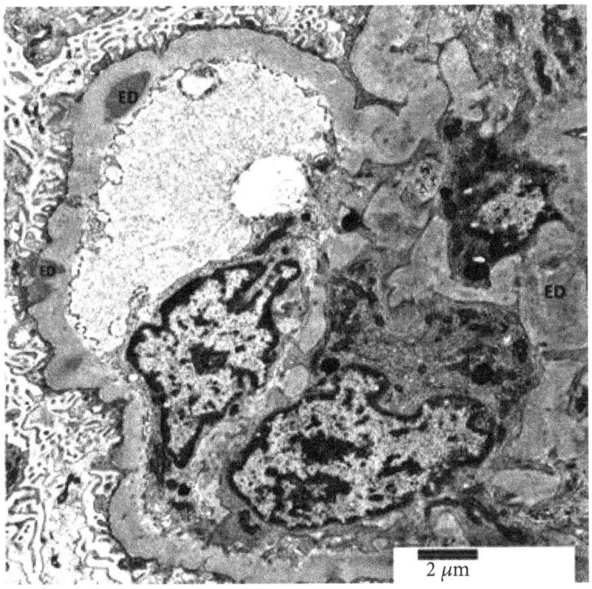

FIGURE 6: There is mesangial hypercellularity and mild thickening of glomerular basement membrane along with electron dense deposits (ED) in mesangial, subendothelial, and subepithelial locations (electron microscopy, x 8000).

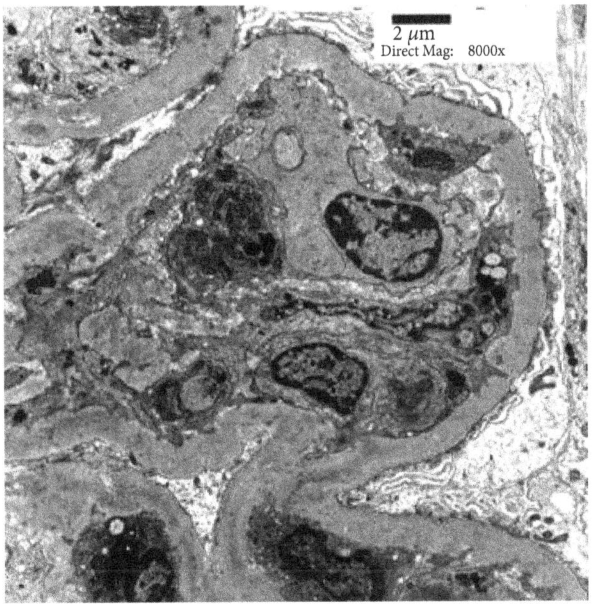

FIGURE 7: There are endocapillary cell hypercellularity and several small electron dense deposits within the glomerular basement membrane (electron microscopy, x 8000).

With these biopsy results in the setting of worsening kidney function, she was diagnosed with immune complex RPGN secondary to IgAN.

She subsequently received intravenous methylprednisolone 500 mg daily for three days and five rounds of plasmapheresis. Unfortunately, her renal function continued to deteriorate, and she was started on hemodialysis. She was discharged with instructions to take prednisone 60 mg daily for one month with a taper. Her clinical symptoms showed mild improvement, however, there was no significant recovery in kidney function, and she was declared to have end-stage renal disease (ESRD).

3. Discussion

Renal disease is a common complication in patients with SLE and can affect up to 50% of the population. While LN must be kept high on the differential in SLE patients presenting with renal dysfunction, it is important to consider these patients are not exempt from renal diseases which affect the general population. Our patient with SLE had known CKD stage IIIa which had been attributed as a complication of T2DM and hypertension, but she was ultimately found to have concomitant IgAN. In addition, the biopsy-proven RPGN of IgAN was without characteristics classically seen in LN.

As the most common cause of primary glomerulonephritis, IgAN was initially seen to run a benign course. However, it is now recognized almost half of the patients affected progress to ESRD. There are several clinical factors which have been known to be markers for progression and severe disease: elevated serum creatinine, hypertension, and persistent proteinuria above 1000/day [6]. Our patient demonstrated all three of these markers upon diagnosis as she presented with blood pressure ranging from 150 to 180/70-80 with a known history of hypertension. She also had a baseline serum creatinine of 1.1 mg/dL with a calculated eGFR of 44 mL/min/1.73m^2. In addition, her urine spot protein-creatinine ratio was 1.48 to suggest approximately protein excretion of 1480 mg per day. Other notable risk factors for progression of disease include obesity, hypertriglyceridemia, hyperuricemia, and smoking [7–9]. Our patient was only notable to be a former smoker who had quit smoking in the remote past.

Lastly, specific histological predictors have been shown to be associated with more severe disease. These include mesangial hypercellularity, endocapillary hypercellularity, segmental glomerulosclerosis, tubular atrophy, and crescent formation. Formally, this is known by the Oxford Classification of IgA nephropathy as the MEST score (or MEST-C score if accounting for crescents). The MEST score with clinical data at the time of biopsy has been shown to provide the same predictive power as monitoring clinical data for two years [10]. Based on histopathological results, our patient would be classified as M1, E0, S0, T1, and C1, with each metric having specific prognostic utility.

The patient was also found to have immune complex RPGN which is clinically and histologically correlated with the rapid progressive loss of renal function with crescent formation and biopsy-proven IgAN. Untreated RPGN typically progresses to end-stage renal disease over a period of weeks to a few months. The treatment for RPGN specifically in patients with IgAN has not been studied in randomized clinical trials; however, observational data suggests regimens used like those of idiopathic crescentic glomerulonephritis may provide possible benefit. This includes intravenous pulse methylprednisolone followed by plasmapheresis, oral prednisone, or cyclophosphamide (either oral or intravenous) [11]. Our patient was treated with intravenous methylprednisolone for three days followed by five days of plasmapheresis and continued oral prednisone. Although her clinical symptoms slightly improved, her renal function continued to deteriorate, and she was declared ESRD.

A previous study analyzed 251 SLE patients with ESRD using United States surveillance data. The results of the study showed that 21.1% of patients had ESRD attributed to a cause other than SLE. The majority of this subset was due to hypertension and diabetes. However, only 3.1% of the total study population had ESRD attributed to a non-SLE glomerulonephritis [12], and this is the subset which our patient fits into. Furthermore, she presented with crescentic IgA nephropathy, which although is the most commonly observed glomerulonephritis globally, it rarely presents with RPGN.

To our knowledge there is a large void of studies which report patients with SLE who develop non-LN-related crescentic glomerulonephritis. This is a case of a patient with known SLE and CKD who presented with acute kidney injury ultimately diagnosed with RPGN of IgA nephropathy without lupus nephritis. This highlights the importance renal biopsy to guide diagnosis and treatment in a patient with multiple risk factors for renal disease.

References

[1] S. Almaani, A. Meara, and B. H. Rovin, "Update on lupus nephritis," *Clinical Journal of the American Society of Nephrology*, vol. 12, no. 5, pp. 825–835, 2017.

[2] J. J. Weening, V. D. D'Agati, and M. M. Schwartz, "The classification of glomerulonephritis in systemic lupus erythematosus revisited," *Journal of the American Society of Nephrology*, vol. 15, no. 2, pp. 241–250, 2004.

[3] R. N. Verma et al., "Lupus Nephritis–light, electron and immunofluorescent Microscopy (a Clinicopathological Study," *Indian Journal of Pathology & Microbiology*, vol. 32, no. 4, pp. 246–551, 1989.

[4] G. D'Amico, "Natural history of idiopathic IgA nephropathy: role of clinical and histological prognostic factors," *American Journal of Kidney Diseases*, vol. 36, no. 2, pp. 227–237, 2000.

[5] J. Lv, Y. Yang, H. Zhang et al., "Prediction of outcomes in crescentic IgA nephropathy in a multicenter cohort study," *Journal of the American Society of Nephrology*, vol. 24, no. 12, pp. 2118–2125, 2013.

[6] G. D'Amico, "Influence of Clinical and Histological Features on Actuarial Renal Survival in Adult Patients With Idiopathic IgA Nephropathy, Membranous Nephropathy, and Membranoproliferative Glomerulonephritis: Survey of the Recent Literature," *American Journal of Kidney Diseases*, vol. 20, no. 4, pp. 315–323, 1992.

[7] F. Bonnet, C. Deprele, A. Sassolas et al., "Excessive body weight as a new independent risk factor for clinical and pathological progression in primary IgA nephritis," *American Journal of Kidney Diseases*, vol. 37, no. 4, pp. 720–727, 2001.

[8] J. Syrjänen, J. Mustonen, and A. Pasternack, "Hypertriglyceridaemia and hyperuricaemia are risk factors for progression of IgA nephropathy," *Nephrology Dialysis Transplantation* , vol. 15, no. 1, pp. 34–42, 2000.

[9] R. Yamamoto, Y. Nagasawa, T. Shoji et al., "Cigarette Smoking and Progression of IgA Nephropathy," *American Journal of Kidney Diseases*, vol. 56, no. 2, pp. 313–324, 2010.

[10] H. Trimarchi, J. Barratt, D. C. Cattran et al., "Oxford Classification of IgA nephropathy 2016: an update from the IgA Nephropathy Classification Working Group," *Kidney International*, vol. 91, no. 5, pp. 1014–1021, 2017.

[11] D. Roccatello and et al., "Report on intensive treatment of extracapillary glomerulonephritis with focus on crescentic IgA

nephropathy," *Nephrology Dialysis Transplantation*, vol. 10, no. 11, pp. 2054–2094, 1995.

[12] L. C. Plantinga, C. Drenkard, S. O. Pastan, and S. S. Lim, "Attribution of cause of end-stage renal disease among patients with systemic lupus erythematosus: the georgia lupus registry," *Lupus Science & Medicine*, vol. 3, no. 1, Article ID e000132, 2016.

17

Iatrogenic Infective Endocarditis in Hemodialysis Patients: A Case Report and Review of the Literature

Ali Oullaï, Edouard Cubilier, Mohamed Tayeb Salaouatchi, Maxime Taghavi, Yasmin Zouggari, Joëlle Nortier, and Maria Do Carmo Filomena Mesquita

Department of Nephrology, Brugmann University Hospital, Université Libre de Bruxelles, Brussels, Belgium

Correspondence should be addressed to Maria Do Carmo Filomena Mesquita; maria.mesquita@chu-brugmann.be

Academic Editor: Anja Haase-Fielitz

Foreign bodies such as implanted cardiac devices are susceptible to infections and may be involved in infective endocarditis. Exposure to pathogens, by frequent use of intravascular accesses for hemodialysis (i.e., catheters or fistulas), combined with high rates of degenerative heart valve diseases in hemodialysis patients, both favor the development of infective endocarditis in this population. The mitral and aortic valves are predominantly implicated in endocardial infections. The involvement of both mitral and tricuspid valves is rare in the general population but can occur in hemodialysis patients with implanted cardiac devices. Infective endocarditis is associated with high morbidity and mortality rates among hemodialysis patients, mostly because of the complications of septic emboli. Prevention, prophylaxis, and early diagnosis of endocarditis can be lifesaving in this fragile population. We report a case of right and left heart methicillin-sensitive *Staphylococcus aureus* endocarditis with cerebral septic emboli in an elderly hemodialysis patient carrier of an arteriovenous fistula and an ipsilateral nonleadless pacemaker.

1. Introduction

Cardiovascular diseases and infections are the two main causes of mortality in hemodialysis (HD) patients [1]. The prevalence of infective endocarditis (IE) in chronic HD patients is 2.9% [2], and its incidence is 50 to 60 times higher than in the general population [3].

HD patients are at higher risk of IE due to their intrinsic fragility related to older age and multiple comorbidities, such as cardiovascular diseases and hyperuricemia-induced immunosuppression [4], in addition to a high exposure to pathogenic microorganisms during HD sessions due to repeated manipulations of their vascular access [1]. Moreover, mortality rates of IE in the HD population reach 25 to 77%, which is higher than the general population [1]. Sadeghi et al. reported in-hospital IE death rates and long-term death rates as 45.6% and 29.5% of cases, respectively [2].

Other risk factors for IE in the general population include the presence of implanted cardiac devices as well as the absence of antibiotic prophylaxis during dental and surgical procedures [5]. Methicillin-sensitive *Staphylococcus aureus* (MSSA) is the main pathogen involved in IE as reported by several previous studies [6]. IE is often associated with several complications such as systemic embolism, among which brain septic emboli are the most common, with an incidence of 65% in MSSA-related IE. Such complications were associated with longer ICU stays and higher mortality rates [7].

2. Case Presentation

We report a case of a 77-year-old hemodialyzed man with a medical history of congenital anomalies of the kidney and urinary tract (CAKUT)-related ESRD requiring HD. He underwent a left brachial radio-radial AVF and began dialysis sessions in our center 6 years ago. The patient was also known for a severe chronic obstructive pulmonary disease (COPD) (Gold IV) due to smoking and chronic alcoholism. Moreover, he benefitted, two years ago, from a dual chamber St Jude Assarity Magnetic Resonance Imaging (MRI) PM placement for an auriculoventricular block of 2 : 1, with leads

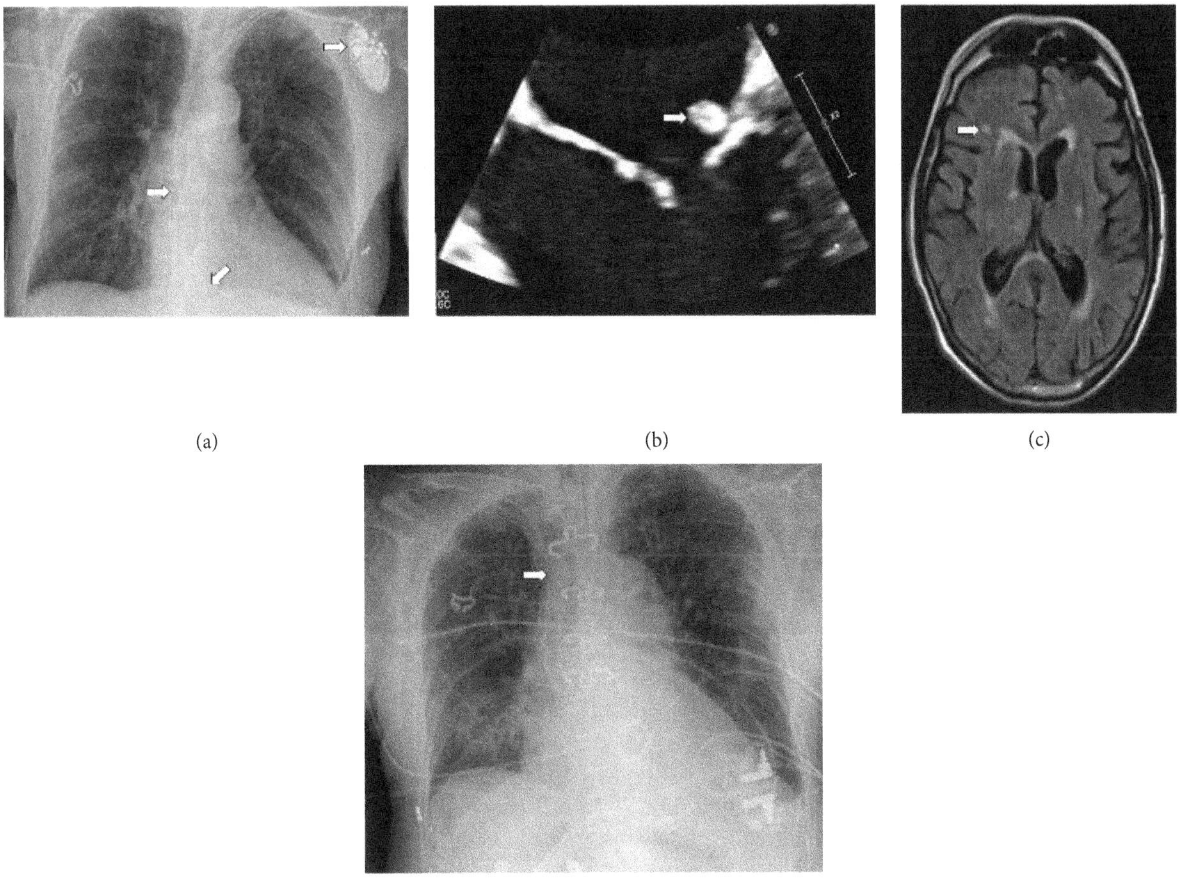

(a) (b) (c) (d)

FIGURE 1: (a) Chest radiography with implanted pacemaker, (b) transesophagal echography, (c) MRI cerebral showed the emboli, and (d) chest radiography with external pacemaker.

placed in the right heart via the left jugular vein in the right atrium and right ventricle, respectively (Figure 1(a)).

The patient was admitted to the emergency room for fever. A clinical examination revealed a debilitated patient with a fever (40°C) and chills. Examination of the AVF showed no sign of infection, and an oral examination did not show decayed teeth. No invasive dental, respiratory, gastrointestinal, or genitourinary procedures were performed for the last year.

Relevant laboratory findings displayed an elevated inflammatory marker C-Reactive Protein of 408 mg/L (reference values (RF): ≤0.5 mg/dL), a leukocytosis of 11 260/μL (RF: 3.50–11.00 [×103/μL]) with 10.360/μL neutrophils (RF: 1.50–6.70 [×103/μL]), ion disorders hyperkaliemia at 5.6 mmol/L (RF: 3.4–4.5 mmol/L), hypercalcemia at 2.56 mmol/L (RF: 2.20–2.55 mmol/L), and hyperphosphatemia at 2.27 mmol/L (RF: 0.75–1.39 mmol/L). Four sets of blood cultures were collected, all of which were positive for Gram-positive cocci identified as MSSA.

The thoracic-abdominal computed tomography (CT) scan performed did not show any acute abnormalities, despite COPD lung lesions, polycystic kidneys, and non-inflammatory diverticulosis.

Initial antibiotic treatment consisted in intravenous (IV) ceftazidime and vancomycin, prior to blood culture results, and was then switched to IV flucloxacillin sodium according to the antibiotic sensitivity spectrum, with an adjusted dose for HD patients (2 g four times a day). Antibiotic doses were then increased to six times a day, because of increased laboratory inflammatory markers and persisting bacteremia five days after admission.

The trans-esophageal echocardiography (TEE) showed vegetations on the tricuspid valve (18 × 10 mm), on the mitral valve's posterior leaflet (8 mm), and on the atrium lead of the PM (<10 mm) (Figure 1(b)).

Four days after admission, the patient presented with delirium and left upper limb paresis. A cerebral MRI was performed and showed multiple ischemic lesions with embolic features (Figure 1(c)).

The pacemaker box and its leads were removed on the 10th day and a temporary external pacemaker was placed (Figure 1(d)). There were no signs of infection on direct examination. The whole device was put into culture and the results were negative. The patient was then transferred to the cardiology unit for cardiac monitoring.

Despite two weeks of a well-conducted antibiotic therapy, the control of TEE showed an increase in the size of the mitral vegetation (15 mm), in addition to the appearance of an abscess of the aortic annulus, which required cardiac surgery.

On the 17th day after admission, the patient underwent a mitral valve replacement by bioprosthesis and a tricuspid valvuloplasty. The surgical report described a residual vegetation on the posterior valve of the tricuspid valve where the ventricular lead used to be in place and a massive invasion of the mitral valve by a voluminous vegetation. The patient was then transferred to the intensive care unit (ICU) for postoperative monitoring. During the ICU stay, the patient presented with hemodynamic instability due to a global cardiac dysfunction which culminated in an acute pulmonary edema, and a sepsis related to a *Pseudomonas aeruginosa* ventilator-associated pneumonia (VAP). HD was continued thrice a week and supplementary HD was administered whenever necessary.

After clinical stabilization, the patient was transferred back to the cardiology ward with a temporary pacemaker in await for the definitive leadless PM which had been ordered. Unfortunately, the patient died on the 29th day of hospitalization because of recurrent cardiogenic shocks. The timeline of clinical course, diagnostics, interventions and outcome are shown in Figure 2.

3. Discussion

The risk factors for endocarditis in HD patients are well known. Nevertheless, prevention and rapid diagnosis are essential for optimal management in these fragile patients.

Chronic HD patients are vulnerable to IE because of frequent valvular degeneration secondary to the cardiovascular complications of ESRD [1]. These complications imply fluid overload, uremic cardiomyopathy, secondary hyperparathyroidism, anemia, altered lipid metabolism, myocardial hemodynamic stress due to HD, and accumulation of gut microbiota uremic toxins like trimethylamine N-oxidase [8]. HD patients often present with arterial hypertension, which raises mechanical stress on the valves of the left heart by increasing cardiac postcharge, thus accelerating valve deterioration [1]. Moreover, valve damage can result from "jet lesions" due to turbulent blood flow during HD or by repeated IV drugs that are commonly given during dialysis sessions [9]. Indeed, our patient, who underwent HD for 6 years, had known calcifications on both the aortic and mitral valves.

In HD patients, the mitral and aortic valves are predominantly involved in IE, with a respective prevalence of 80 and 100% of IE cases [1]. The left heart is a high-pressure system that tends to deteriorate the mitral and aortic valves faster, which therefore promotes valve calcification in the context of frequent calcium-phosphate disorders, as seen in ESRD patients. Right-sided IE is rare and its incidence varies from 0% to 26% depending on different studies, with a predominant implication of the tricuspid valve [1]. In our patient, we observed simultaneous right (tricuspid) and left (mitral) involvement. As the leads of the PM were in the right heart and were infected, the formation of vegetation on the tricuspid valve could have followed. The left heart involvement may have occurred as a result of an embolus via the pulmonary circulation.

The principal source of infections in HD patients is their vascular access, which can be either a catheter or an AVF [10]. AVF induces fewer infectious complications compared to other accesses. AVF-related infection occurs in 2–4% of this population, with an incidence of 0.018/100 per access day [11]. Clinical examination of the AVF by the patient, nursing staff, and medical staff should be routinely done. In our patient, on admission and thereafter, meticulous examination of the AVF showed no sign of infection. Nonetheless, its repeated punctures during HD sessions could have been the portal of entry.

Cardiac implantable devices such as PM, implantable cardiovascular defibrillators, or cardiac resynchronization therapy devices are vulnerable to infections [12]. PM-related infections have been estimated to be 0.77% for their initial implantation and 2.08% for revision or replacement procedures [13]. Device infection can occur because of skin infections which may colonize the pocket of the device or by hematogenous implantation of bacteria [13]. In our patient, the insertion site of the PM bared no sign of infection and there was no report of any infectious complication related to the device since its installation two years ago.

In HD patients, cardiac devices should be placed on the contralateral side of the vascular access due to the increased risk of venous stenosis and infection of the device [14]. Unfortunately, our patient's PM was placed on the ipsilateral side of the AVF because puncture of the contralateral jugular vein was not technically possible. He had a left radio-radial AVF, and the leads of PM were introduced through the left cephalic vein in the right side of the heart. This setup increases the risk of hematogenous bacterial colonization on the device because of the direct vascular contact of the microbes with the PM. Indeed, we hypothesized that repeated punctures of the AVF could have silently brought bacteria to the PM.

In our patient, PM was removed a week before surgery. We observed an increase in the size of the mitral valve vegetation despite two weeks of adequate antibiotic therapy. The vegetations seen on the valves were much bigger than those seen on the leads of the PM. The bacteria were probably more adherent to the endothelium of the sick valve than to the biofilm of the lead. This could explain the bigger lesions on the mitral valve compared to the flat surface of the lead of the PM [15].

Blood cultures obtained before the beginning of any antibiotic treatment are an important part of the diagnostic procedure. They must be repeated daily until they come back negative to determine the first day of the 6 weeks of antibiotic therapy [16]. In addition to antibiotics, device removal is indicated if it is infected, or in the case of IE, or a Gram-positive bacteremia [17]. Leadless PM reduces the risk of device infection and central venous stenosis because no invasive intravascular intervention is needed to install the leads, and leadless PM infections are very rare [13]. This could be due to the absence of a subcutaneous pocket and transvenous leads, the small surface area of this device, and the parylene coating of the leadless PM [13]. In fact, parylene reduces bacterial adherence and has antibacterial properties compared to either polyurethane or bare titanium which

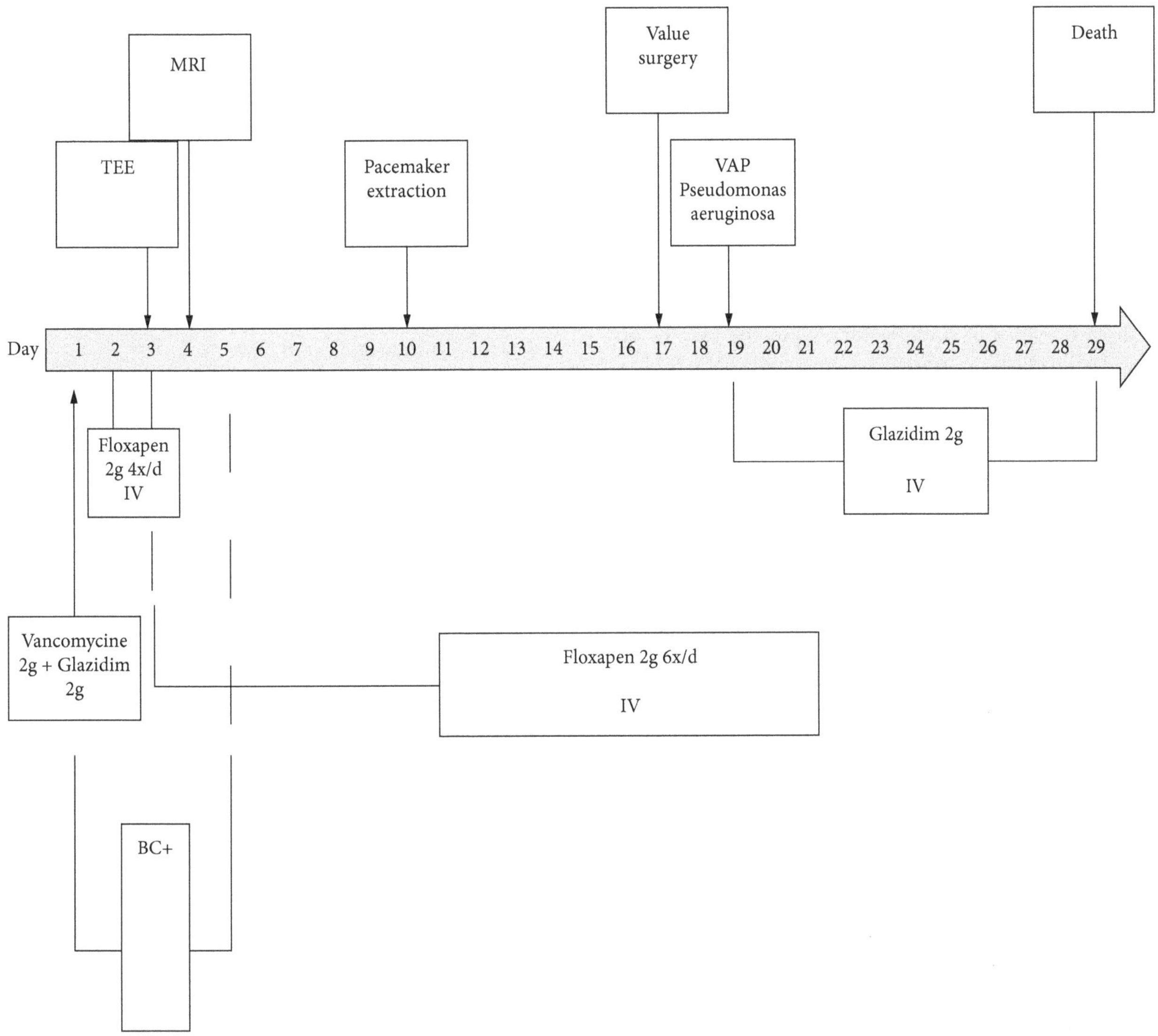

FIGURE 2: Time line of clinical course, diagnostics, interventions, and outcomes. BC: blood culture, TEE: transoesophageal echography, MRI: magnetic resonance imaging, and VAP: ventilator-associated pneumonia.

composes the pulse generators of traditional PM [13]. Our patient did not benefit from this novel device at that time because leadless PM was not available two years ago in our center.

IE can have local and distant complications. Heart failure in IE can occur because of a valvular dysfunction directly caused by the vegetation [18] or a peri-annular extension of the infection which then urges the need for surgical procedures and raises mortality rates [18]. Distant IE complications on a remote site occur via septic emboli. The destination of septic emboli depends on the heart valve involved; right-side IE frequently causes pulmonary septic emboli, whereas left-side IE causes systemic septic emboli [7]. In a multinational study, 44.4% of patients with IE had major embolic events, predominantly in the brain (26.3%), as it occurred in our patient [18].

General septic emboli are best diagnosed by fluorodeoxyglucose positron emission tomography (FDG PET-CT), but this exam cannot detect cerebral emboli because of the intense cerebral capture of the FDG [19]. MRI is therefore the gold standard for the diagnosis of cerebral septic emboli because of its high sensitivity compared to CT-scan [20].

Treatment of IE in an HD population should combine preventive strategies such as reducing hospital-acquired bacteremia, good oral hygiene, antibiotic prophylaxis according to the local guidelines when required, especially for dental and other surgical procedures, and the use of antibacterial coating materials in implantable devices when available. Special attention is required in patients with implanted cardiac devices that could be silently infected. In order to improve diagnosis, a high index of systematic clinical suspicion of device infection is required. These patients should therefore be educated on related signs and symptoms, an adequate microbiological assessment must be made rapidly in order to start empiric treatment, and a TEE must be scheduled hastily. Optimal management of these fragile patients with the help of an IE-devoted team is advisable. Tailored antibiotic therapy and early surgery when required, as well as monitoring for complications, are necessary in order to face the challenges of the dreaded IE complications [5].

Unfortunately, our patient died on the 29th day of hospitalization and 12 days after cardiac surgery. The in-hospital mortality rate of HD patients with IE is up to 45.6% [2]. The prognosis of patients with IE is determined by four main factors: patient characteristics, the occurrence of IE-related cardiac and noncardiac complications, the infecting organism, and the echocardiographic findings. In patients with three or more of these factors, as in the case of our patient, the in-hospital mortality rate reaches 79% [21].

In addition, our patient had signs of persistent infection as he presented with a fever and persistent positive blood cultures for five days after starting the antibiotics. The persistence of positive blood cultures after 48–72 h of antibiotic therapy has been recently associated with a higher risk of hospital mortality [22], which suggests, in fact, that early surgery should have been considered in our patient.

Early surgery was indeed considered in our patient, but the occurrence of symptomatic septic emboli and the clinical stability of the patient motivated our cardiac team to delay the surgery. In patients with a good response to antibiotics, surgery can be postponed for 2–4 weeks under close monitoring of the aortic abscess by serial TEE [23].

Finally, the control of TEE after two weeks of antibiotics in our patient showed an increase in the size of the mitral vegetation, in addition to the appearance of an abscess of the aortic annulus, which indicates locally uncontrolled infection and then urged the need for surgical procedure. However, it is known that the results of surgery when the reason for the procedure is uncontrolled infection are worse than when surgery is performed for other reasons [21].

4. Conclusion

Awareness about IE is crucial in clinical practice given its high morbidity and mortality in HD patients. In this population, the risk of IE increases because of high rates of valvular damage as a consequence of metabolic and cardiovascular complications of ESRD. Vascular access is often the source of IE even in the absence of clinical signs of infection.

Implanted cardiac devices are risk factors for endocarditis and should be placed on the contralateral side of HD patients' vascular access whenever possible. Leadless PM should be considered in HD patients, but the cost, the availability, and the expertise can limit its prescription.

Regular planning of antibiotic prophylaxis during dental and different surgical procedures should be in the good practice guidelines of all the dialysis centers.

For optimal management of IE, a devoted IE team of nurses and clinicians is advised in order to prevent and treat IE.

Endocarditis in hemodialysis: key points

- Clinical suspicion and early diagnosis are necessary
- Careful monitoring of the vascular access sites is important
- Antibiotic prophylaxis in the case of dental and all surgical procedures is recommended
- If an implantable cardiac device is required:
  - Implant on the contralateral side of the device when possible
  - Use a leadless pacemaker if available
  - Remove the device if MSSA bacteremia, valvular, or device infection occurs
- Look for septic emboli and discuss appropriate treatment
- Work with a dedicated IE team

Consent

The patient's next of kin provided consent to publish this case study.

References

[1] Y. Bentata, "Physiopathological approach to infective endocarditis in chronic hemodialysis patients: left heart versus right heart involvement," *Renal Failure*, vol. 39, no. 1, pp. 432–439, 2017.

[2] M. Sadeghi, S. Behdad, and F. Shahsanaei, "Infective endocarditis and its short and long-term prognosis in hemodialysis patients: a systematic review and meta-analysis," *Current Problems in Cardiology*, vol. 46, no. 3, Article ID 100680, 2021.

[3] G. Nucifora, L. P. Badano, P. Viale et al., "Infective endocarditis in chronic haemodialysis patients: an increasing clinical challenge," *European Heart Journal*, vol. 28, no. 19, pp. 2307–2312, 2007.

[4] N. D. Vaziri, M. V. Pahl, A. Crum, and K. Norris, "Effect of uremia on structure and function of immune system," *Journal of Renal Nutrition*, vol. 22, no. 1, pp. 149–156, 2012.

[5] L. M. B. Thomas J. Cahill, G. Habib, H. Bruno et al., "Challenges in infective endocarditis," *Journal of the American College of Cardiology*, vol. 69, no. 3, pp. 325–344, 2017.

[6] A. M. Georgescu, L. Azamfirei, K. Szalman, and E. Szekely, "Fatal endocarditis with methicilin-sensible *Staphylococcus aureus* and major complications: rhabdomyolysis, pericarditis, and intracerebral hematoma: a case report and review of the literature," *Medicine (Baltimore)*, vol. 95, no. 41, Article ID e5125, 2016.

[7] S. P. Stawicki, M. S. Firstenberg, M. R. Lyaker et al., "Septic embolism in the intensive care unit," *International Journal of Critical Illness and Injury Science*, vol. 3, no. 1, p. 58, 2013.

[8] S. Ahmadmehrabi and W. H. W. Tang, "Hemodialysis-induced cardiovascular disease," *Seminars in Dialysis*, vol. 31, no. 3, pp. 258–267, 2018.

[9] V. Jain, M.-H. Yang, G. Kovacicova-Lezcano, A. F. B. Leah S Juhle, L. G. Winston, and L. G. Winston, "Infective endocarditis in an urban medical center: association of individual drugs with valvular involvement," *Journal of Infection*, vol. 57, no. 2, pp. 132–138, 2008.

[10] T. F. Saad, D. M. Hentschel, B. Koplan et al., "Cardiovascular implantable electronic device leads in CKD and ESRD

patients: review and recommendations for practice," *Seminars in Dialysis*, vol. 26, no. 1, pp. 114–123, 2013.

[11] L. Kumbar and J. Yee, "Current concepts in hemodialysis vascular access infections," *Advances in Chronic Kidney Disease*, vol. 26, no. 1, pp. 16–22, 2019.

[12] D. M. Charytan, A. R. Patrick, J. Liu et al., "Trends in the use and outcomes of implantable cardioverter-defibrillators in patients undergoing dialysis in the United States," *American Journal of Kidney Diseases*, vol. 58, no. 3, pp. 409–417, 2011.

[13] M. F. El-Chami, M. Bonner, R. Holbrook et al., "Leadless pacemakers reduce risk of device-related infection: review of the potential mechanisms," *Heart Rhythm*, vol. 17, no. 8, pp. 1393–1397, 2020.

[14] C. S. Tan, C. Jie, J. Joe et al., "The impact of transvenous cardiac devices on vascular access patency in hemodialysis patients," *Seminars in Dialysis*, vol. 26, no. 6, pp. 728–732, 2013.

[15] T. L. Holland, L. M. Baddour, A. S. Bayer, B. Hoen, J. M. Miro, and V. G. Fowler Jr., "Infective endocarditis," *Nature Reviews Disease Primers*, vol. 2, no. 1, Article ID 16059, 2016.

[16] L. M. Baddour, W. R. Wilson, A. S. Bayer et al., "Infective endocarditis in adults: diagnosis, antimicrobial therapy, and management of complications: a scientific statement for healthcare professionals from the American heart association," *Circulation*, vol. 132, no. 15, pp. 1435–1486, 2015.

[17] F. M. Kusumoto, M. H. Schoenfeld, B. L. Wilkoff et al., "2017 HRS expert consensus statement on cardiovascular implantable electronic device lead management and extraction," *Heart Rhythm*, vol. 14, no. 12, pp. e503–e551, 2017.

[18] H. Erdem, E. Puca, Y. Ruch et al., "Portraying infective endocarditis: results of multinational ID-IRI study," *European Journal of Clinical Microbiology & Infectious Diseases*, vol. 38, no. 9, pp. 1753–1763, 2019.

[19] M. R. Sohail and L. M. Baddour, "Role of PET imaging in management of implantable electronic device infection," *Journal of the American College of Cardiology: Cardiovascular Imaging*, vol. 9, no. 3, pp. 291–293, 2016.

[20] N. Mgbojikwe, S. R. Jones, T. M. Leucker, and D. J. Brotman, "Infective endocarditis: beyond the usual tests," *Cleveland Clinic Journal of Medicine*, vol. 86, no. 8, pp. 559–567, 2019.

[21] G. Habib, P. Lancellotti, M. J. Antunes et al., "2015 ESC guidelines for the management of infective endocarditis: the task force for the management of infective endocarditis of the European society of cardiology (ESC). Endorsed by: European association for cardio-thoracic surgery (EACTS), the European association of nuclear medicine (EANM)," *European Heart Journal*, vol. 36, no. 44, pp. 3075–3128, 2015.

[22] J. Lopez, T. Sevilla, I. Vilacosta et al., "Prognostic role of persistent positive blood cultures after initiation of antibiotic therapy in left-sided infective endocarditis," *European Heart Journal*, vol. 34, no. 23, pp. 1749–1754, 2013.

[23] D. H. Kang, "Timing of surgery in infective endocarditis," *Heart*, vol. 101, no. 22, pp. 1786–1791, 2015.

18

Cabazitaxel Induced Thrombotic Microangiopathy in a Patient with Prostate Cancer

Yannick Nlandu, Franck Pourcine, Ly van phach Vong, Jonathan Chelly, Sebastien Jochmans, Sandie Mazerand, and Mehran Monchi

Groupe Hospitalier Sud Ile-De-France, Centre Hospitalier de Melun, 77000 Melun, France

Correspondence should be addressed to Yannick Nlandu; yannicknlandu@yahoo.fr

Academic Editor: Ze'ev Korzets

Cancer-associated thrombotic microangiopathy (TMA) refers to a group of disorders characterized by microangiopathic haemolytic anemia, thrombocytopenia, and ischemic organ damage. TMA manifestations can be induced by cancer or by chemotherapy. We report the case of a 64-year-old man with metastatic prostate cancer who experienced a Cabazitaxel-induced TMA manifestation. TMA responds to conservative therapy, dialysis without plasmaphoresis, with progressive recovered renal function.

1. Introduction

Thrombotic microangiopathy (TMA) is a clinical association of thrombocytopenia, microangiopathic haemolytic anaemia and organ dysfunction related to microvascular thrombosis [1, 2]. TMA is associated with significant mortality and morbidity including acute renal failure [3], a common feature caused by high susceptibility of renal vessels to endothelial damage [3]. In the course of cancer, TMA can be secondary to malignancy or to direct chemotherapy toxicity [4]. Al-Nouri et al. have established a list of anti-cancer agents associated with TMA with evidence of definitive causality, including a taxane drug, Docetaxel [5]. We report a case of TMA induced by Cabazitaxel, a newly integrated taxane drug in the treatment of advanced prostate cancer.

2. Case Report

A 64-year-old male, is treated since 2005 for metastatic (spine and sub-diaphragmatic lymph nodes) and hormone-resistant prostate cancer. The patient was previously treated with Docetaxel and currently with Cabazitaxel every 3 weeks since 13th june 2018. The level of Prostate-specific antigen (PSA) in March 2019 was 25.00 ng/mL for free PSA, and 898 ng/mL for total PSA. The patient who had previously received 18 cycles of Cabazitaxel at 25 mg/m^2 (50 mg) and blood samples on 28th January 2019 showed a thrombocytopenia at 82 G/L and an elevated creatinine up to 328 μmol/L with spontaneous normalization of creatinine and platelet count 7 weeks later after its discontinuation (Hb 9 g/dL, platelets 439G/L, creatinine 77 μmol/L). Another injection of Cabazitaxel at lower dose (40 mg) was given on 21th march 2019, with appearance 24 hours later of oliguria and asthenia. The file chart doesn't mention acute kidney injury (AKI) at the moment of reinjection. The clinical examination was unremarkable except for moderate hypertension at 150/90 mmHg. Blood samples on 26th march showed an anemia with haemoglobin at 5 g/dL, thrombocytopenia at 17 G/L, schizocytes at more than 15% on blood smear, LDH at 4597 IU/L, haptoglobin <0.1 g/L, and normal INR at 1.14. The Coombs test was negative and there was renal insufficiency with creatinine at 1022 μmol/L, urea 62 mmol/L. The profile of this renal failure was parenchymal with urinary sodium-potassium ratio >1. An ultrasound ruled out a post-renal AKI. The serum potassium was 5.7 mmol/L. Etiological investigations of this thrombotic microangiopathy showed 75% ADAMST13 activity, C4 at 0.45 g/L (0.10–0.40), C3 at 1.60 g/L (0.9–1.8), CH50 141% (70–130), 137% of factor H (65–140) and 180% factor I (60–130). The anti-factor H antibody was negative. The TMA aetiology looks as if associated with Cabazitaxel and chronologically compatible. Simultaneously to drug interruption, the patient had six

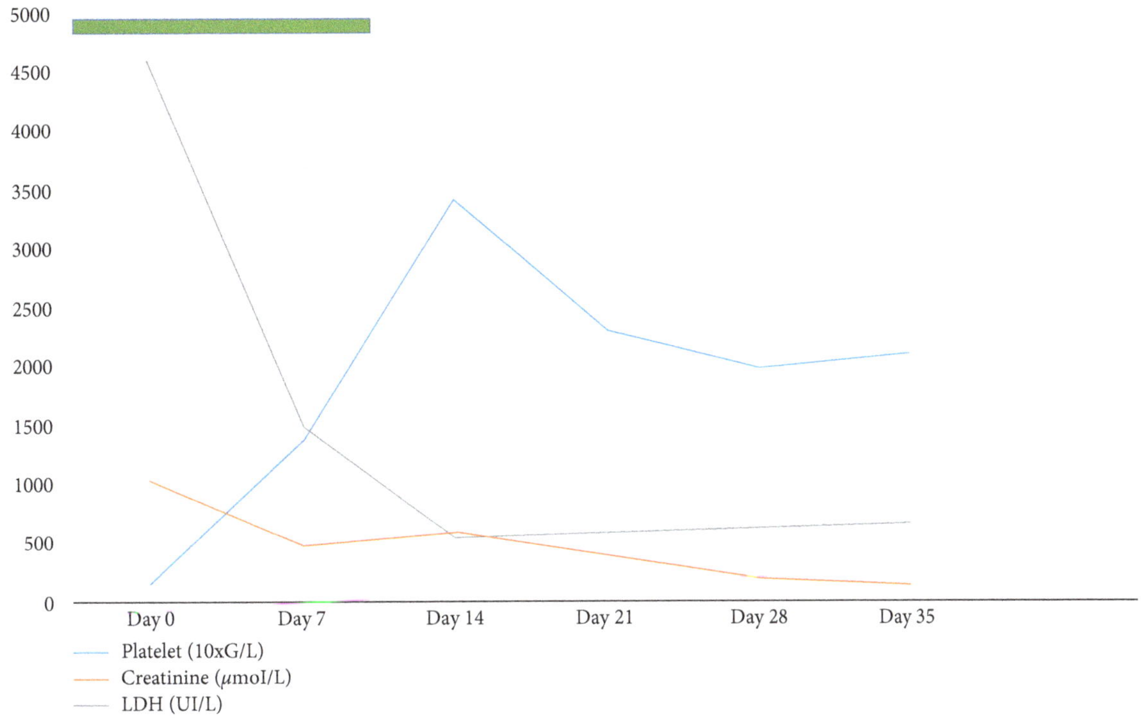

FIGURE 1: Laboratory parameters. Treatment period by haemodialysis is indicated by a coloured green bar. Day 0 represents TMA manifestations.

dialysis sessions without plasmaphoresis. The evolution was characterized by progressive disappearance of biological signs of haemolysis and improvement of renal function (Figure 1). On May 3, 2019, haemoglobin level was 8.6 g/dL without schizocytes, platelets count at 209 G/L, creatinine at 137 μmol/L, urea at 9 mmol/L, LDH at 661 IU/L and haptoglobin at 2.5 g/L. In this context, renal biopsy was not performed. The patient survived to the AKI KDIGO 3 episode with creatinine at 95 μmol/L (eGFR 73 ml/min/1.73 m^2) at 6 month.

3. Discussion

In a cancer patient, it is often difficult to distinguish chemotherapy-induced TMA from TMA caused by cancer [6]. Tumor-related TMA occurs in poorly controlled carcinomas, whereas chemotherapy-associated TMA is more common in disease remission or in minimal tumoral burden [7]. TMA induced by chemotherapy occurs by two main mechanisms: an immune-mediated reaction involving the development of drug-dependent antibodies or a direct endothelial damage [5, 6]. Direct toxicity is dose dependent in case of acute toxicity [5, 8]. The main anticancer agents associated with TMA are bleomycin, and mitomycin C [9, 10, 11]. In a systematic review, AL-Nouri et al. reported 22 drugs that had evidences for association with TMA, including Docetaxel, a taxane class molecule [5].They defined the typical clinical manifestations of an immune reaction by the onset of symptoms within 21 days for a drug administered daily or in the hours following exposure (within 24 hours) for a drug taken intermittently [5]. Direct toxicity was defined either by the acute onset of symptoms after exposure to the offending drug or by the progressive development of toxicity in the form of acute renal failure [5]. Cabazitaxel is used for prostatic cancer [12] in combination with prednisolone. Renal insufficiency following treatment with Cabazitaxel is very rare, but cases of nephrotoxicity in patients have been reported [13]. Most of the cases of renal insufficiency described are associated with sepsis, dehydration or obstructive uropathy, without evidence for a direct nephrotoxicity [13]. Tumma et al. reported a case of TMA, 48 hours after the first dose of Cabazitaxel, with a fatal renal failure [7]. In our case, the occurrence after 18 cycles of Cabazitaxel and the regression of TMA after withdrawal of the treatment suggests a cumulative dose nephrotoxicity of this new treatment. The taxanes have significant antiangiogenic properties in vitro and in vivo [14]. They inhibits endothelial function and angiogenesis and shows a dose-dependent vascular toxicity [14]. In this context, taxane can impair renal vasculature and cause TMA. Our patient had already received 18 injections of Cabazitaxel with a first episode suggesting TMA in January 2019 (platelets at 82 G/L and creatinine at 328 μmol/L with normalization in February, at distance from injections). The current episode was following an injection on march 21, 2019 (haemoglobin 9 g/dL, platelet 439 G/L, creatinine 77 μmol/L before the injection).

4. Conclusion

We report a case of thrombotic microangiopathy due to Cabazitaxel, a toxoid used in the treatment of advanced prostate cancer.

Consent

Informed consent was obtained from the patient.

Acknowledgments

The authors gratefully thank the staff of the Intensive Care Unit at the Hospital of Melun for their commitment to always provide the utmost care to our patients.

References

[1] J. L. Moake, "Thrombotic microangiopathies," *New England Journal of Medicine*, vol. 347, no. 8, pp. 589–600, 2002.

[2] J. N. George and C. M. Nester, "Syndromes of thrombotic microangiopathy," *New England Journal of Medicine*, vol. 371, no. 7, pp. 654–666, 2014.

[3] V. Brocklebank, K. M. Wood, and D. Kavanagh, "Thrombotic microangiopathy and kidney," *Clinical Journal of American Society of Nephrology*, vol. 13, no. 2, pp. 300–317, 2018.

[4] K. G. Babu and G. R. Bhat, "Cancer-associated thrombotic microangiopathy," *Ecancermedicalscience*, vol. 10, p. 649, 2016.

[5] Z. L. Al-Nouri, J. A. Reese, D. R. Terrell, S. K. Vesely, and J. N. George, "Drug-induced thrombotic microangiopathy: a systematic review of published reports," *Blood*, vol. 125, no. 4, pp. 616–618, 2015.

[6] H. Izzedine and M. A. Thrombotic Perazella, "Microangiopathy cancer drugs," *American Journal of Kidney Diseases*, vol. 66, no. 5, pp. 857–868, 2015.

[7] A. Tumma and S. F. Lee, "Atypical haemolytic uraemic syndrome associated with cabazitaxel in advanced prostate cancer," *Medical Case Reports*, vol. 2, p. 3, 2016.

[8] J. N. George, "Systemic malignancies as a cause of unexpected microangiopathic haemolytic anemia and thrombocytopenia," *Oncology (Williston Park)*, vol. 25, no. 10, pp. 908–914, 2011.

[9] N. Lameire, "Nephrotoxicity of recent anti-cancer agents," *Clinical Kidney Journal*, vol. 7, pp. 11–22, 2014.

[10] J. Gradishar, E. Vokes, K. Ne, and R. Panje, "Chemotherapy-related hemolytic uremic syndrome after the treatment of head and neck cancer: a case report," *Cancer*, vol. 66, no. 9, pp. 1914–1918, 1990.

[11] M. A. Perazella, "Onco-nephrology: renal toxicities of chemotherapeutic agent," *Clinical Journal of American Society of Nephrology*, vol. 7, no. 10, pp. 1713–1721, 2012.

[12] G. Nightingale and J. Ryu, "Cabazitaxel (jevtana) a novel agent for metastatic castration-resistant prostate cancer," *Pharmacy and Therapeutics*, vol. 37, no. 8, pp. 440–448, 2012.

[13] F. Mahmood, M. Matar, and A. Davis, "Renal failure and hypocalcaemia secondary to cabazitaxel treatment for prostate cancer: a rare but potentially lethal side effect," *Journal of Clinical Diagnosis and Research*, vol. 2, p. 106, 2014.

[14] A. Soultati, G. Mountzios, C. Avgerinou et al., "Vascular toxicity from chemotherapeutic agents: preclinical evidence and clinical implications," *Cancer Treatment Reviews*, vol. 438, pp. 473–483, 2012.

19

Ineffectiveness of Intermittent Hemodialysis in a Critically Ill COVID-19 Patient: A Case of Persistent Heparin-Induced Hyperkalemia

Yannick M. Nlandu,[1,2] Yannick M. Engole,[1,2] Marie-France I. Mboliassa,[1,2] Théodore-Junior M. Sakaji,[1] Patrick U. Kobo,[1,3] Patrick M. Boloko,[1,3] Pally K. Mafuta,[1,3] Joseph P. Tsangu,[1,3] Karel Van Echkout,[1] Jean-Pierre M. Kanku,[1] Golan Kalifa,[1] Rodolphe Ahmed,[1] and Justine B. Bukabau[1,2]

[1]*Intensive Care Unit, Centre Médical de Kinshasa, Kinshasa, Democratic Republic of the Congo*
[2]*Nephrology Unit, Kinshasa University Hospital, Kinshasa, Democratic Republic of the Congo*
[3]*Intensive Care Unit, Kinshasa University Hospital, Kinshasa, Democratic Republic of the Congo*

Correspondence should be addressed to Yannick M. Nlandu; yannicknlandu@yahoo.fr

Academic Editor: Hern n Trimarchi

Heparin is widely used in the intensive care unit despite the risk of bleeding it can cause. Although it is rarely reported, hyperkalemia is one of the side effects associated with heparin therapy (unfractionated or fractionated heparin). It would be secondary to hypoaldosteronism by blocking the biosynthesis of aldosterone in the adrenal gland and often appears in context of prolonged heparin therapy or inappropriate renin production in elderly, diabetic, and kidney insufficiency patients. We report a case of persistent hyperkalemia in a diabetic COVID-19 patient treated with curative heparin in the context of severe COVID-19.

1. Introduction

Hyperkalemia is a potentially life-threatening electrolyte disorder [1]. Factors associated with its development include altered renal clearance of potassium and release from the intracellular space, as well as altered transfer to the intracellular space. [1]. During acute kidney injury (AKI) and particularly in hemodialysis (HD), hyperkalemia can be persistent in some situation such as rhabdomyolysis or tumor lysis syndrome [1]. We report the case of a refractory hyperkalemia to intermittent hemodialysis (IHD) in a COVID-19 patient without any situation of continuous potassium release.

2. Case Presentation

A 72-year-old European man presented to the Centre Médical de Kinshasa (CMK) for progressive respiratory distress since June 29, 2021, associated with generalized weakness. His past medical history was remarkable for diabetes mellitus type II, hypertension, and unspecified arrhythmia for the past ten years. His medications included the oral antidiabetic drug repaglinide and the antihypertensive drugs ibesartan, hydrochlorothiazide, manidipine, and flecainide. A nasopharyngeal swab sample was positive for COVID-19 mRNA by reverse transcriptase-PCR (RT-PCR), and the patient was initially managed at home with azithromycin, rivaroxaban, vitamin C, vitamin D, prednisone, and oxygen for six days. The course was marked by worsening dyspnea, and the patient visited CMK on July 7, 2021. On hospital admission, he was dyspneic with a respiratory rate of 33 breaths per minute. His blood pressure was 145/74 mmHg, and peripheral oxygen saturation was 75% despite the 15 L/min of oxygen. Pulmonary auscultation was marked by crackling rales, and the patient also had lower limb edema. The blood sample revealed elevated cardiac and inflammatory biomarkers and respiratory alkalosis with hypoxemia. The chest CT scan argues for a very significant COVID-19 pneumonia stage 5 without pulmonary embolism. There was no kidney dysfunction, significant proteinuria, or hyperkalemia. Initial laboratory assessment and selected trends are depicted in Table 1.

A diagnosis of severe COVID-19 was made, and the patient was managed with a noninvasive ventilation with high level of oxygen, dexamethasone, vitamin C, vitamin D, empirical antibiotic (ceftriaxone plus ofloxacin was used as the first line of antibiotic, and imipenem, amikacin, and vancomycin were used as the second line), and curative anticoagulation dose (1 mg/kg) of enoxaparin subcutaneously every 12 h started at admission. Anti-Xa activity of enoxaparin was not available. Ten days after his admission, he experienced a respiratory degradation with severe hypoxemia, shock, and acute kidney injury (AKI) which required, respectively, intubation with mechanic ventilation and vasoactive drugs (norepinephrine and dobutamine). On July 21, the patient started hemodialysis consecutively to the worsening of AKI with progressive anuria associated with hypervolemia and hyperkalemia refractory to medical strategy (insulin-dextrose, $\beta 2$ agonist, and sodium polystyrene sulfonate). Ibesartan was stopped for suspected drug-induced hyperkalemia. Even during hemodialysis (was made every day) combined to medical strategy, hyperkalemia remained persistent in the absence of rhabdomyolysis, tumoral lysis syndrome, or metabolic acidosis and was associated to hyponatremia. The patient had a total of 7 sessions (one by day) of combined hemodiafiltration (4) to classic hemodialysis (3), 3 to 4 hours per day with a plasma and dialysate flow rates in order of 200–250 and 400–500 mL/min, respectively. The daily KT/V by online clearance measurement varied between 0.6 and 0.7. The dialyzer used was made of polysulfone or high-flux membrane, and the dialysate had a lower potassium concentration of 2 mmol/L and a high bicarbonate concentration of 36 mmol/L. Unfractionated heparins were used for anticoagulation during the hemodialysis session. On July 28, the patient was transferred abroad. One day after, he died in context of a severe hypoxemia.

3. Discussion

SARS-CoV-2 infection is currently recognized to be a multivisceral disease, which can affect several organs due to the wide distribution of angiotensin-converting enzyme 2 (ACE2) receptors, the entry point of the virus into the human cell [2]. In the kidney, the SARS-CoV-2 virus can be responsible for various lesions, including the proximal tubulopathy responsible for hypokalemia [3]. In the AKI context, hyperkalemia is the most expected complication. However, during dialysis, its incidence is reduced and gradually decreased with the kidney function recovery. The persistence of hyperkalemia during dialysis is most often associated with a situation of continuous release of potassium from the intracellular to the extracellular space such as in rhabdomyolysis or tumor lysis syndrome [1]. The improvement of kidney replacement therapy (KRT) is favorable to better potassium clearance. Indeed, the potassium dialysance depends not only on its gradient between the plasma and the dialysate, on their respective flow rates, or on the characteristics of the dialyzer but also on the different dialysis modalities (hemodialysis, hemofiltration, or hemodiafiltration) [1]. The potassium mass transfer depends on the time of dialysis as well as on the intracellular potassium kinetics described according to a multi-compartimental model, explaining the phenomenon of rebound in postdialysis significantly reduced by continuous dialysis techniques [1]. The use of intermittent dialysis, therefore, requires, on one hand, high plasma and dialysate flow rates and, on the other hand, the extension of its duration in the context of uncontrolled hyperkalemia cause such as rhabdomyolysis and tumor lysis syndrome [1]. The persistence of hyperkalemia in a COVID-19 patient was also reported by Siddharth et al. and could be explained by the use of IHD [4]. However, even for a prolonged sustained low-efficiency dialysis (SLED), Ramanand et al. reported a higher incidence of hyperkalemia in the COVID-19-AKI group compared to the AKI group of other causes [5]. According to them, refractory hyperkalemia was secondary to a continuous release of intracellular ions from the damaged tissues associated with the COVID-19 cytokine storm as shown by the correlation between potassium, phosphorus, and elevated lactate dehydrogenase (LDH) levels reported in their cohort as well as the use of a non-continuous dialysis technique. The reverse kinetic in our patient of LDH with normal creatine kinase (CK) and uric acid level compared to the occurrence of a concomitant episode of hyperkalemia at the beginning of dialysis suggests another hypothesis than tissue damage. Acidemia causes an extracellular shift of potassium and can, thus, explain hyperkalemia in our patient. However, respiratory acidosis rarely causes clinically significant hyperkalemia [6]. Indeed, during respiratory acidosis, rapid cell entry of CO_2 will acidify intracellular pH that, by stimulating Na^+ entry by Na^+-H^+ exchange, tends to enhance Na^+/K^+-ATPase activity and oppose a net loss of intracellular K^+. Heparin therapy may be the cause of this hyperkalemia. Indeed, the prothrombotic profile of the severe COVID-19 patient associated with a significant incidence of thromboembolic events justifies the use of curative anticoagulation [7]. Hyperkalemia secondary to heparin is a rarely reported side effect. It is secondary to a state of hypoaldosteronism following a reduction in the number and the affinity of angiotensin II receptors in the glomerular zone of the adrenals and, therefore, responsible for an increase in kidney retention of potassium [8]. This process is strongly pronounced in the elderly, diabetic patients, and patients with kidney failure who were unable to adequately increase renin production [9]. The risk is even greater for large and prolonged doses of

Table 1: Summary of laboratory evaluations and relevant trend during hospitalization.

Date	Reference	July 7, 2021	July 9, 2021	July 10, 2021	July 12, 2021	July 14, 2021	July 17, 2021*	July18, 2021	July 19, 2021	July 20,2021**	July 21,2021	July 22, 2021	July 23, 2021	July 24, 2021	July 25, 2021	July 26,2021
Arterial pH	7.35–7.45	7.62	7.45	7.50	7.50	7.45	7.5	7.41	7.44	7.29	7.33	7.36	7.37	7.38	7.35	7.16
pCO2 (mmHg)	35–45	27.4	47.8	49.7	43.3	43	27	44.7	52.9	61.3	53	48	83	84	88	63
HCO3 (mmol/L)	22–32	27.4	33.7	39.4	33.8	30.6	27	28	32.8	24.9	25	28	28	26	26	25.8
Hemoglobin (g/dl)	12.5–15			15.9		16.3	14.8	14.4		14.3		13.6				12.0
White blood cell count (elements/ mm^3)	4,000–10,000	13870		13080		14940	24370	18100		18.500		25.570				27.150
Glycated hemoglobin (%)	4–5.6	7.1														
Fibrinogen (g/L)	2–4	5.5														
D-dimer (ng/mL)	220–500	>10000			1224.2											
Procalcitonin (ng/ mL)	<0.15	0.18		0.25	0.17	0.10	0.28			0.74			0.41			0.98
CRP (mg/L)	<6	147		66	41	23	105			297			71			132
Blood urea (mmol/L)	2.5–7.5	10.6			14	14.3	18.6	19.5	14.9	19.8	26.4		25.8			20.3
Serum creatinine (μmol/L)	53–120	69			95	75	126	123	94	170	292		336			290
Sodium (mmol/L)	135–145	129	139	138	139	131	129	134		134	136	134	135	135	134	137
Potassium (mmol/L)	3.0–5.0	4	4.5	4.8	4.7	4.8	4.2	4.5		5.1	6.6	6.4	6.0	6.0	6.4	5.9
Ionized calcium (mmol/L)	1.15–1.30	1.09			1.20											
Aspartate amino transferase (UI/L)	6–34	32									45					
Alanin amino transferase (UI/L)	8–38	29									41					
Uric acid (μmol/L)	150–420	320									332					
Phosphorus (mmol/ L)	0.97–1.45	1.10									1.7					
LDH (UI/L)	140–280	936				674	450				441					
CK (UI/L)	22–198	101					97				82					
Troponin (Abbot) (ng/mL)	0–0.4	258.3	138.2													
Brain natriuretic peptide (pg/mL)	<300	2071	770			2179	4334	3232	1040	1027	2169					
PCR-COVID-19		+				—										—
Antigen/IgG COVID-19		—														
Antigen/IgM COVID-19		+														

*Day of intubation. **Start of hemodialysis.

heparin [7]. The pathophysiological mechanisms of hyponatremia among patients with COVID-19 are diverse, including syndrome of inappropriate antidiuretic hormone secretion (SIADH), digestive loss of sodium ions, reduced sodium ion intake, or use of diuretic therapy. Hyponatremia in our context can be associated to the hypoaldosteronism state. The trend of acid-base alterations in our COVID-19 patient with pneumonia is in line to lung disease that cause abnormalities in alveolar gas exchange without an alveolar hypoventilation and are characterized by a ventilation stimulation due to hypoxia responsible of a respiratory alkalosis. Hypercapnia typically occurs late in the disease process with severe pulmonary disease or when respiratory muscle fatigue occurs. The lack of the metabolic acidosis component in the context of an anuric patient is exceptional but can be explained in our context by the daily dialysis with an optimal dialysate bicarbonate concentration.

4. Conclusions

Hyperkalemia is associated with morbidity and mortality and requires identifying possible causes in order to provide appropriate care to patients. We report a case of heparin-induced hyperkalemia in critically ill COVID-19 patients.

Consent

The information collected during the history and clinical examination respected the confidentiality and privacy of the patient, and the National Ethics committee of Health, Democratic Republic of Congo (N°225/CNES/BN/PMMF/2020), authorized the present research project on COVID-19 in which this patient was included.

Disclosure

This work was performed as part of the authors' employment at the Kinshasa Medical Center (CMK).

Acknowledgments

The authors gratefully thank the staff of the Kinshasa Medical Center (CMK) for their commitment to the provision of excellent care to their patients.

References

[1] F. Dépret, W. F. Peacock, K. D. Liu, Z Rafique, P Rossignol, and M Legrand, "Management of hyperkalemia in the acutely ill patient," *Annals of Intensive Care*, vol. 9, Article ID 32, 2019.

[2] M. Gheblawi, K. Wang, A. Viveiros et al., "Angiotensin-converting enzyme 2: SARS-CoV-2 receptor and regulator of the renin-angiotensin system," *Circulation Research*, vol. 126, no. 10, pp. 1456–1474, 2020.

[3] J. Morelle, A. Wérion, L. Belkhir, Z. Chen, M. Jadoul, and O. Devuyst, "L'infection à SRAS-COV-2 cause une dysfonction tubulaire proximale du rein," *Louvain Medical*, vol. 139, no. 8, pp. 496–499, 2020.

[4] M. Siddharth, P. Rohan, S. Shantanu, S. Jagmeet, and P. Rajvee, "Hemodialysis refractory hyperkalemia in a case of SARS-COV-2 infection," in *Proceedings of the Presented at: Kidney Week 2020 Reimagined*, San Diego, CA, USA, October 2020.

[5] A. Ramanand, V. Varghese, Y. Wen, M. Mohamed, and J. C. Velez, "Refractoriness of hyperkalemia and hyperphophatemia in dialysis-dependent AKI associate with COVID-19," in *Proceedings of the Presented at: Kidney Week 2020 Reimagined*, San Diego, CA, USA, October 2020.

[6] P. S. Aronson and G. Giebisch, "Effects of pH on potassium: new explanations for old observations," *Journal of the American Society of Nephrology*, vol. 22, no. 11, pp. 1981–1989, 2011.

[7] Y. Sakr, M. Giovini, M. Leone et al., "Pulmonary embolism in patients with coronavirus disease-2019 (COVID-19) pneumonia: a narrative review," *Annals of Intensive Care*, vol. 10, Article ID 124, 2020.

[8] G. Bengalorkar, P. Venkatrathnamma, N. Sarala, and T. Kumar, "Effect of heparin and low-molecular weight heparin on serum potassium and sodium levels," *Journal of Pharmacology and Pharmacotherapeutics*, vol. 2, no. 4, pp. 266–269, 2011.

[9] K. Sodhi, S. Garg, B. Singh, A. Shrivastava, and M. K. Singla, "Refractory hyperkalemia related to heparin abuse," *Indian Journal of Critical Care Medicine: Peer-Reviewed, Official Publication of Indian Society of Critical Care Medicine*, vol. 17, no. 6, pp. 388–391, 2013.

20

Renal Involvement of CD20-Negative Intravascular Large B Cell Lymphoma with Neurological Manifestations

Faten Aqeel,[1] **Serena M. Bagnasco**,[2] **and Duvuru Geetha**[1]

[1]*Division of Nephrology, Johns Hopkins Hospital, Baltimore, MD, USA*
[2]*Department of Pathology, Johns Hopkins Hospital, Baltimore, MD, USA*

Correspondence should be addressed to Faten Aqeel; faqeel1@jh.edu

Academic Editor: Yoshihide Fujigaki

The involvement of hematological tumors such as lymphoma in the kidneys is a well-recognized phenomenon. Some of the distinct reported pathological processes resulting in kidney dysfunction include minimal change disease, lymphocytic invasion of the parenchyma, immune complex disposition, immunotactoid glomerulopathy, membranous glomerulopathy, and acute tubular injury. We report a rare case of CD20-negative intravascular lymphoma found on a kidney biopsy in a male with primary angiitis of the central nervous system (CNS) who presented with acute kidney injury and proteinuria. After the initiation of rituximab, cyclophosphamide, doxorubicin hydrochloride, vincristine sulfate, and prednisone (R-CHOP), kidney function improved and proteinuria resolved.

1. Introduction

Intravascular large B cell lymphoma (IVLBCL) is a rare subtype of extranodal non-Hodgkin lymphoma. It is characterized by the tendency of malignant cells to proliferate in the intraluminal space of small and medium vessels, sparing surrounding tissues [1]. The incidence rate of IVLBCL is 0.095 cases per 1,000,000 in the United States, with increasing incidence in recent years due to increased recognition [2]. The median age of diagnosis is between 60 and 70 years old with no clear sex preference [3]. The nervous system and skin have the highest incidence of involvement [4]. Renal involvement is rare, with only case reports published in the literature describing its manifestation.

We describe a patient with primary angiitis of the central nervous system, on treatment with intravenous rituximab and corticosteroids, who presented with acute kidney injury and proteinuria. Kidney biopsy showed findings consistent with IVLBCL. Improvement in serum creatinine and proteinuria ensued the following therapy with R-CHOP.

2. Case Report

A 59-year-old man presented with acute kidney injury and proteinuria. He has a history of primary angiitis of the central nervous system (CNS) diagnosed one year before his presentation. His primary angiitis of the CNS initially manifested with recurrent admissions for various neurological deficits, including vertigo, gait instability, expressive aphasia, and cranial nerve palsies. Magnetic resonance imaging (MRI) of the brain showed multiple subacute ischemic strokes. A formal 4-vessel cerebral angiogram showed several fusiform aneurysmal dilations of cerebral arteries in the posterior fossa concerning for vasculitis. Brain biopsy revealed nonspecific focal leptomeningeal acute inflammation. Immunostaining for beta-amyloid highlighted scattered neocortical deposition and was negative in the vascular walls. No other stains were done. A lumbar puncture revealed a high total protein of 122 mg/dL (reference value 15–45 mg/dL) but was otherwise unremarkable. Serological studies were negative, including antineutrophilic cytoplasmic autoantibodies (ANCA) and antinuclear antibodies (ANA). The diagnosis of primary angiitis of the CNS was made based on his imaging findings, and treatment with intravenous rituximab and corticosteroids ensued. He received intravenous rituximab (two doses of 1 g, two weeks apart) in addition to intravenous pulse methylprednisolone 1 g for 5 days with improvement in his cognition. This was followed by 100 mg oral prednisone daily for 1.5 months and a slow taper. Four months later, he presented with worsening neurological symptoms while on 20 mg prednisone daily. Rituximab was administered again (two doses of 1 g, two weeks apart) with significant improvement. At six months and one year of treatment initiation, he remained on 5 mg prednisone daily with no recurrence of neurological symptoms.

One year into his diagnosis of primary angiitis of the CNS, routine laboratory testing showed a serum creatinine level 1.57 mg/dL from a normal baseline (reference value 0.4–1.2 mg/dL), blood urea nitrogen 18 mg/dL (reference value 7–25 mg/dL), serum albumin 4.2 g/dL (reference value 3.6–5.1 g/dL), hemoglobin 10.3 g/dL (reference value 13.9–16.3 g/dL), lactate dehydrogenase 351 U/L (reference value 100–190 U/L), haptoglobin 90 mg/dL (reference value 43–212 mg/dL), and normal complement levels (C3 and C4). Urinalysis showed 2^+ proteinuria without any hematuria or pyuria. Urine protein-to-creatinine ratio (UPCR) was 500 mg/g. Serological workup including serum protein electrophoresis (SPEP), immunofixation, and kappa/lambda ratio was negative for monoclonal gammopathy. Anti-neutrophilic cytoplasmic autoantibody (ANCA) was negative. Renal ultrasound showed the right kidney measuring 11.1 cm and the left kidney measuring 12.0 cm with normal echogenicity. There was no evidence of masses, hydronephrosis, or stones.

A percutaneous kidney biopsy was performed. Light microscopy showed nine glomeruli, two partially sclerosed with mild tubulointerstitial scarring. Several glomeruli appeared enlarged and hypercellular (Figure 1). The glomerular capillary lumen showed atypical cells with large nuclei, prominent nucleoli, and rare mitotic figures. Occasionally, these atypical cells were noted within the tubular epithelial walls and in rare peritubular capillaries. The atypical cells showed positive staining for CD45, Mum-1, CD79a, and KI-67 and negative staining for CD3, CD5, CD10, CD20, CD30, CD56, CD138, ALK, BCl-6, Pax-5, and HHV8. No immune deposits were detected by immunofluorescence and electron microscopy.

Based on the immunophenotype of CD10-negative, BCl-6-negative, and MUM-1-positive and the diagnosis of intravascular large B cell lymphoma, nongerminal center B cell subtype was made per the Hans classification [5].

A referral to hematology/oncology was made. Positron emission tomography-computed tomography (PET-CT) scan revealed increased fluorodeoxyglucose (FDG) uptake in the kidneys bilaterally (Figure 2), left C2 and right C4, C5 concerning the perineural invasion of nerve roots. There was no evidence of skin rash, but a skin biopsy was done which did not show evidence of lymphoma. Intravascular large B cell lymphoma with renal and central nervous system involvement was diagnosed. Serum creatinine level and proteinuria peaked at 2.2 mg/dL and 700 mg/g, respectively, before the initiation of chemotherapy. His Eastern Cooperative Oncology Group (ECOG) performance status was 2 at that time. After three cycles of R-CHOP and intrathecal chemotherapy over two months, serum creatinine improved to 1.3 mg/dL with complete resolution of proteinuria and improvement in neurological symptoms. After six cycles of R-CHOP and intrathecal chemotherapy over four months, serum Cr was 1.1 mg/dL with no proteinuria. Unfortunately, new neurological deficits were noted with widespread cranial nerve involvement on PET-CT concerning the relapsed disease. He was started on high-dose methotrexate plus rituximab and ultimately received chimeric antigen receptor therapy (CAR-T). Unfortunately, his clinical status deteriorated, and he expired three months later.

3. Discussion

The diagnosis of IVLBCL has been increasingly recognized in recent years. Despite that, it remains a diagnostic challenge given the variability in clinical presentations and the delay in diagnosis without a tissue biopsy. Previously, two clinical variants were widely accepted: A Western variant, characterized by the CNS and skin involvement; and an Asian variant, characterized by fevers, multiorgan involvement, and hepatosplenomegaly [6]. Most recently, three different variant types, classical (characterized by organ-involved symptoms), cutaneous, and hemophagocytic syndrome-associated, have been described given differences in outcomes [7]. The most common presentation is fever (90%), cytopenias (90%), and confusion (50%) [8]. IVLBCL involving the kidney directly has been only described in case reports. A review of 43 published case reports concluded that the most common renal manifestation is proteinuria (90.0%), followed by renal failure (60.5%) and nephrotic syndrome (21.0%) [9]. Despite significant improvement in outcomes with chimeric anti-CD20 monoclonal antibody (rituximab-based) chemotherapy, relapses are still common.

In our patient, the findings in light microscopy and the immunophenotypic pattern met the diagnostic criteria for IVLBCL. Compared to the case reports published in the literature, this case is unusual given the lack of significant symptom burden on presentation and negative CD20 cells. At the time of the kidney biopsy, our patient was treated with intravenous rituximab for his primary angiitis of the CNS, which likely eliminated CD20-positive cells, leading to a unique presentation.

Quintero Vega et al. [10] described a case of a patient who initially presented with fevers, dyspnea, arthralgia, and headaches and was found to have anemia and an elevated level of lactate dehydrogenase. A bone marrow biopsy was negative for neoplasm or hemophagocytic syndrome. Rapid onset of nephrotic syndrome with an unclear degree of proteinuria ensued and warranted a kidney biopsy, which showed atypical lymphocytes located in the glomerulus and tubules, making the diagnosis of IVLBCL. Another case of IVLBCL confirmed with a kidney biopsy had a similar presentation with fevers and dyspnea followed by rapid onset of nephrotic syndrome with UPCR 4.94 g/g and normal kidney function with negative bone marrow biopsy

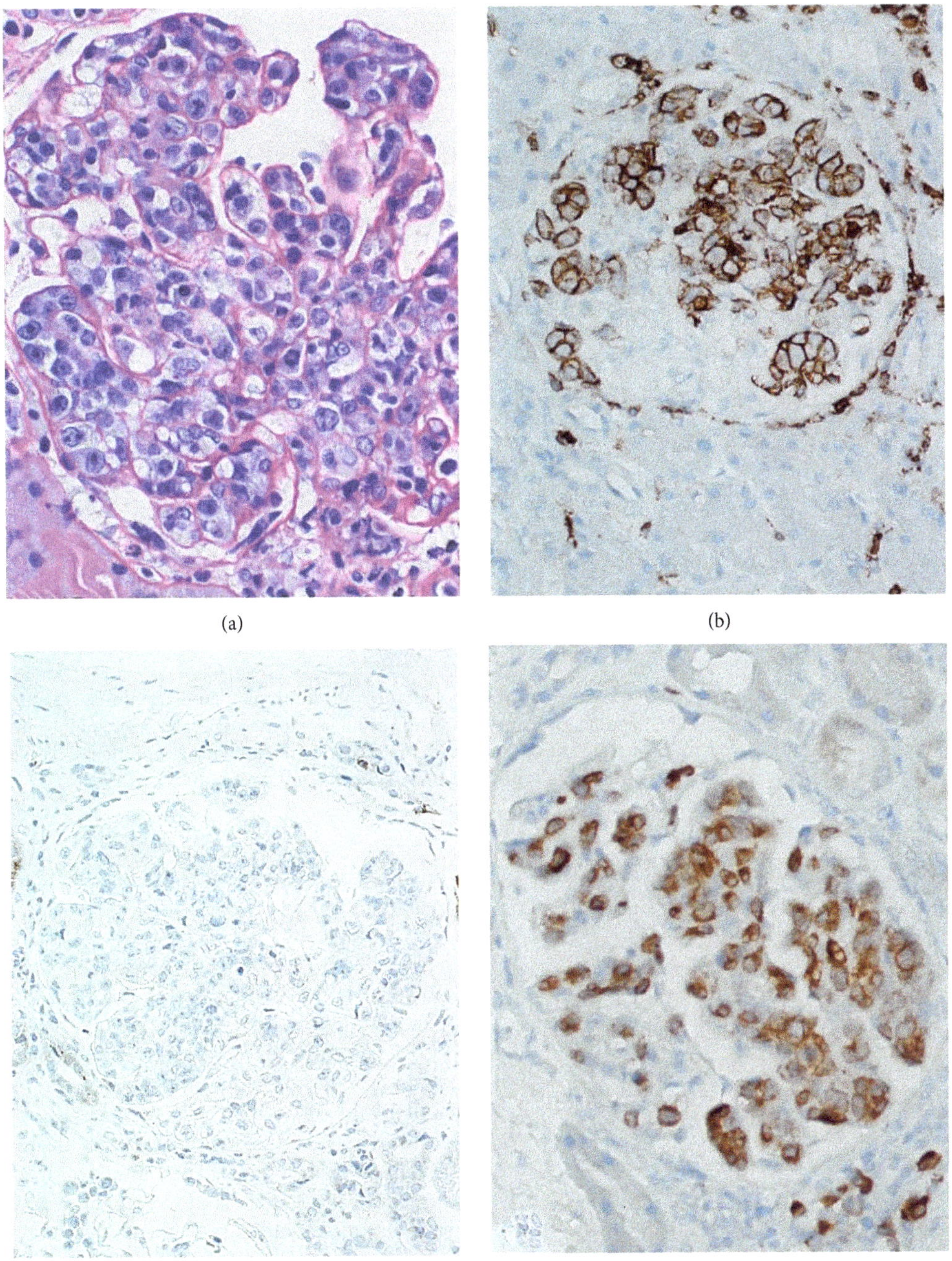

(a) (b)

(c) (d)

FIGURE 1: Continued.

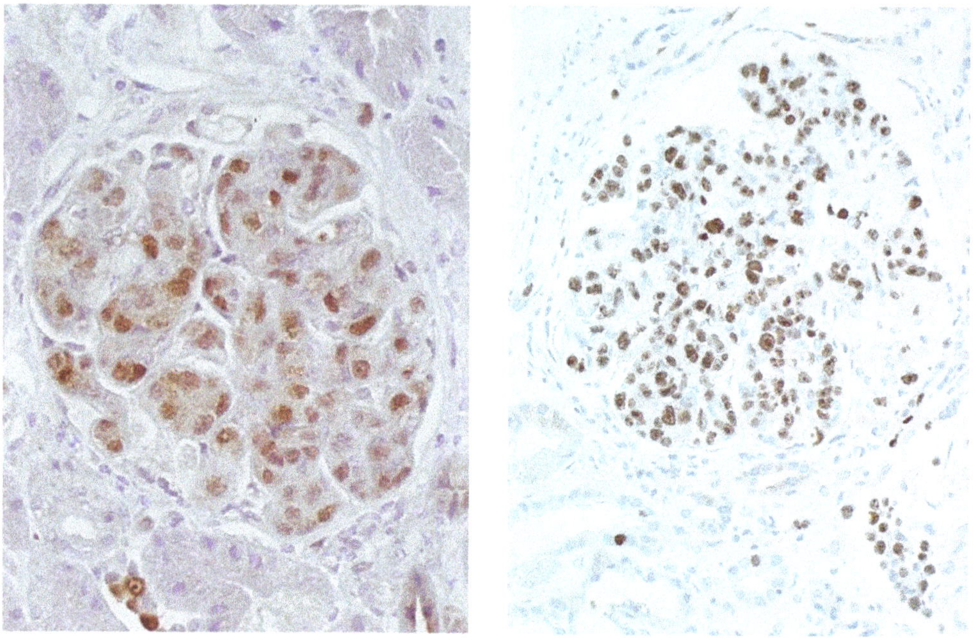

(e) (f)

Figure 1: Intraglomerular lymphoma cells. (a) PAS large atypical cells obstructing the glomerular capillary lumen (magnification 600x). (b) Intracapillary glomerular cells positive for CD45 (magnification 400x). (c) Intracapillary glomerular cells negative for CD20 (magnification 400x). (d) Intracapillary glomerular cells positive for CD79A (magnification 400x). (e) Intracapillary glomerular cells positive for MUM-1 (magnification 400x). (f) Intracapillary glomerular cells highly positive for KI-67 (magnification 400x).

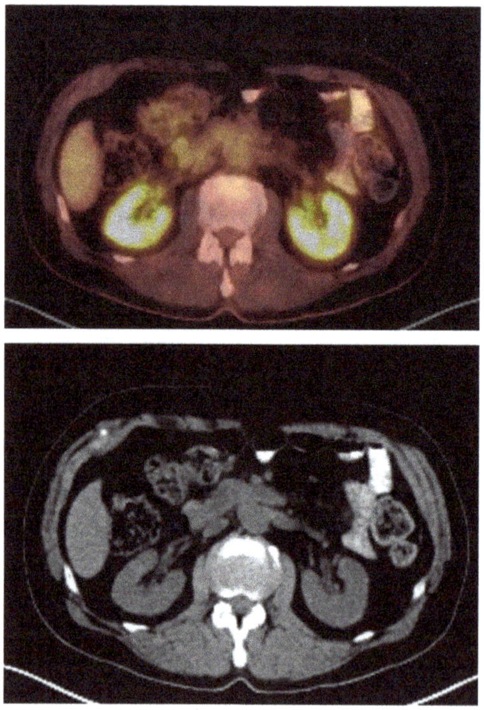

Figure 2: Diffuse symmetric fluorodeoxyglucose (FDG) uptake within the bilateral renal parenchyma on positron emission tomography-computed tomography (PET-CT) scan.

results [9]. Similarly, another case proved the diagnosis of IVLBCL with a kidney biopsy but negative bone marrow biopsy results [11]. This raises the question of the utility of bone marrow biopsies when there is evidence of other organ involvement.

Histologically, atypical cells usually express B cell markers such as CD20, CD79a, BCl-2, BCl-6, and MUM-1 and variable expressions of CD50 and CD10. Of the 43 cases of IVLBCL with renal involvement reviewed by Kim et al. [9], 35 patients exhibited infiltration of the malignant cells within the glomerular capillaries, with or without peritubular and interstitial involvement. The tumor cells were localized in peritubular capillaries without glomerular involvement in four cases. The remaining three cases received a presumptive diagnosis of intrarenal IVLBCL given kidney dysfunction ± bilateral kidney enlargement on imaging, with a tissue diagnosis of IVLBC made by means other than a kidney biopsy [9].

In terms of imaging, enlargement of the kidneys on radiologic evaluation can be seen in 34.3% of the cases [9]. In our case, a PET-CT scan revealed increased (FDG) uptake in the kidneys bilaterally without marked enlargement and swelling, as seen in some other case reports [12, 13]. In a case series of ten patients, a skin biopsy was performed on three patients with cutaneous lesions, making the diagnosis of IVLBCL. For those who did not have skin lesions or cytopenias, the diagnosis of IVLBCL was made by bone marrow biopsies after increased FDG uptake was noted on PET/CT. Therefore, PET/CT may be helpful for early diagnosis of IVLBCL [8].

CNS vasculitis is characterized histologically by inflamed cerebral vessel walls and is a heterogeneous group of primary and secondary disorders. A diagnosis of primary angiitis of the CNS is a diagnosis of exclusion and other etiologies will need to be considered first. These etiologies include systemic vasculitis (Wegener's granulomatosis, polyarteritis nodosa, and eosinophilic granulomatosis with polyangiitis), infections such as tuberculosis and aspergillus, intravascular lymphoma, which can be intraluminal or infiltrating the vessel walls, cerebral amyloid characterized by heavy beta-amyloid deposition, and substance abuse such as cocaine or amphetamine [14].

In conclusion, with the increased recognition of renal involvement of IVLBCL, a high index of suspicion of this disease entity is required. This patient's diagnosis of IVLBCL was established while he was on rituximab and corticosteroids to treat his primary angiitis of the CNS, which was likely the CNS manifestation of his lymphoma rather than a separate primary vasculitis disease. Despite thorough workup with brain imaging, lumbar puncture, and brain biopsy, this diagnosis of IVLBCL with renal and CNS involvement was only made with a kidney biopsy and the pathology findings were unusual, showing negative CD20 in the atypical lymphoid cells after treatment with rituximab. The case highlights the extranodal manifestations and diffuse nature of this disease. Early recognition is critical as treatment with rituximab-based therapies, such as R-CHOP, intrathecal chemotherapy, and high-dose methotrexate, has significantly improved survival rates, though relapses remain common.

References

[1] H. Itami, H. Nakamine, M. Kubo et al., "Diffuse large B-cell lymphoma (DLBCL) with significant intravascular invasion. Close resemblance of its clinicopathological features to intravascular large B-cell lymphoma, but not to DLBCL-not otherwise specified," *Journal of Clinical and Experimental Hematopathology*, vol. 61, no. 3, pp. 20066–20161, 2021.

[2] D. J. Rajyaguru, C. Bhaskar, A. J. Borgert, A. Smith, and B. Parsons, "Intravascular large B-cell lymphoma in the United States (US): a population-based study using surveillance, epidemiology, and end results program and national cancer database," *Leukemia and Lymphoma*, vol. 58, no. 9, pp. 2080–2088, 2017.

[3] K. Shimada, K. Matsue, K. Yamamoto et al., "Retrospective analysis of intravascular large B-cell lymphoma treated with rituximab-containing chemotherapy as reported by the IVL study group in Japan," *Journal of Clinical Oncology*, vol. 26, no. 19, pp. 3189–3195, 2008.

[4] T. P. Baumann, N. Hurwitz, E. Karamitopolou-Diamantis, A. Probst, R. Herrmann, and A. J. Steck, "Diagnosis and treatment of intravascular lymphomatosis," *Archives of Neurology*, vol. 57, no. 3, p. 374, 2000.

[5] A. Ichiki, J. Carreras, M. Miyaoka et al., "Clinicopathological analysis of 320 cases of diffuse large B-cell lymphoma using the Hans classifier," *Journal of Clinical and Experimental Hematopathology*, vol. 57, no. 2, pp. 54–63, 2017.

[6] M. Ponzoni, A. J. Ferreri, E. Campo et al., "Definition, diagnosis, and management of intravascular large B-cell lymphoma: proposals and perspectives from an international consensus meeting," *Journal of Clinical Oncology*, vol. 25, no. 21, pp. 3168–3173, 2007.

[7] M. Ponzoni, E. Campo, and S. Nakamura, "Intravascular large B-cell lymphoma: a chameleon with multiple faces and many masks," *Blood*, vol. 132, no. 15, pp. 1561–1567, 2018.

[8] Y. C. Ong, H. W. Kao, W. Y. Chuang et al., "Intravascular Large B-cell lymphoma: a case series and review of literature," *Biomedical Journal*, vol. 44, no. 4, pp. 479–488, 2021.

[9] M. Kim, H. Chung, W. I. Yang, and H. J. Jeong, "Renal intravascular large B cell lymphoma: the first case report in Korea and a review of the literature," *J Pathol Transl Med*, vol. 54, no. 5, pp. 426–431, 2020.

[10] G. E. Quintero Vega, D. Osorio, J. A. de la Hoz Valle, and D. Rodríguez Feria, "Limited renal intravascular lymphoma: a case report and review of the literature," *Case Reports in Oncological Medicine*, vol. 2020, Article ID 7052536, 7 pages, 2020.

[11] M. Sekulic, S. Martin, A. Lal, and A. Weins, "Intravascular large B-cell lymphoma of the kidney," *Kidney International Reports*, vol. 3, no. 6, pp. 1501–1505, 2018.

[12] X. Bai, X. Li, L. Wan, G. Wang, N. Jia, and J. Geng, "Intravascular large B-cell lymphoma of the kidney: a case report," *Diagnostic Pathology*, vol. 86, 2011.

[13] A. Desclaux, E. Lazaro, J. B. Pinaquy, M. Yacoub, and J. F. Viallard, "Renal intravascular large B-cell lymphoma: a case report and review of the literature," *Internal Medicine*, vol. 56, no. 7, pp. 827–833, 2017.

[14] R. A. Hajj-Ali and L. H. Calabrese, "Diagnosis and classification of central nervous system vasculitis," *Journal of Autoimmunity*, vol. 48-49, pp. 149–152, 2014.

21

Concomitant Nephrotic Syndrome and Cryoglobulinemia in a Case of Malignant Mesothelioma

Kei Nagai,[1,2] **Hiroaki Tachi**,[3] **Kohei Inoue**,[1] **and Atsushi Ueda**[1]

[1]*Department of Nephrology, Hitachi General Hospital, 2-1-1 Jonan-cho, Hitachi, Ibaraki 317-0077, Japan*
[2]*Department of Nephrology, Faculty of Medicine, University of Tsukuba, 1-1-1 Tennodai, Tsukuba, Ibaraki 305-8575, Japan*
[3]*Department of Respiratory Medicine, Hitachi General Hospital, 2-1-1 Jonan-cho, Hitachi, Ibaraki 317-0077, Japan*

Correspondence should be addressed to Kei Nagai; knagai@md.tsukuba.ac.jp

Academic Editor: Kouichi Hirayama

Malignant pleural mesothelioma is rarely associated with nephrotic syndrome. Cryoglobulinemia is found in various pathological statuses, such as hepatitis C virus infection but rarely in malignant neoplasms. We recently encountered a patient with malignant mesothelioma coincident with nephrotic syndrome and cryoglobulinemia in the course of chemotherapy. A 60-year-old man employed as a building painter was diagnosed with malignant mesothelioma by lung biopsy two years earlier and was started on chemotherapy. Nivolumab seemed effective in controlling mesothelioma, but skin immune-related adverse events occurred during the course of treatment. After discontinuation of nivolumab and administration of gemcitabine as an alternative therapy, the patient was referred to a nephrologist because of the subsequent development of edema, renal injury, and proteinuria. Following the investigation, he was diagnosed with nephrotic syndrome and cryoglobulinemia with C4-dominant cold activation. However, a percutaneous renal biopsy could not be performed due to persistent severe cough induced by pleural involvement. The patient died a little over three years after the pathological diagnosis of pleural mesothelioma. Our case had three key features nephrotic syndrome was possibly associated with malignant mesothelioma; cryoglobulinemia occurred in malignant mesothelioma; and concomitant nephrotic syndrome and cryoglobulinemia occurred after chemotherapy. Unfortunately, our rare case lacks a basis in renal pathology or evidence of links between the pathogenesis of malignant mesothelioma, cryoglobulinemia, and nephrotic syndrome. This case does not provide a causal mechanism, but may be worth adding to the case list as one of the rare renal involvement in a patient with malignant mesothelioma.

1. Introduction

Nephrotic syndrome is rarely associated with malignant pleural mesothelioma but is well-known to be induced as a paraneoplastic syndrome [1]. Although not leading to any cohort studies or case series, sporadic cases of nephrotic syndrome associated with malignant mesothelioma have been reported [2–16]. While most cases are assumed to represent nephrotic syndrome secondary to cancer, nephrotic syndrome may develop during the treatment of mesothelioma, and a mechanism specifically related to chemotherapy has also been postulated [15].

Cryoglobulinemia is found in various pathologic statuses. Before the appearance of specific antiviral treatments, the main etiology was chronic hepatitis C virus (HCV) infection, and currently, cryoglobulinemia is mainly associated with systemic autoimmune diseases, malignant neoplasms, and cases without an identified etiology (i.e., essential cryoglobulinemia) [17, 18]. Malignant mesothelioma with the development of cryoglobulinemia is very rare but has been reported in some cases [19].

In addition to such rare cases, we recently encountered a patient with malignant mesothelioma with concomitant nephrotic syndrome and cryoglobulinemia during the course of chemotherapy.

2. Case Presentation

A 60-year-old man visited a nephrologist due to edema, renal injury, and proteinuria. The man was a building painter and had developed massive lateral pleural effusions three years earlier. He was finally diagnosed with malignant

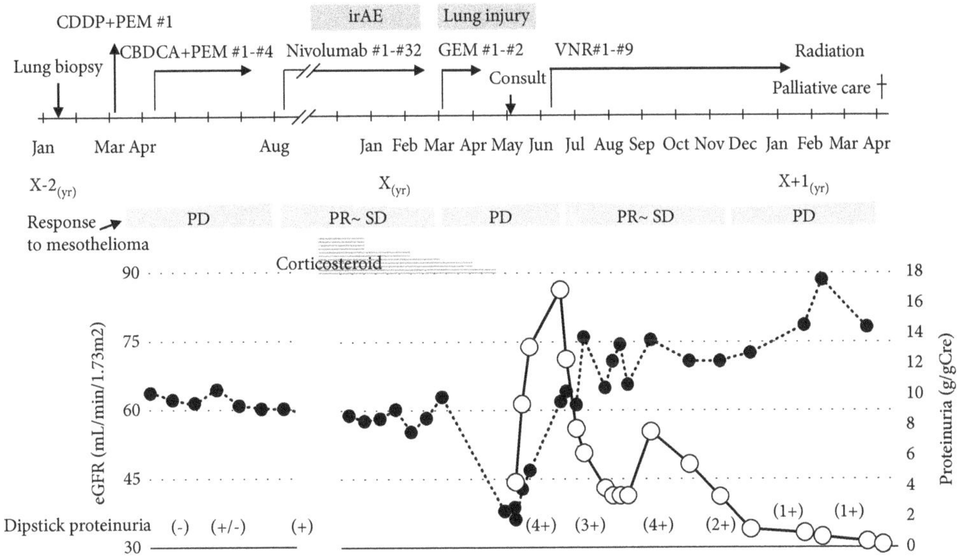

Serum albumin (g/dL)	2.9	4.2	2.4	2.0	1.5	2.5	3.4	3.3	2.1	
Cryoglobulin	N.A.	N.A.	(+)	(+)	(-)	(-)			(-)	(Normal range)
Immunoglobulin G (mg/dL)	1322	656	2288	1964	1173	1629			1401	(917 - 2011)
Immunoglobulin A (mg/dL)	211	141	455	392	268	312			216	(106 - 442)
Immunoglobulin M (mg/dL)	88	75	94	152	58	59			38	(49 - 287)
Complement C3 (mg/dL)	200	153	170	207	210	249			154	(50 - 98)
Complement C4 (mg/dL)	43	30	17	28	46	47			35	(18 - 49)
CH50 (U/mL)	85	N.A.	57	69	82	99			83	(23 - 46)

··●·· eGFR (mL/min/1.73m2)

—○— Proteinuria (g/gCre)

Figure 1: The clinical course of the patient. Two years earlier, the patient had been diagnosed with malignant mesothelioma by lung biopsy and treated with chemotherapy. Cisplatin plus pemetrexed (CDDP + PEM) and carboplatin plus pemetrexed (CBDCA + PEM) were determined to result in an insufficient response, and nivolumab was considered to have induced immune-related adverse events and was discontinued. After starting the administration of gemcitabine (GEM), drug-induced lung injury occurred. He was also referred to a nephrologist because of the subsequent development of edema, renal injury, and proteinuria. After investigations and careful consideration, vinorelbine (VNR) was administered to treat the nephrotic syndrome with cryoglobulinemia due to the progression of malignant mesothelioma. Response of chemotherapy to malignant mesothelioma is presented as partial response (PR), stable disease (SD), and progressive disease (PD). Palliative care was subsequently provided, along with radiation therapy for metastatic bone lesions and antibiotics against bacterial pneumonia. The patient died a little over 3 years after the pathological diagnosis of mesothelioma without recurrence of nephrotic syndrome in the end-stage of cancer.

mesothelioma from a thoracoscopic lung biopsy 2 years earlier and was started on chemotherapy (Figure 1). Cisplatin plus pemetrexed (CDDP + PEM) was administered as first-line therapy, followed by carboplatin plus pemetrexed (CBDCA + PEM) as second-line treatment. This regimen proved ineffective and the disease progressed, so the patient was switched to nivolumab. Nivolumab seemed effective in controlling mesothelioma, but skin immune-related adverse events (irAEs) occurred during the course of treatment. Prednisolone (20 mg/day) was given to alleviate irAEs and was gradually tapered. After discontinuation of nivolumab and administration of gemcitabine (GEM) as fourth-line therapy, drug-induced lung injury occurred and GEM was also discontinued. The patient was referred to a nephrologist after edema, renal injury and proteinuria developed.

At the first visit, as shown in Table 1, laboratory data showed massive proteinuria (4.3 g/day) and hypoalbuminemia (2.4 g/day), suggesting nephrotic syndrome. Notable findings were newly developed polyclonal gammopathy (IgG 2,288 mg/dL, IgA 455 mg/dL, and IgM 94 mg/dL) and characteristic low complementemia (C3 170 mg/dL, C4 17 mg/dL, and CH50 57 U/mL), suggesting C4-dominant cold activation. Cryoglobulins were qualitatively found to be positive. Other causes of secondary cryoglobulinemia, such as hepatitis B virus and HCV chronic infections were serologically excluded. Since cryoglobulin might occur with antigens from malignant disease, the patient was administered another line of chemotherapy for nephrotic syndrome with cryoglobulinemia due to the progression of malignant mesothelioma after careful consideration and informed consent. Nephrotic syndrome gradually improved along with the administration of vinorelbine (VNR) as the fifth-line treatment (Figure 1). Low serum C4, cryoglobulinemia, and nephrotic range of

Table 1: Laboratory findings.

Urinalysis		Blood chemistry tests (cont.)	
Gravity	1.009	Sodium	136 mmol/L
Protein	3+	Chloride	104 mmol/L
Sugar	Negative	Potassium	3.0 mmol/L
Blood	1+	Corrected calcium	10.0 mg/dL
Sediment		Phosphate	3.0 mg/dL
Red blood cells	5–9/HPF	Total bilirubin	0.3 mg/dL
White blood cells	10–19/HPF	Aspartate aminotransferase	22 U/L
Urinary biochemical tests	Alanine aminotransferase	26 U/L	
Daily urinary protein	4.3 g/24 hr	Lactate dehydrogenase	292 U/L
Selectivity index	0.09	Alkaline phosphatase	167 U/L
Bence-Jones protein	Negative	Creatine kinase	73 U/L
Complete blood count	Total cholesterol	197 mg/dL	
White blood cells	10600/mL	LDL cholesterol	129 mg/dL
Neutrophils	58%	Triglyceride	191 mg/dL
Eosinophils	12%	Glucose	103 mg/dL
Basophils	3%	Hemoglobin A1c	5.1%
Lymphocytes	15%	Serology	
Monocytes	11%	C-reactive protein	3.38 mg/dL
Hemoglobin	11.0 g/dL	HBs antigen	Negative
Platelets	57.3 × 104/mL	Anti-HCV antibody	Negative
Coagulation tests	Immunoglobulin G	2288 mg/dL	
PT-INR	1.13	Immunoglobulin A	455 mg/dL
APTT	28.5 sec	Immunoglobulin M	94 mg/dL
APTT, ctrl	33.5 sec	Complement 3	170 mg/dL
Fibrinogen	760 mg/dL	Complement 4	17 mg/dL
von Willebrand factor	341% (60–170%)	CH50	57.0 U/mL
Blood chemistry tests	Rheumatoid factor	33 IU/mL	
Total protein	7.2 g/dL	Antinuclear antibody	x40 >
Albumin	2.4 g/dL	Anti-dsDNA-Ab	< 10 U/mL
Uric acid	10.1 mg/dL	PR3-ANCA	< 1.0 U/mL
Urea nitrogen	14.2 mg/dL	MPO-ANCA	< 1.0 U/mL
Creatinine	1.59 mg/dL	Cryoglobulin	(+)

HPF: high-power field; PT-INR: prothrombin time-international normalized ratio; APTT: activated partial thromboplastin time; CH50:50% hemolytic unit of complement; LDL: low-density lipoprotein; HBs: hepatitis B surface; HCV: hepatitis C virus; dsDNA-Ab: double-strand deoxyribonucleic acid antibody; PR3-ANCA: proteinase-3-antineutrophil cytoplasmic antibodies; MPO-ANCA: myeloperoxidase-antineutrophil cytoplasmic antibodies.

proteinuria had disappeared after VNR therapy. Percutaneous renal biopsy could not be performed due to persistent severe cough induced by pleural involvement. The clinical diagnosis was thought to be nephrotic syndrome with cryoglobulinemia due to the progression of malignant mesothelioma. Thereafter, palliative care was provided, along with radiotherapy for metastatic bone lesions and antibiotics against bacterial pneumonia. The patient died a little over three years after pathological diagnosis of mesothelioma without recurrence of nephrotic syndrome in the end-stage of cancer.

3. Discussion

The present case showed three features newly developed nephrotic syndrome was possibly associated with malignant mesothelioma; cryoglobulinemia occurred in malignant mesothelioma; and concomitant transient nephrotic syndrome and cryoglobulinemia occurred after the use of nivolumab or GEM, but not VNR. Unfortunately, this case lacked a basis in renal pathology or evidence of links between the pathogenesis of malignant mesothelioma, cryoglobulinemia, and nephrotic syndrome. However, we discuss here the causal relationship between the three events based on the literature as much as possible.

We reviewed 15 publications presenting cases of nephrotic syndrome with malignant mesothelioma at various sites [2–16]. Seven cases included information on complement levels, all of which were within the normal range. A description of cryoglobulins was absent in all previous cases (Table 2). Most of the renal pathology involved minimal-change disease in patients with malignant mesothelioma and nephrotic syndrome [12], accounting for 9 of the 15 cases (60%) in Table 2. Three cases of membranous nephropathy were identified, followed by one case each of focal segmental glomerulosclerosis and mesangial proliferative nephritis, but no reports of membranous proliferative glomerulonephritis, which may occur in cryoglobulinemia. Meanwhile, definitively assessing the pathological characteristics of this case is difficult because renal biopsy could not be performed at the moment of nephrotic syndrome due to the condition of the patient. Nevertheless, the result of the high selectivity of proteinuria (index, 0.09; Table 1) suggests the possibility of minimal-change disease, consistent with previous cases.

Table 2: The literature review of cryoglobulin and renal diseases in malignant mesothelioma.

First Author	Year	Disease site	Complement	Cryoglobulin	Chemotherapy for mesothelioma	Renal Pathology
Schroeter	1986	Pleura	Normal	NA	Cyclophosphamide, doxorubicin, hydrochloride, and decarbonize	MCNS
Venzano	1990	Pleura	NA	NA	NA	MCNS
Absy	1992	Pleura	NA	NA	Carboplatin	FSGS
Tanaka	1994	Pleura	Normal	NA	Carboplatin, etoposide	MesPGN
Galesic	2000	Pleura	Normal	NA	None (corticosteroid)	MN
Sakamoto	2000	Pleura	NA	NA	None (surgery)	MN
Farmer	2001	Pleura and brain metastasis	NA	NA	None (corticosteroid)	MCNS
Bacchetta	2009	Testis	Normal	NA	Cisplatin and pemetrexed	MCNS
Li	2010	Pleura	Normal	NA	Gemcitabine and carboplatin	MCNS
Dogan	2012	Pleura	NA	NA	None (surgery)	Not examined
Suzuki	2014	Pleura	Normal	NA	None (conservative)	MCNS
Tsukamoto	2015	Pleura, pulmonary, and skull metastasis	NA	NA	Carboplatin, pemetrexed, and gemcitabine	MCNS
Pu	2016	Pleura	NA	NA	Cisplatin and pemetrexed	MN
Bickel	2016	Pleura	NA	NA	Carboplatin, pemetrexed, vinorelbine, and pembrolizumab	MCNS
Yildiz	2016	Pleura	Normal	NA	None (corticosteroid)	MCNS
Nagai	Present case	Pleural mesothelioma and bone metastasis	Low C4	Positive	Cisplatin, pemetrexed, carboplatin, nivolumab, gemcitabine, and vinorelbine	Not examined

MCNS: minimal-change nephrotic syndrome; FSGS: focal segmental glomerulosclerosis; MesPGN: mesangial proliferative glomerulonephritis: MN: membranous nephropathy.

Cryoglobulinemia-associated glomerulonephritis is most commonly seen in the context of hepatitis C infection and occasionally seen in relation to lymphoma and malignant neoplasm [18, 20–22]. In contrast with renal disease associated with HCV, renal involvement in patients with cryoglobulinemia not associated with HCV has only been poorly described, and few cases have been reported [23]. In an analyzed series of 20 cases without HCV-associated cryoglobulinemia, renal involvement was characterized by nephrotic range proteinuria in 75% of patients and renal failure in 85% of patients (mean glomerular filtration rate, 46 mL/min/1.73 m^2) [23]. Membranoproliferative glomerulonephritis with subendothelial deposits was observed in all kidney specimens [23]. Generally, therapeutic options for the disease include removal of circulating cryoglobulin by plasmapheresis, immunosuppression, and pharmacological treatment to address the underlying cause of protein production. After excluding the possibility of any infectious diseases, including viral hepatitis, and careful consideration, we tried suppression of cancer progression by next-line chemotherapy with VNR after the diagnosis of nephrotic syndrome. In this case, cryoglobulin disappeared without apheresis or immunosuppressive drugs, suggesting that one of the relevant mechanisms was anticancer therapy reducing the tumor burden as an antigen against cryoglobulin.

Another possibility for the pathogenesis was that the concomitant nephrotic syndrome and cryoglobulinemia were driven by chemotherapy. In terms of the time course, in this case, the suspect drug was nivolumab or GEM, but not VNR. Only one study suggested that anti-PD-1-related cryoglobulinemia during nivolumab treatment in a patient with lung cancer [24]. He was treated with prednisone and cryoprecipitates disappeared after 26 days of steroid therapy. The patient continued to receive nivolumab for a total of eight cycles with no recurrence of cryoglobulinemia [24]. Nivolumab is also known as a rare cause of nephrotic syndrome during cancer therapy, represented by minimal-change disease [25], membranous nephropathy [26], membranoproliferative glomerulonephritis [27], and renal vasculitis [28]. A hemolytic uremic syndrome is the most perilous adverse effect of gemcitabine, with an incidence of approximately 0.15% based on reported cases [29]. GEM-induced secondary thrombotic microangiopathy may be diagnosed as a nephrotic syndrome [30]. Membranous nephropathy as a cause of nephrotic syndrome was also found in a case treated using GEM [31]. Collectively, both nivolumab and GEM could cause nephrotic syndrome, while no previous reports have shown any association between GEM and cryoglobulinemia. Therefore, if we consider nephrotic syndrome and cryoglobulinemia to represent linked complications rather than coincidences, the suspect drug is most likely nivolumab, not GEM.

To the best of our knowledge, this represents the first description of concomitant nephrotic syndrome and cryoglobulinemia in a case of malignant mesothelioma. Although no causal mechanisms or pathological findings were identified, this case may be worth adding to the case list as a rare coincidence in a patient with malignant mesothelioma.

Acknowledgments

The authors declare that they have no conflicts of interest for this article. The corresponding author is employed by the University of Tsukuba.

References

[1] K. D. Jhaveri, H. H. Shah, K. Calderon, E. S. Campenot, and J. Radhakrishnan, "Glomerular diseases seen with cancer and chemotherapy: a narrative review," *Kidney International*, vol. 84, no. 1, pp. 34–44, 2013.

[2] N. J. Schroeter, D. A. Rushing, J. P. Parker, and E. Beltaos, "Minimal-change nephrotic syndrome associated with malignant mesothelioma," *Archives of Internal Medicine*, vol. 146, no. 9, pp. 1834–1836, 1986.

[3] C. Venzano, E. Di Marco, M. Garbero, P. Forno, A. Marchese, and R. Borghesi, "Nephrotic syndrome associated with pleural mesothelioma. An unusual paraneoplastic event," *Recenti Progressi in Medicina*, vol. 81, no. 5, pp. 325-326, 1990.

[4] M. Absy, B. Gazzawi, and E. Amoah, "Focal and segmental glomerulosclerosis associated with malignant mesothelioma," *Nephron*, vol. 60, no. 2, p. 250, 1992.

[5] S. Tanaka, H. Oda, H. Satta et al., "Nephrotic syndrome associated with malignant mesothelioma," *Nephron*, vol. 67, no. 4, pp. 510-511, 1994.

[6] K. Galesic, B. Bozic, R. Heinzl, M. Scukanec-Spoljar, and V. Bozikov, "Pleural mesothelioma and membranous nephropathy," *Nephron*, vol. 84, no. 1, pp. 71–74, 2000.

[7] K. Sakamoto, H. Suzuki, and T. Jojima, "Membranous glomerulonephritis associated with diffuse malignant pleural mesothelioma: report of a case," *Surgery Today*, vol. 30, no. 12, pp. 1124–1126, 2000.

[8] C. K. T. Farmer and D. J. Goldsmith, "Nephrotic syndrome and mesenteric infarction secondary to metastatic mesothelioma," *Postgraduate Medical Journal*, vol. 77, no. 907, pp. 333-334, 2001.

[9] J. Bacchetta, D. Ranchère, F. Dijoud, and J. P. Droz, "Mesothelioma of the testis and nephrotic syndrome: a case report," *Journal of Medical Case Reports*, vol. 3, no. 1, p. 7248, 2009.

[10] J. Y. Li, T. Y. Yong, B. J. Kuss, S. Klebe, D. Kotasek, and J. A. Barbara, "Malignant pleural mesothelioma with associated minimal change disease and acute renal failure," *Renal Failure*, vol. 32, no. 8, pp. 1012–1015, 2010.

[11] M. Dogan, G. Ozal, B. Savas et al., "Malign peritoneal mesothelioma with nephrotic syndrome," *Bratislava Medical Journal*, vol. 113, no. 01, pp. 43–45, 2012.

[12] S. Suzuki, M. Toyoshima, F. Nihashi et al., "An autopsy case of malignant pleural mesothelioma associated with nephrotic syndrome," *Internal Medicine*, vol. 53, no. 3, pp. 243–246, 2014.

[13] Y. Tsukamoto, T. Otsuki, H. Hao et al., "Epithelioid pleural mesothelioma concurrently associated with miliary pulmonary metastases and minimal change nephrotic syndrome-a hitherto undescribed case," *Pathology, Research & Practice*, vol. 211, no. 12, pp. 1014–1019, 2015.

[14] X. Pu, Y. Dou, D. Liu et al., "Membranous nephropathy associated with malignant pleural mesothelioma in an adult patient: a case report," *Molecular and Clinical Oncology*, vol. 5, no. 4, pp. 407–410, 2016.

[15] A. Bickel, I. Koneth, A. Enzler-Tschudy, J. Neuweiler, L. Flatz, and M. Früh, "Pembrolizumab-associated minimal change disease in a patient with malignant pleural mesothelioma," *BMC Cancer*, vol. 16, no. 1, p. 656, 2016.

[16] H. Yildiz, S. I. Andreea, D. Hoton, and J. C. Yombi, "Minimal change disease associated with malignant pleural mesothelioma: case report and review of the literature," *BMJ Case Reports*, vol. 2016, Article ID bcr2016217958, 2016.

[17] S. Retamozo, L. Quartuccio, and M. Ramos-Casals, *Medicina Clínica*, vol. 158, no. 10, pp. 478–487, 2022.

[18] M. Ramos-Casals, J. H. Stone, M. C. Cid, and X. Bosch, "The cryoglobulinaemias," *The Lancet*, vol. 379, no. 9813, pp. 348–360, 2012.

[19] A. I. Cetingil, M. A. Ozen, and O. M. Sandalci, "Mesothelioma associated with cryoglobulinemia," *The American Journal of Medicine*, vol. 31, no. 4, pp. 640–646, 1961.

[20] R. Misiani, P. Bellavita, D. Fenili et al., "Hepatitis C virus infection in patients with essential mixed cryoglobulinemia," *Annals of Internal Medicine*, vol. 117, no. 7, pp. 573–577, 1992.

[21] A. H. Bryce, R. A. Kyle, A. Dispenzieri, and M. A. Gertz, "Natural history and therapy of 66 patients with mixed cryoglobulinemia," *American Journal of Hematology*, vol. 81, no. 7, pp. 511–518, 2006.

[22] B. Moulin, P. M. Ronco, B. Mougenot, A. Francois, J. P. Fillastre, and F. Mignon, "Glomerulonephritis in chronic lymphocytic leukemia and related B-cell lymphomas," *Kidney International*, vol. 42, no. 1, pp. 127–135, 1992.

[23] M. Matignon, P. Cacoub, M. Colombat et al., "Clinical and morphologic spectrum of renal involvement in patients with mixed cryoglobulinemia without evidence of hepatitis C virus infection," *Medicine (Baltimore)*, vol. 88, no. 6, pp. 341–348, 2009.

[24] B. Pellegrino, A. Musolino, and M. Tiseo, "Anti-PD-1-related cryoglobulinemia during treatment with nivolumab in NSCLC patient," *Annals of Oncology*, vol. 28, no. 6, pp. 1405-1406, 2017.

[25] E. Vaughan, E. Connolly, M. Hui, and S. Chadban, "Minimal change disease in a patient receiving checkpoint inhibition: another possible manifestation of kidney autoimmunity?" *Cancer Reports*, vol. 3, no. 5, Article ID e1250, 2020.

[26] K. Wakabayashi, S. Yamamoto, S. Hara et al., "Nivolumab-induced membranous nephropathy in a patient with stage IV lung adenocarcinoma," *CEN Case Reports*, vol. 11, no. 2, pp. 171–176, 2022.

[27] J. Cruz-Whitley, N. Giehl, K. Y. Jen, and B. Young, "Membranoproliferative glomerulonephritis associated with nivolumab therapy," *Case Reports in Nephrology*, vol. 20204 pages, 2020.

[28] A. J. Gallan, E. Alexander, P. Reid, F. Kutuby, A. Chang, and K. J. Henriksen, "Renal vasculitis and pauci-immune glomerulonephritis associated with immune checkpoint inhibitors," *American Journal of Kidney Diseases*, vol. 74, no. 6, pp. 853–856, 2019.

[29] M. W. Saif and P. J. McGee, "Hemolytic-uremic syndrome associated with gemcitabine: a case report and review of literature," *JOP*, vol. 6, no. 4, pp. 369–374, 2005.

[30] D. Katagiri and F. Hinoshita, "Gemcitabine-induced thrombotic microangiopathy with nephrotic syndrome," *CEN Case Reports*, vol. 7, no. 2, pp. 217–220, 2018.

[31] A. Ata, I. Gürses, A. Kıykım, and A. Arıcan, "Nephrotic syndrome associated with gemcitabine use in a patient with ovarian cancer," *The American Journal of Case Reports*, vol. 13, pp. 268–270, 2012.

22

Incidentally Diagnosed Alport Syndromeina Patient with Drug-Induced Vasculitis

D. Lai,[1,2] N. Dave,[1,2,3] and R. Raghavan[1,2,3]

[1]*Baylor College of Medicine, Houston, TX 77030, USA*
[2]*Department of Medicine, Baylor College of Medicine, Houston, TX 77030, USA*
[3]*Selzman Institute for Kidney Health, Baylor College of Medicine, Houston, TX 77030, USA*

Correspondence should be addressed to D. Lai; derian.lai@bcm.edu

Academic Editor: Salih Kavukcu

A 53-year-old woman is admitted with a serum creatinine of 16 mg/dl. Seven months earlier, she was diagnosed with heart failure and started on several medications, including Hydralazine. Laboratory studies revealed the presence of dual Anti-Neutrophil Cytoplasmic Antibodies (anti-MPO and anti-PR3), anti-nuclear and anti-histone antibodies. The clinical diagnosis was Drug-Induced ANCA Vasculitis (DIAV). Kidney histology, however, did not reveal crescents, but showed characteristic features of Alport's syndrome.

1. Clinical History and Initial Laboratory Data

A 53-year-old woman with Stage 3 Chronic Kidney Disease (CKD) and a baseline serum creatinine of 2.3mg/dl presented to the hospital with 2 weeks of generalized malaise and vomiting. Her past medical history was significant for hypertension, heart failure, and paroxysmal atrial fibrillation. Seven months prior to this presentation, the patient was started on carvedilol, Hydralazine, isosorbide mononitrate, and furosemide, to treat her cardiac disease. Prior to this she had not had consistent follow-up with a physician. At presentation, she reported 100% compliance with these medications. Her family history is significant for end-stage kidney disease (ESKD) in her 38-year-old brother, diagnosed 2 years earlier, of unknown etiology.

Laboratory values on presentation are listed in Table 1. Most notably, the serum creatinine was 16.6 mg/dl and there was active urinary sediment. Laboratory findings were concerning for rapidly progressive glomerulonephritis, and the history suggested a drug-induced etiology. Hydralazine was the suspected culprit and was immediately discontinued. The patient was started on pulse dose corticosteroid therapy. A noncuffed temporary dialysis catheter was placed. The patient received two hemodialysis treatments, one therapeutic plasma exchange (PLEX), and these interventions were followed by a kidney biopsy to confirm the diagnosis.

On Day 4 of the patient's hospitalization, the kidney biopsy revealed minimal inflammation and the absence of necrotizing vasculitis or crescent formation. The immunofluorescence did not show a "full house" pattern, despite high titers of both ANA and double-stranded DNA. Surprisingly, the electron microscopy revealed the characteristic features of Alport's syndrome (Figure 1). There was only 1 crescent out of 13 glomeruli, and no glomerular necrosis or immune deposition. The degree of interstitial fibrosis and tubular atrophy was 60%. There was loss of staining for alpha 3 and 5 chains of type 4 collagen. Due to the significant fibrosis and lack of active inflammation, both corticosteroids and PLEX were discontinued. Her renal function never recovered and she opted to pursue peritoneal dialysis.

2. Discussion

The rapidly declining renal function, double positive ANCA serologies, and recent initiation of Hydralazine led to the suspected clinical diagnosis of Drug-Induced ANCA Vasculitis (DIAV). Nearly 20 drugs have been reported to induce ANCA antibodies, but the more common culprits include Propylthiouracil, Hydralazine, Allopurinol, and Minocycline

Table 1: Laboratory values on presentation.

	Patient values	Reference range
Sodium	150	135-148 meq/L
Potassium	4.9	3.6-5.5 meq/L
Total CO2	13	24-32 meq/L
BUN	189	10-26 mg/dL
Creatinine	16.66	0.50-1.2 mg/dL
Albumin	3.6	3.5-5 g/dL
Hemoglobin	5.8	12-15 g/dL
Anti-nuclear antibody	1:2,560	Negative
Anti-dsDNA	Negative	Negative
Anti-PR3	2.7 AI	<1 AI
Anti-MPO	>800 AI	<1 AI
Anti-histone	7.1 U	<1 U
Anti-glomerular basement Membrane Titer	Negative	Negative
Anti-streptolysin O	Negative	Negative
C3	71 mg/dL	82-193 mg/dL
C4	23 mg/dL	15-57 mg/dL
Serum electrophoresis	No monoclonal spike	
Urine drug screen	Negative	

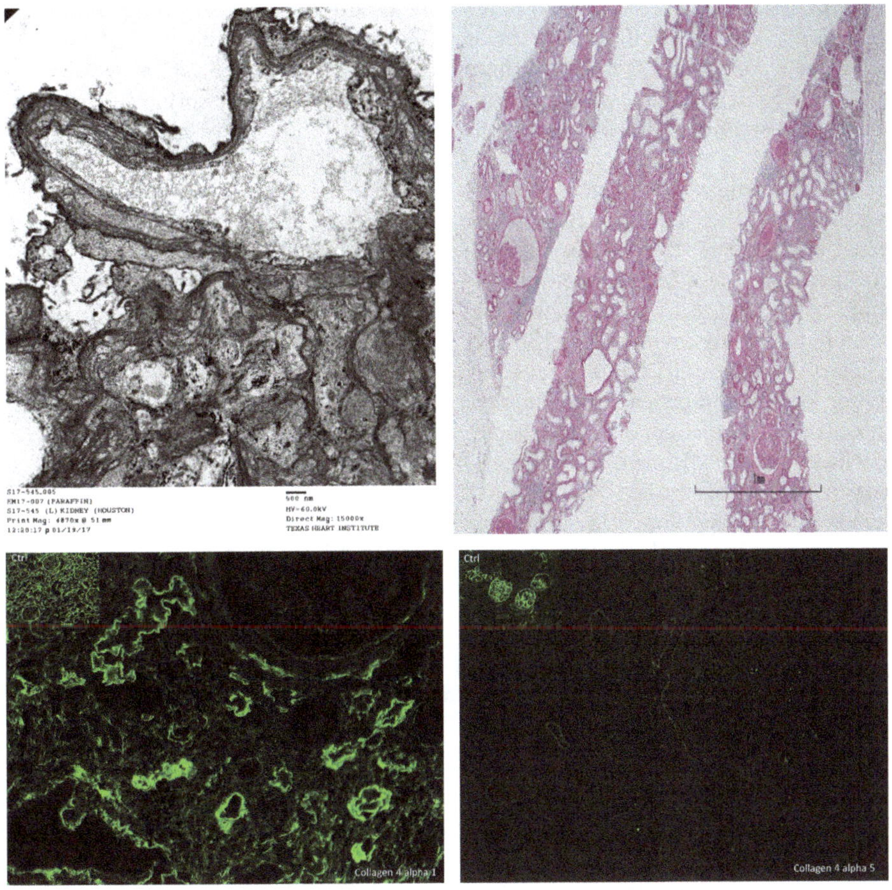

Figure 1: *Kidney Biopsy*. Electron microscopy identifying a split lamina densa (top left). Light microscopy demonstrating significant tubular atrophy and interstitial fibrosis (top right). Immunofluorescence highlighting absent staining for the a5 chain of type 5 collagen in the patient and no immune deposits (bottom row).

Immunologic features that characterize Drug Induced ANCA Vasculitis (DIAV) include: high titers of anti-MPO, dual positive anti-MPO and anti-PR3, anti-histone, and/or anti-nuclear antibodies
Alport's syndrome is diagnosed with the absence of alpha5 chain of type 4 collagen on immunofluorescence and splitting / lamellation of the glomerular basement membrane on electron micrography.
Even in the absence of proteinuria, renin-angiotensin-aldosterone system (RAAS) inhibition can slow the progression of kidney disease in Alport's syndrome.

Box 1: Key Teaching Points.

[1, 2]. The presence of antibodies directed against both MPO and PR3 antigens is not a common finding, but when present, it is highly suggestive of DIAV [3, 4]. The B-cells activated in DIAV can also produce other antibodies including anti-nuclear, anti-histone, anti-double-stranded DNA, anti-elastase, anti-lactoferrin, and anti-phospholipid antibodies [5]. Hence, the finding of multiple neutrophilic antibodies in a patient should raise suspicion for drug-induced injury. The classic kidney biopsy finding in DIAV is necrotizing or crescentic glomerulonephritis with a pauci-immune immunofluorescence. However, there are reports of patients with DIAV and minimal histologic changes on kidney biopsy [6]. Some patients have been shown to have immune complex deposition in contrast to the classic cases [6]. The role of these immune complexes is unclear. They may be directly pathogenic, a benign immune phenomenon induced by the drug or due to a secondary disease process all together.

DIAV has a better prognosis compared to primary ANCA Associated Vasculitis (AAV) [1]. The first line treatment is to remove the suspected culprit drug. If the biopsy shows severe inflammation or there is a severe decline in estimated GFR, then immunosuppressive therapy is warranted, though its use is largely based on published case reports. The Kidney Disease Improving Global Outcomes (KDIGO) guidelines recommend consideration of PLEX in patients with rapidly rising serum creatinine or diffuse alveolar hemorrhage. Importantly, the guidelines do not distinguish treatment of DIAV from primary AAV. Patients treated with plasma exchange (PLEX) were found to have lower incidence of end-stage kidney disease requiring dialysis, but there was no difference in mortality on long-term follow-up when compared to patients not treated with PLEX [7, 8]. A small study of 7 patients was able to show that plasma exchange decreased the levels of MPO and PR-3 antibody titers in all patients treated. However, the study was not designed to follow the patient's long-term clinical outcome. There is mixed evidence on whether MPO and PR-3 antibody titers correlate with disease severity or likelihood or relapse [9, 10].

Alport's syndrome can manifest with varying glomerular pathology including focal segmental, then diffuse glomerular sclerosis in an increasing number of glomeruli. There is no reported association between Alport's syndrome and necrotizing vasculitis. The hallmark lesion is diffuse thickening and splitting of the Glomerular Basement Membrane (GBM) with strikingly irregular outer and inner contours [11].

Alport syndrome (AS) is a hereditary disease of the GBM. Patients often present with hematuria, and it is associated with sensorineural deafness and ocular abnormalities. It accounts for 0.3 to 2.3% of all patients reaching end-stage kidney disease [11]. The disease is genetically heterogeneous and is associated with mutations in the genes: *COL4A3*, *COL4A4*, or *COL4A5*. These genes encode the $\alpha3$(IV), $\alpha4$(IV), and $\alpha5$(IV) chains of type IV collagen, respectively [11, 12].

Genetic testing may be utilized in patients in whom the diagnosis of Alport's syndrome is suspected but biopsy results show nondiagnostic histologic findings. Genetic testing can provide prognostic information on the likelihood of progression to early renal failure or deafness based on the specific type of mutation identified. Genetic sequencing can also provide the patient with more information on the risk of his or her offspring inheriting the disease [13]. The decision to undergo genetic testing must be individualized because there is currently no disease-modifying treatment to alter the course of Alport's syndrome. Furthermore, test results have the potential to cause psychological harm [14]. The patient in this vignette was never previously treated with a RAAS inhibitor and elected not to pursue genetic testing.

The primary treatment for patients with Alport's is inhibition of the Renin-Angiotensin Aldosterone System (RAAS). Studies demonstrate that RAAS inhibition slows the progression of renal impairment even in patients without proteinuria [15]. Impaired activity of the nuclear 1 factor (erythroid-derived 2)–related factor 2 (Nrf2) transcription factor is implicated in chronic kidney disease by increasing oxidative stress and inflammation. The synthetic drug Bardoxolone Methyl activates the Nrf2 pathway and holds promise to suppress proinflammatory cytokine production [16]. The BEACON investigators studied Bardoxolone methyl in advanced diabetic kidney disease, but this study was terminated early due to increased cardiovascular events [17]. An ongoing clinical trial (CARDINAL) is underway to assess the safety and efficacy of Bardoxolone methyl in patients with Alport's syndrome.

3. Conclusion

To summarize, clinicians must be aware of the rare but serious consequence of drug-induced vasculitis in patients who are taking Hydralazine. When the decline in renal function is more rapid than expected, clinicians should search for multiple etiologies of kidney disease that may be superimposed on one another.

Alport's syndrome provided an explanation for our patient's chronic renal impairment. Clinicians must consider hereditary kidney disorders in patients with unexplained kidney disease and a positive family history. Because of the late diagnosis, there was a missed opportunity to intervene earlier with RAAS inhibitors.

A summary of our key teaching points can be found in Box 1.

References

[1] Y. Gao and M.-H. Zhao, "Review article: Drug-induced anti-neutrophil cytoplasmic antibody-associated vasculitis," *Nephrology*, vol. 14, no. 1, pp. 33–41, 2009.

[2] W. F. Pendergraft and J. L. Niles, "Trojan horses: drug culprits associated with antineutrophil cytoplasmic autoantibody (ANCA) vasculitis," *Current Opinion in Rheumatology*, vol. 26, no. 1, pp. 42–49, 2014.

[3] H. K. Choi, P. A. Merkel, A. M. Walker, and J. L. Niles, "Drug-associated antineutrophil cytoplasmic antibody-positive vasculitis: prevalence among patients with high titers of antimyeloperoxidase antibodies," *Arthritis & Rheumatology*, vol. 43, no. 2, pp. 405–413, 2000.

[4] M. M. McGrath, T. Isakova, H. G. Rennke, A. M. Mottola, K. A. Laliberte, and J. L. Niles, "Contaminated cocaine and antineutrophil cytoplasmic antibody-associated disease," *Clinical Journal of the American Society of Nephrology*, vol. 6, no. 12, pp. 2799–2805, 2011.

[5] N. Yokogawa and F. B. Vivino, "Hydralazine-induced autoimmune disease: comparison to idiopathic lupus and ANCA-positive vasculitis," *Modern Rheumatology*, vol. 19, no. 3, pp. 338–347, 2009.

[6] F. Yu, M. Chen, Y. Gao et al., "Clinical and pathological features of renal involvement in propylthiouracil-associated ANCA-positive vasculitis," *American Journal of Kidney Diseases*, vol. 49, no. 5, pp. 607–614, 2007.

[7] A. S. Bomback and G. B. Appel, "Glomerular disease: ANCA associated GN- to PLEX or not to PLEX?" *Nature Reviews Nephrology*, vol. 9, no. 8, pp. 436–438, 2013.

[8] M. Walsh, F. Catapano, W. Szpirt et al., "Plasma exchange for renal vasculitis and idiopathic rapidly progressive glomerulonephritis: a meta-analysis," *American Journal of Kidney Diseases*, vol. 57, no. 4, pp. 566–574, 2011.

[9] Y. Gao, M. Chen, H. Ye, F. Yu, X.-H. Guo, and M.-H. Zhao, "Long-term outcomes of patients with propylthiouracil-induced anti-neutrophil cytoplasmic auto-antibody-associated vasculitis," *Rheumatology*, vol. 47, no. 10, pp. 1515–1520, 2008.

[10] D. R. W. Jayne, G. Gaskin, C. D. Pusey, and C. M. Lockwood, "ANCA and predicting relapse in systemic vasculitis," *QJM: An International Journal of Medicine*, vol. 88, no. 2, pp. 127–133, 1995.

[11] L. Heidet and M. Gubler, "The renal lesions of Alport syndrome," *Journal of the American Society of Nephrology*, vol. 20, no. 6, pp. 1210–1215, 2009.

[12] J. P. Jais, B. Knebelmann, I. Giatras et al., "X-linked Alport syndrome: Natural history and genotype-phenotype correlations in girls and women belonging to 195 families: A "European community alport syndrome concerted action study," *Journal of the American Society of Nephrology*, vol. 11, no. 4, pp. 649–657, 2000.

[13] J. Adam, T. M. Connor, K. Wood et al., "Genetic testing can resolve the diagnostic confusion in Alport Syndrome," *Clinical Kidney Journal*, vol. 7, no. 2, pp. 197–200, 2014.

[14] L. Copelovitch and B. S. Kaplan, "Is genetic testing of healthy pre-symptomatic children with possible Alport Syndrome ethical?" *Pediatric Nephrology*, vol. 21, no. 4, pp. 455-456, 2006.

[15] O. Gross, C. Licht, H. J. Anders et al., "Early angiotensin converting enzyme inhibition in Alport syndrome delays renal failure and improves life expectancy," *Kidney International*, vol. 81, no. 5, pp. 494–501, 2012.

[16] M. P. Chin, S. A. Reisman, G. L. Bakris et al., "Mechanisms contributing to adverse cardiovascular events in patients with type 2 diabetes mellitus and stage 4 chronic kidney disease treated with bardoxolone methyl," *American Journal of Nephrology*, vol. 39, no. 6, pp. 499–508, 2014.

[17] D. de Zeeuw, T. Akizawa, P. Audhya et al., "Bardoxolone methyl in type 2 diabetes and stage 4 chronic kidney disease," *The New England Journal of Medicine*, vol. 369, no. 26, pp. 2492–2503, 2013.

23

Beer Potomania: Why Initial Fluid Resuscitation May be Harmful

Zhuo Lin Yu[1] **and Lisa Fisher**[2]

[1]*Stony Brook University Hospital, 101 Nicolls Rd, Stony Brook, NY 11794, USA*
[2]*Northport VA Medical Center, 79 Middleville Rd, Northport, NY 11768, USA*

Correspondence should be addressed to Zhuo Lin Yu; zhuo.yu@stonybrookmedicine.edu

Academic Editor: Rumeyza Kazancioglu

Beer potomania is one of the less common causes of hyponatremia that we encounter. Patients usually have a recent history of binge drinking along with poor diet. The low solute content in alcoholic beverages limits daily urine output, and ingestion of extra fluid will cause dilutional hyponatremia as a result. Blindly providing intravenous fluid without an underlying cause of the hyponatremia can be detrimental, such as in patients with beer potomania. In our case, a patient presented to the emergency department due to poor oral intake from jaw pain and was found to be hyponatremic from alcohol intake. He initially received 2 liters of fluid, which caused overcorrection of his sodium, requiring more free water to lower his sodium as a result.

1. Background

Our case occurs at a university hospital in Long Island, New York.

2. Objective

Our case discusses the underlying pathophysiology of beer potomania, and the reason that beer potomania patients are prone to overcorrection of sodium levels with intravenous fluid infusion.

2.1. Patient Information. The patient is a 53-year-old man with a past medical history of metastatic squamous cell carcinoma of the head and neck treated with laser ablation and multiple oral surgeries in the past, alcohol abuse, and nicotine dependence. He presented to the hospital due to worsening jaw pain and decreased oral intake. The patient reported feeling fatigued but had no fever or chills. He was not taking any medications at home. Due to jaw pain, he also had not been eating much, but instead had been drinking two six-packs of beer and one pint of vodka daily.

2.2. Physical Exam. On presentation, he was afebrile with a temperature of 36.9 C, heart rate 89, blood pressure 92/60, and saturated 95% on room air. On physical exam, he appeared thin and cachectic but comfortable without signs of distress. He had bitemporal wasting, dry mucous membrane, and a large irregular mass extending from the lower jaw to the submandibular region. His cardiac and pulmonary exams were unremarkable. There was no focal neurologic deficit observed.

2.3. Diagnostic Assessment. Initial laboratory tests showed the following: WBC 10.02 k/μL, RBC 4.18 k/μL, hemoglobin 13.3 g/dL, hematocrit 39%, sodium 113 mmol/L, chloride 70 mmol/L, potassium 4 mmol/L, CO_2 34 mmol/L (27 mmol/L 4 hours later and stayed within normal range on subsequent labs), AG 9, BUN 8 mg/dL, Cr 0.43 mg/dL, magnesium 1.4 mg/dL, ALT 19 IU/L, AST 44 IU/L, alkaline phosphate 152 IU/L, and albumin 3.2 g/dL. The rest of the biochemical analysis including calcium, phosphorus, and glucose were within normal range.

Given the patient's low serum sodium, we obtained more labs for further workup of his hyponatremia. Further tests

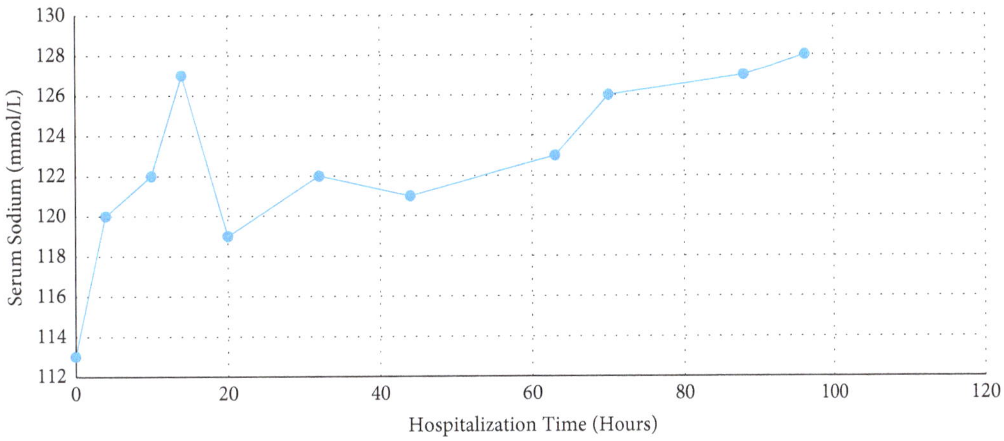

FIGURE 1: The Patient's sodium level throughout his hospital stay. He presented initially with a sodium level of 113 mmol/L at hour 0, then corrected to 127 mmol/L after receiving 2 liters of normal saline, which prompted a nephrology consult. The patient then received D5W and DDAVP, and sodium was able to lower to 119 mmol/L at hour 20.

showed plasma osmolality 258 mOsm/kg (275–300 mOsm/kg), sodium in the urine sample was <15 mmol/L, and urine osmolality 94 mOsm/kg. On urine analysis, the sample was negative for nitrite or leukocyte esterase, but specific gravity was low at 1.002.

2.4. Treatment. While in the emergency department, the patient received 2 liters of normal saline, along with supplementation of magnesium. Repeat labs four hours later showed an increase in sodium from 113 to 120 and continued to increase to 127 fourteen hours later. The patient denied neurologic symptoms. Given overcorrection of sodium within the first 14 hours with a concern of osmotic demyelination syndrome from overcorrection [1,2], nephrology was consulted urgently. They recommended lowering the sodium level by giving 500 cc of D5W over 2 hours, DDAVP 2mcg intravenously immediately, and then starting a D5W infusion at 100 cc/hour. The free water deficit formula based on weight was used to calculate the amount of free water needed to bring the patient back down to his target. After the above sodium lowering interventions, the repeat sodium level 20 hours after the initial presentation resulted at 119. The patient then received a small volume of normal saline in a controlled amount per nephrology's recommendation throughout his hospital stay, and his sodium was able to correct appropriately.

Given the patient's labs and history, he was diagnosed with hypo-osmolar hyponatremia from low solute intake, likely beer potomania given his history of binge drinking.

3. Discussion

To diagnose the underlying cause of hypo-osmolar hyponatremia, we require the help of urine electrolytes. We first look at urine osmolality, since urine osmolality is the nearest window to the body's ADH activity. ADH activation will increase the resorption of free water in the renal collecting duct, resulting in concentrated urine with high urine osmolality. Also, the opposite stays true; ADH suppression will result in low urine osmolality as a result [3].

In order to understand beer potomania and why it corrects rapidly with fluid, we first discuss the underlying pathophysiology. In the setting of hyponatremia, dilute urine with urine osmolality <100–200 mOsm/kg indicates that ADH is not activated. Several etiologies are known to cause hypo-osmolar hyponatremia without activation of ADH: tea-toast syndrome, primary polydipsia, and beer potomania. In our case, the patient had a urine osmolality of 94 and a history of binge drinking, pointing towards a diagnosis of beer potomania.

The cause of hyponatremia in beer drinking is related to the low solute in alcoholic beverages and protein insufficiency [4–6]. In a person with normal renal function, his or her kidney can maximally dilute urine to 50 mOsm/kg (or 50 mmol/L) [1, 6, 7] and maximally concentrate urine to 1200 mOsm/kg (or 1200 mmol/L). The amount of daily urine output will depend on a person's daily solute intake [2]; daily solute ingested will equal solute excreted under normal conditions. For example, if a 70 kg person ingests 10 mOsm/kg/day, his or her solute load will be 700 mOsm/day, which is excreted in the urine. A solute load of 700 mOsm/day divided by a maximally diluted urine concentration of 50 mmol/L will equal 14 L of urine output, and a solute load of 700 mOsm/day divided by maximally concentrated urine of 1200 mmol/L will equal around 0.6 L of urine output daily. In the same person, if he or she ingests 15 L of water, that extra 1 L will not be able to be excreted and sodium level will fall due to a dilutional effect [6]. In beer potomania patients, they usually have poor diet with low daily solute intake [8]. In our patient who has been drinking 12 cans of beer daily with poor diet due to jaw pain, we estimate that his daily solute intake is about 150 mOsm per day, which indicates that if his fluid intake is greater than 3 L per day, dilutional hyponatremia will result.

Beer potomania patients are highly prone to rapid sodium correction with intravenous fluid. Each liter of normal saline consists of 308 mOsm of solute, so the patient can now generate 6 L of urine from that one liter of fluid. This can cause rapid correction of sodium as he or she now has the capacity to produce six extra liters of urine, effectively lowering the blood sodium level as a result [2, 9]. As a result, it can be dangerous to give fluids without first delineating the underlying cause of hyponatremia, as in our case.

References

[1] D. Kujubu, "Beer potomania—an unusual cause of hyponatremia," *The Permanente Journal*, vol. 50, 2015.
[2] S. R. Sanghvi, P. S. Kellerman, and L. Nanovic, "Beer potomania: an unusual cause of hyponatremia at high risk of complications from rapid correction," *American Journal of Kidney Diseases*, vol. 50, no. 4, pp. 673–680, 2007.
[3] R. Joshi and S. Y. Chou, "Beer potomania: a view on the dynamic process of developing hyponatremia," *Cureus*, vol. 10, 2018.
[4] M. Hettema, "Beer drinker's hyponatraemia: a case report," *The Netherlands Journal of Medicine*, vol. 54, no. 3, pp. 105–107, 1999.
[5] S. M. Joyce and R. Potter, "Beer potomania: an unusual cause of symptomatic hyponatremia," *Annals of Emergency Medicine*, vol. 15, no. 6, pp. 745–747, 1986.
[6] M. U. Lodhi, T. S. Saleem, A. R. Kuzel et al., ""Beer potomania"—a syndrome of severe hyponatremia with unique pathophysiology: case studies and literature review," *Cureus*, vol. 9, 2017.
[7] H. Rafei, R. Yunus, and P. Khurana, "Beer potomania: a challenging case of hyponatremia," *Journal of Endocrinology and Metabolism*, vol. 6, no. 4, pp. 123–126, 2016.
[8] S. Thaler, I. Teitelbaum, and T. Berl, ""Beer potomania" in non-beer drinkers: effect of low dietary solute intake," *American Journal of Kidney Diseases*, vol. 31, no. 6, pp. 1028–1031, 1998.
[9] T. Imam, "Taking alcohol with a (large) pinch of salt: understanding the osmoles in "beer potomania" and "starvation potomania"," *Indian Journal of Nephrology*, vol. 24, no. 4, p. 203, 2014.

24

Pleuroperitoneal Leak as an Uncommon Cause of Pleural Effusion in Peritoneal Dialysis: A Case Report and Literature Review

Minh Huan Dang, Mathew Mathew, and Rajesh Raj

Department of Nephrology, Launceston General Hospital, Launceston, Tasmania, Australia

Correspondence should be addressed to Minh Huan Dang; huandg341@gmail.com

Academic Editor: Hiro Matsukura

Pleural effusions are frequently seen in patients on dialysis. A pleuroperitoneal leak or communication is a rare but important cause of pleural effusion in patients on peritoneal dialysis. This diagnosis can be made with a combination of biochemical tests and radiological modalities, in the absence of a gold standard diagnostic test. In addition to thoracocentesis, treatment often involves cessation of peritoneal dialysis and transition to hemodialysis. We describe a case of an 80-year-old man who presented with unilateral right-sided pleural effusion. He underwent therapeutic thoracocentesis and was subsequently diagnosed with a pleuroperitoneal leak through pleural fluid analysis. Peritoneal dialysis was ceased, and he transitioned temporarily to hemodialysis. He was subsequently treated with talc pleurodesis and successfully recommenced on peritoneal dialysis at six weeks after operation. In our report, we also review diagnostic imaging modalities, as well as advantages and disadvantages of each modality. A pleuroperitoneal leak is a rare but important complication of peritoneal dialysis and needs consideration in any patient on peritoneal dialysis presenting with unilateral pleural effusion.

1. Introduction

Pleural effusions are common in patients on peritoneal dialysis (PD). Determining their etiology can be challenging for clinicians since there are a wide variety of differential diagnoses. Among these, a pleuroperitoneal leak causing a pleural effusion is a rare but dramatic cause. Delays in diagnosis can lead to worsening of pleural effusions, particularly if a mistaken suspicion of fluid overload leads to the escalating use of high osmolar peritoneal dialysate fluids and volumes with the aim to achieve better ultrafiltration.

We present a case of pleuroperitoneal leak in an elderly gentleman who presented with unilateral pleural effusion after a recent change of PD mode from continuous ambulatory peritoneal dialysis (CAPD) to automated peritoneal dialysis (APD). In this report, we review the literature on this topic, explore mechanisms, and discuss treatment options.

2. Case Presentation

An 80-year-old gentleman on treatment with PD was admitted with increasing dyspnea and progressive reduction in ultrafiltration volumes over the previous week. His end-stage kidney disease was secondary to hypertension; he had also previously had a left nephrectomy for cancer. His comorbidities included systemic hypertension, stroke, glaucoma, prostatic hypertrophy, and osteoarthritis. He had started PD 3 months prior to admission. During the previous 2 weeks, he had switched from CAPD with daytime exchanges to nocturnal cycler-assisted automated peritoneal dialysis (APD).

On initial assessment, he was tachypneic and hypoxic. The jugular venous pressure was elevated; there was also peripheral edema. On auscultation, he had reduced breath sounds over the right lower hemithorax, with dullness on percussion. His electrocardiogram (ECG) and initial blood tests were unremarkable. The chest X-ray showed a large right pleural effusion (Figure 1).

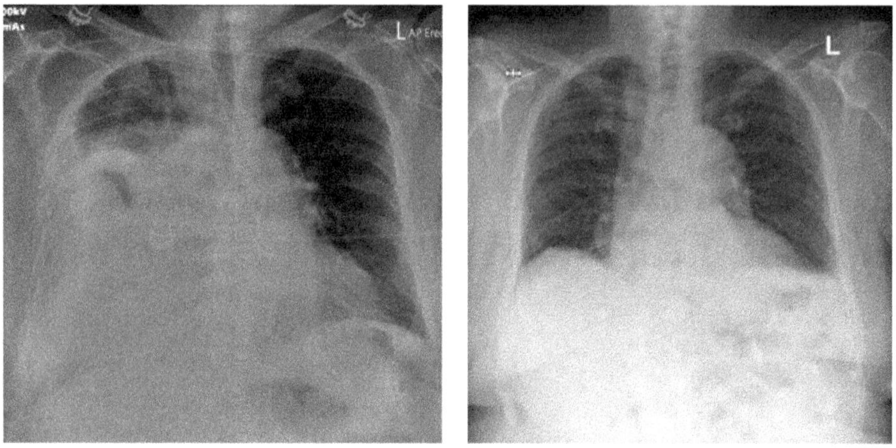

(a) (b)

Figure 1: Chest X-ray on presentation (a) and after thoracentesis (b).

Therapeutic thoracentesis was performed. 3 litres of fluid were drained; his clinical status improved markedly. A repeat chest X-ray showed complete resolution of pleural effusion (Figure 1).

Biochemical analysis of pleural fluid showed high concentrations of sugar and creatinine, and negligible protein, consistent with peritoneal dialysate fluid (Table 1).

Treatment was changed temporarily to hemodialysis via a tunneled central venous catheter. He underwent video-assisted thoracoscopic surgery and talc pleurodesis, which he tolerated well. At the time of the procedure, most pleural fluids had been drained. There was no fresh drainage of fluid into the pleural space. Some pleural thickening was described.

4 weeks later, PD was recommenced, in CAPD mode, with small fill volumes and avoidance of nightly dwells. He subsequently tolerated CAPD without complications and was recommenced on APD. Hemodialysis was successfully discontinued.

Table 1: Serum and pleural biochemical markers.

	Serum	Pleural
Glucose (mmol/L)	8.0	12.1
Creatinine (μmol/L)	527	509
Protein (g/L) (RR 60–80)	67	3
LDH (U/L)	417	60

Table 2: Etiology of pleural effusions.

Pleural fluid	Differential diagnoses
Transudative	Fluid overload
	Heart failure
	Pericardial diseases
	Pulmonary embolism
	Nephrotic syndrome
	Liver cirrhosis
	Pleuroperitoneal leak
	Hypothyroidism
Exudative	Pneumonia and other systemic infections
	Uremic pleuritis
	Malignancy
	Tuberculosis
	Chylothorax
	Connective tissue disorders
	Esophageal perforation
	Drug reactions

3. Discussion

The incidence of pleural effusions in the dialysis population has been reported to be as high as 80% [1]. The most common causes are hypervolemia, parapneumonic effusions, and uremic pleuritis (Table 2). However, in a patient undergoing peritoneal dialysis who develops reduced ultrafiltration and pleural effusion, special consideration must be given to a possible pleuroperitoneal leak.

Pleuroperitoneal leaks are uncommon complications of peritoneal dialysis, with an estimated incidence of less than 2% [2]. The first case of a pleuroperitoneal leak was described by Edwards and Unger in 1967 [3]. Patients often present with acute dyspnea, cough, or pleuritic chest pain [4].

There are multiple predisposing mechanisms for pleuroperitoneal leaks including diaphragmatic muscular hypotonia, congenital diaphragmatic defects, pleuroperitoneal pressure gradients, and lymphatic drainage disorders [4]. A known risk factor for a pleuroperitoneal leak is polycystic kidney disease, where the high intra-abdominal pressure could lead to an increased pleuroperitoneal pressure gradient. Patients with previous episodes of peritonitis are also more likely to develop this complication, possibly related to weakened diaphragm [5].

Cases occurring within the first month of initiation of PD likely represent congenital diaphragmatic defects leading to a pleuroperitoneal communication. This leads to the development of hydrothorax, almost always on the right side once PD is started. A study of 50 patients with this complication showed 88% of cases occurring on the right side, 8% on the left, and 4% bilaterally [2]. It was suggested that the right-sided predominance occurs since the left side of the

TABLE 3: Radiological modalities in diagnosing peritoneal-pleural leak.

Modality	Advantages	Disadvantages
Ultrasound	(i) Readily available (ii) Effective in confirming pleural effusion	(i) Limited value in determining etiology
Plain X-ray	(i) Readily available (ii) Effective in confirming pleural effusion	(i) Limited value in determining etiology
Peritoneal scintigraphy	(i) Safe and rapid way to diagnose	(i) Difficult to locate site of leak (ii) Requires PD-trained nurse for intraperitoneal administration of contrast
CT peritoneography	(i) Provides better resolution of anatomical details (including location and extent of extraperitoneal fluid) and can potentially locate the defect	(i) Potential nephrotoxicity with systemic absorption of contrast medium (ii) Requires PD-trained nurse for intraperitoneal administration of contrast
MR peritoneography	(i) Effective in diagnosing pleuroperitoneal leak	(i) Risk of nephrogenic systemic fibrosis with gadolinium (if used as contrast medium) (ii) More expensive and not readily available

diaphragm is protected by the situation of the heart on this side [5].

There is no definitive test to confirm the diagnosis; most cases require both biochemical and radiological assessment. Biochemically, the nature of the pleural fluid is transudative [6]. Although there is no widely accepted threshold for pleural glucose concentration to diagnose the condition, a pleural glucose concentration higher than serum is highly suggestive of a pleuroperitoneal connection [7, 8].

Radiological assessment can aid diagnosis, but tests are plagued by relatively low sensitivity (Table 3). Both ultrasound and X-ray can confirm the presence of effusion, but not the source of the fluid. Peritoneal scintigraphy is considered an excellent modality to diagnose a pleuroperitoneal leak, but the sensitivity has been reported to be only 40% to 50%, and its utility in locating the site of the pleuroperitoneal communication is limited [4, 7, 9]. In a case report, Kang and Kim suggested that CT peritoneography with intraperitoneal contrast could confirm and locate the pleuroperitoneal fistula [10]. However, another study by Tang et al. showed that only 33% of patients with a pleuroperitoneal leak actually show contrast passing into the pleural cavity [11]. Documenting the appearance of methylene blue in the pleural fluid after it has been added to peritoneal dialysate has been suggested as an alternative to contrast studies; however, the test has low sensitivity, and cases of chemical peritonitis have been described [7, 11–13].

In the short term, the management of a pleuroperitoneal leak often requires discontinuation of peritoneal dialysis and a switch to hemodialysis. Thoracentesis will be required for diagnostic evaluation or symptomatic relief of large effusions. Our patient tolerated large volume thoracocentesis, with 3 L of fluid removed. Pulmonary edema has been described after large volume thoracocentesis [14]. However, our patient did not develop any complications; we suspect that this was because of rather rapid detection and treatment of his pleural effusion. Absence of adequate ultrafiltration and increasing dyspnea alerted us to the possibility early in the clinical course.

The long-term management of a pleuroperitoneal leak depends on its severity. With conservative treatment (stopping PD and continuing on hemodialysis) for six weeks to three months, the success rate is approximately 50% [15]. Alternately, for instance, in circumstances where patients have a significant residual renal function or in individuals who will be receiving a renal transplant soon, one could continue peritoneal dialysis with smaller exchange volumes, performed in Semi-Fowler's position (head and upper body inclined at 30–45 degrees to the horizontal) [16]. Surgical or chemical pleurodesis, with agents such as talc or tetracycline, are successful in ameliorating the pleuroperitoneal communication in 67–90% of cases [17, 18]. When successful, this procedure may also allow patients to return to PD therapy.

This case highlights pleuroperitoneal communication as a rare but important differential diagnosis for pleural effusions in patients on peritoneal dialysis, and especially in those with a unilateral right-sided effusion.

Consent

The patient has provided informed consent to publish this case.

References

[1] H. A. M. Mahmoud, A. A. Mahmoud, I. S. Mobark, and A. T. Hassan, "Pleural complications in patients with chronic and end-stage renal disease," *European Respiratory Journal*, vol. 44, no. Suppl 58, p. P597, 2014.

[2] Y. Nomoto, T. Suga, K. Nakajima et al., "Acute hydrothorax in continuous ambulatory peritoneal dialysis—a collaborative study of 161 centers," *American Journal of Nephrology*, vol. 9, no. 5, pp. 363–367, 1989.

[3] S. R. Edwards and A. M. Unger, "Acute hydrothorax—a new complication of peritoneal dialysis," *JAMA: The Journal of the American Medical Association*, vol. 199, no. 11, pp. 853–855, 1967.

[4] K. A. Alhasan, "Recurrent hydrothorax in a child on peritoneal dialysis: a case report and review of the literature," *Clinical Case Reports*, vol. 7, no. 1, pp. 149–151, 2019.
[5] C. Kennedy, C. McCarthy, S. Alken et al., "Pleuroperitoneal leak complicating peritoneal dialysis: a case series," *International Journal of Nephrology*, vol. 2011, Article ID 526753, 4 pages, 2011.
[6] K. Tapawan, E. Chen, N. Selk, E. Hong, S. Virmani, and R. Balk, "A large pleural effusion in a patient receiving peritoneal dialysis," *Seminars in Dialysis*, vol. 24, no. 5, pp. 560–563, 2011.
[7] Y. Cho, V. D'Intini, and D. Ranganathan, "Acute hydrothorax complicating peritoneal dialysis: a case report," *Journal of Medical Case Reports*, vol. 4, no. 1, p. 355, 2010.
[8] K. M. Chow, C. C. Szeto, T. Y.-H. Wong, and P. K.-T. Li, "Hydrothorax complicating peritoneal dialysis: diagnostic value of glucose concentration in pleural fluid aspirate," *Peritoneal Dialysis International: Journal of the International Society for Peritoneal Dialysis*, vol. 22, no. 4, pp. 525–528, 2002.
[9] M. Chavannes, A. P. Sharma, R. N. Singh, R. H. Reid, and G. Filler, "Diagnosis by peritoneal scintigraphy of peritoneal dialysis-associated hydrothorax in an infant," *Peritoneal Dialysis International: Journal of the International Society for Peritoneal Dialysis*, vol. 34, no. 1, pp. 140–143, 2014.
[10] T. W. Kang and C. K. Kim, "Pleuroperitoneal communication of peritoneal dialysis demonstrated by multidetector-row CT peritoneography," *Abdominal Imaging*, vol. 34, no. 6, pp. 780–782, 2009.
[11] S. Tang, W. H. Chui, A. W. C. Tang et al., "Video-assisted thoracoscopic talc pleurodesis is effective for maintenance of peritoneal dialysis in acute hydrothorax complicating peritoneal dialysis," *Nephrology Dialysis Transplantation*, vol. 18, no. 4, pp. 804–808, 2003.
[12] D. G. Nolan, "Inflammatory peritonitis with ascites after methylene blue dye chromopertubation during diagnostic laparoscopy," *The Journal of the American Association of Gynecologic Laparoscopists*, vol. 2, no. 4, pp. 483–485, 1995.
[13] M. Macia, E. Gallego, I. Garcia-Cobaleda, J. Chahin, and J. Garcia, "Methylene blue as a cause of chemical peritonitis in a patient on peritoneal dialysis," *Clinical Nephrology*, vol. 43, no. 2, pp. 136-137, 1995.
[14] E. P. Cantey, J. M. Walter, T. Corbridge, and J. H. Barsuk, "Complications of thoracentesis," *Current Opinion in Pulmonary Medicine*, vol. 22, no. 4, pp. 378–385, 2016.
[15] K. M. Chow, C. C. Szeto, and P. K.-T. Li, "Review articles: management options for hydrothorax complicating peritoneal dialysis," *Seminars in Dialysis*, vol. 16, no. 5, pp. 389–394, 2003.
[16] F. Christidou and G. Vayonas, "Recurrent acute hydrothorax in a CAPD patient: successful management with small volumes of dialysate," *Peritoneal Dialysis International: Journal of the International Society for Peritoneal Dialysis*, vol. 15, no. 4, p. 389, 1995.
[17] C. D. Sudduth and S. A. Sahn, "Pleurodesis for nonmalignant pleural effusions," *Chest*, vol. 102, no. 6, pp. 1855–1860, 1992.
[18] I. Krivokuca, J.-W. J. Lammers, and J. Kluin, "Peritoneal dialysis—an unusual cause of pleural effusion ("sweet hydrothorax")," *Respiratory Medicine CME*, vol. 2, no. 4, pp. 197–200, 2009.

25

Dialysis Disequilibrium Syndrome and Cerebellar Herniation with Successful Reversal using Mannitol

Anna Curtis,[1] **Christian Lamb**,[2] **Hussain Rao**,[1] **Andrew Williams**,[1] **and Amit Patel**[3]

[1]*School of Medicine, University of Missouri-Kansas City, Kansas City, MO 64108, USA*
[2]*Department of Medicine, Brooke Army Medical Center, San Antonio, TX 78234, USA*
[3]*Department of Medicine—Division of Nephrology, Truman Medical Center, Kansas City, MO 64108, USA*

Correspondence should be addressed to Anna Curtis; akc8bv@mail.umkc.edu and Christian Lamb; christian.lambmd@gmail.com

Academic Editor: Manel Vera

Dialysis disequilibrium syndrome (DDS) is a morbid but rare complication of dialysis. Feared sequalae of this diagnosis are brain herniation and death. This report presents a patient who was diagnosed with DDS with subsequent tonsillar herniation shown on imaging with complete resolution of clinical signs and symptoms, as well as imaging findings of herniation after prompt initiation of intravenous mannitol. This is the first known case of reversal and survival of DDS-induced tonsillar herniation using mannitol.

1. Introduction

Dialysis disequilibrium syndrome (DDS) is a neurological complication of hemodialysis typically seen in individuals receiving therapy for the first time. First described in 1962, symptoms can include mild headache, vomiting, altered sensorium, seizures, arrhythmias, and even death [1]. Current research suggests that the reverse urea effect may be the primary mechanism due to which this syndrome occurs. Urea and other osmotically active solutes are critical in maintaining intravascular volume. During hemodialysis, these intravascular solutes are removed rapidly, creating an osmotic gradient that favors free water influx into the cerebral parenchyma [2]. This brisk expansion of tissue compresses pivotal brain structures and can result in cerebral herniation.

The diagnosis of DDS is one of the exclusions and may be difficult to identify by clinicians due to its vast array of presenting symptoms [3]. Luckily, most cases of DDS are mild and self-resolving, though a myriad of devastating consequences have been reported, including demyelination, posterior reversible encephalopathy syndrome, and most notably, cerebral herniation [4–6]. An extensive literature review yielded thirteen documented reports of patients suffering herniation secondary to DDS with poor outcomes. We present what we believe to be the first reported case of cerebellar tonsillar herniation secondary to DDS which was resolved using intravenous (IV) mannitol with no residual neurologic deficits.

2. Case Presentation

A 47-year-old African-American male with hypertension presented to the emergency department (ED) with complaints of persistent abdominal pain. Upon evaluation, the patient described his pain as vague and periumbilical. He also reported episodes of nonbloody emesis, headache, and possible hematuria since awaking that morning. His vital signs were significant for a blood pressure of 240/161 mmHg, heart rate of 100 beats per minute, respiratory rate of 18 breaths per minute, and oxygen saturation of 100% while he was breathing ambient air. He was afebrile. Physical exam revealed a malnourished-appearing male with an otherwise normal physical exam. Initial laboratory studies were significant for a creatinine of 15.39 mg/dL (reference range 0.90–1.3 mg/dL), blood-urea-nitrogen (BUN) of 155 mg/dL (reference range 8–20 mg/dL), an anion gap metabolic acidosis of 29 mmol/L (reference range 10–20 mmol/L), platelet count of 45 10^3/cmm (reference range 150–400 10^3/cmm), and hemoglobin of 10.1 g/dL (reference range

14.0–18.0 g/dL). Abdominal and pelvic computed tomography (CT) without contrast was performed and showed enteritis involving the jejunum.

The patient denied any history of renal or hematological disease. His home medications included labetalol 30 mg once per day and nifedipine 100 mg twice per day, both of which he admitted using sparingly. The patient was given intravenous (IV) labetalol in the ED with minimal success in lowering the blood pressure. Due to the presence of end-organ damage, hematological and metabolic aberrancies, thrombotic consumptive coagulopathy secondary to malignant hypertension was suspected. The patient was urgently admitted to the Intensive Care Unit (ICU) for further investigation and intervention.

In the ICU, a continuous IV infusion of nicardipine was initiated. Clinicians recommended urgent placement of a central venous catheter in order to initiate hemodialysis given electrolyte abnormalities. Initially, the patient refused all interventions due to holistic reasons. Fifteen hours following admission, the patient continued to deteriorate with worsening thrombocytopenia and encephalopathy; he ultimately agreed to catheter placement. Two units of platelets were transfused prior to the procedure. A right internal jugular vein triple lumen catheter was placed without complication, and the patient was initiated on hemodialysis with the dialysis prescription shown in Table 1.

A low-flux urea membrane was initially ordered by the attending nephrologist, but this option was not available at the facility in which this patient received treatment. Due to the urgency of treatment, hemodialysis was performed without this membrane.

Approximately 20 minutes into the hemodialysis session, the patient became unresponsive. A right eye gaze deviation and right-sided fasciculations of the upper and lower extremities were observed. Hemodialysis was discontinued, and an urgent head CT without contrast was performed. Imaging revealed pontine edema with mass effect and cerebellar tonsillar herniation (Figure 1). The on-call nephrologist initiated intravenous mannitol, and neurosurgery was consulted urgently. The results of complete basic metabolic panels before and after the initiation of hemodialysis are shown in Table 2.

Within 30 minutes of initiation of the mannitol infusion, the patient regained consciousness and remained hemodynamically stable. Follow-up neurological exam showed no focal deficits and complete resolution of the right-sided fasciculations and gaze palsy. Mannitol was continued for 24 hours. The following morning, head magnetic resonate imaging (MRI) was obtained and showed resolution of the midline shift and tonsillar herniation shown on the head CT scan eight hours prior. A diagnosis of Dialysis Disequilibrium Syndrome was made.

Three days following this diagnosis, a low-flux urea filter was obtained from an outside facility and the patient began continuous renal replacement therapy (CRRT). Serial head CT occurring every 48 hours and scheduled hourly neurologic examinations confirmed the patient's tolerance of CRRT with no further progression or recurrence of symptoms related to DDS. The patient was eventually transferred out of the ICU and underwent placement of a long-term hemodialysis fistula. He had complete resolution of symptoms at the 2-year follow-up, but remained on intermittent hemodialysis.

Table 1: Dialysis prescription.

F180 membrane	
Surface area	1.7 m^2
KUf	58 mL/hr/mmHg
Dialysate solution	
Sodium	140 mmol/L
Potassium	4 mmol/L
Calcium	2.5 mmol/L
Bicarbonate	35 mmol/L
Q_D	600 mL/min
Q_B	300 mL/min

3. Discussion

While the mechanism of DDS remains unclear, several risk factors for the syndrome have been proposed, including first dialysis, extremes of age, electrolyte imbalances, metabolic acidosis, hypertensive emergency, pre-existing neurological conditions, cerebral edema, meningitis, and the presence of intracranial tumors [7]. Additionally, the hemodialysis prescription prescribed by the provider may influence a fluid shift into the cerebral parenchyma. Current guidelines recommend limiting the removal of BUN to 40% over the course of two hours. This can be achieved by utilizing low-flux dialysis membranes, setting low flow rates (Qd of 300 and Qb 250, respectively), modulating the dialysate sodium and glucose concentrations, and shortening the duration of therapy. Additional methods, including prophylactic mannitol administration, have been suggested [2, 7, 8].

As described in the case above, our patient had several predisposing risk factors for DDS upon presentation to the ED. He was in hypertensive emergency and had a metabolic acidosis and significantly elevated BUN. This was also his first-time dialyzing. When dialysis was initiated, the duration was shortened to 120 minutes, dialysate sodium was set at 140 mmol/L, and there was an attempt to secure a low-flux dialysis membrane. Unfortunately, even with these adjustments to therapy, the patient cleared 31 mg/dL of BUN or 20% of his total serum BUN in 20 minutes, as seen by comparing the patient's initial metabolic panel to the one drawn thirty minutes after initiation of HD (Table 2). Other interventions, such as the addition of dialysate glucose, increasing dialysate sodium further, utilizing lower Qb and Qd flow rates, and administering prophylactic mannitol, may have been beneficial at reducing the likelihood of DDS occurrence in this patient.

Historically, even with swift intervention, cerebral herniation due to DDS carries a grim prognosis. A case series by Osgood et al. in 2015 highlighted that four patients who all received hemodialysis were diagnosed with DDS and had cerebral herniation confirmed on imaging. Despite intervention with mannitol and hypertonic saline, all patients succumbed to their neurologic injury and were pronounced brain dead [6]. Similarly, a case series published by Kumar

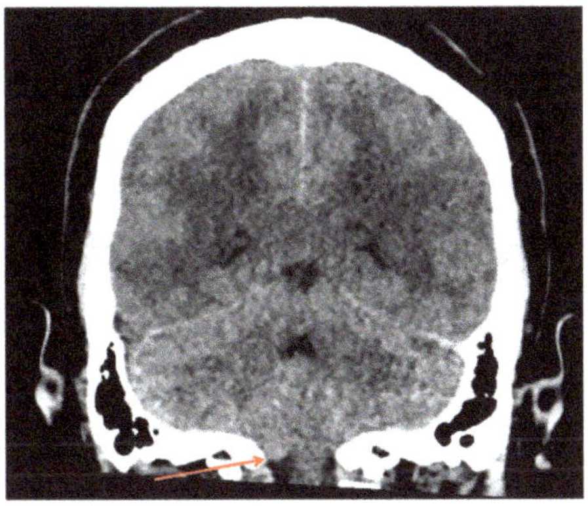

Figure 1: Computed Tomography (CT) showing cerebellar tonsil herniation (red arrow).

Table 2: Results of basic metabolic panels.

	Predialysis	Postdialysis
Sodium	135 mmol/L	137 mmol/L
Potassium	3.2 mmol/L	3.2 mmol/L
Chloride	89 mmol/L	91 mmol/L
Bicarbonate	22 mmol/L	26 mmol/L
Blood-Urea-Nitrogen	152 mg/dL	121 mg/dL
Creatinine	16.25 mg/dL	11.75 mg/dL
Glucose	175 mg/dL	130 mg/dL

et al. in 2014 highlighted a patient suffering from DDS with resultant tonsillar herniation. Despite timely introduction of an infusion of hypertonic saline, the patient died [9]. With the exception of the case reported above, an extensive literature review failed to reveal any other documented cases of survival (with or without return to baseline) among patients with DDS and imaging-confirmed tonsillar herniation.

Guideline-based management of cerebral herniation secondary to DDS currently recommends the cessation of HD, hyperventilation, and elevating the head of the bed. Although numerous studies have shown mannitol's efficacy at treating a variety of neurological conditions, the use of mannitol and other osmotically active infusions for the management of DDS remains controversial [10, 11]. This report is the first known case in which a mannitol infusion successfully reversed DDS-induced tonsillar herniation with a complete return to neurologic baseline.

4. Conclusions

The case reported herein is the first documented account of reversal of the clinical and imaging findings of tonsillar herniation secondary to DDS using intravenous mannitol.

References

[1] A. C. Kennedy, A. L. Linton, and J. C. Eaton, "Urea levels in cerebrospinal fluid after hæmodialysis," *The Lancet*, vol. 279, no. 7226, pp. 410-411, 1962.

[2] N. Patel, P. Dalal, and M. Panesar, "Fellows' forum fellows' forum in dialysis edited by Mark A. Perazella: dialysis disequilibrium syndrome: a narrative review," *Seminars in Dialysis*, vol. 21, no. 5, pp. 493–498, 2008.

[3] A. Muzzammil and U. Bakhsh, "A vanishing complication of haemodialysis: dialysis disequilibrium syndrome," *Journal of the Intensive Care Society*, vol. 21, no. 1, pp. 92–95, 2018.

[4] A. Soomro, R. Al Bahri, N. Alhassan, F. Hejaili, and A. Al Sayyari, "Posterior reversible encephalopathy syndrome with tactile hallucinations secondary to dialysis disequilibrium syndrome," *Saudi Journal of Kidney Diseases and Transplantation: An Official Publication of the Saudi Center for Organ Transplantation, Saudi Arabia*, vol. 25, no. 3, pp. 625–629, 2014.

[5] S. C. Keswani, "Central pontine and extrapontine myelinolysis owing to disequilibrium syndrome," *Journal of Child Neurology*, vol. 19, no. 1, pp. 79-80, 2004.

[6] M. Osgood, R. Compton, R. Carandang, W. Hall, G. Kershaw, and S. Muehlschlegel, "Rapid unexpected brain herniation in association with renal replacement therapy in acute brain injury: caution in the neurocritical care unit," *Neurocritical Care*, vol. 22, no. 2, pp. 176–183, 2014.

[7] K. Mistry, "Dialysis disequilibrium syndrome prevention and management," *International Journal of Nephrology and Renovascular Disease*, vol. 12, pp. 69–77, 2019.

[8] H. Bergman, J. Daugirdas, T. Ing et al., *Handbook of Dialysis*, Lippincott, Williams & Wilkins, Philadelphia, PA, USA, 2001.

[9] A. Kumar, A. Cage, and R. Dhar, "Dialysis-induced worsening of cerebral edema in intracranial hemorrhage: a case series and clinical perspective," *Neurocritical Care*, vol. 22, no. 2, pp. 283–287, 2014.

[10] H. E. Hinson, D. Stein, and K. N. Sheth, "Hypertonic saline and mannitol therapy in critical care neurology," *Journal of Intensive Care Medicine*, vol. 28, no. 1, pp. 3–11, 2011.

[11] D. Zepeda-Orozco and R. Quigley, "Dialysis disequilibrium syndrome," *Pediatric Nephrology*, vol. 27, no. 12, pp. 2205–2211, 2012.

Severe Metabolic Acidosis: A Case of Triple Hit with Ketogenic Diet, Vinegar and Metformin in an Obese Patient

Abdul Mughees Rana,[1] **Kannan Mansoor**,[1] **Salman Assad**,[2] **Mahmoud Abouzid**,[1] **Iheanyichukwu Ogu**,[1] **and Ghassan Salim Issa Bandak**[1]

[1]*Department of Internal Medicine University Huntington, 1249 15th Street Suite 2000, Huntington, WV 25514, USA*
[2]*Department of Neurology Marshall University Joan C. Edwards School of Medicine, 1600 Medical Center Drive Office B561, Huntington, WV, USA*

Correspondence should be addressed to Abdul Mughees Rana; ranaa@marshall.edu

Academic Editor: Ze'ev Korzets

Obesity is an epidemic with high burden of disease. It is directly proportional to increased risk of morbidity and mortality. Ketogenic diet and herbal supplements have recently gained popularity amongst patients struggling with weight loss. There are limited data available for most of these supplements contrary to the claims laid by the mainstream media. Due to lack of awareness, this patient population is at high risk of adverse effects. We present a case of severe acidosis secondary to ketogenic diet and acetic acid (vinegar) ingestion. The use of dietary acetic acid is usually well tolerated; however, in this case, the large quantities and presence of acute renal injury and metformin use may have worsened the acidosis. Severe ketosis in setting of ketogenic diets is a serious complication, which is infrequently reported in literature. Many of these diets and supplements may seem harmless, but as our case illustrates, when combined with other risk factors, patients can face serious adverse effects and even require hospitalization. It is imperative that such dietary practices are physician supervised to avoid complications. With the recent surge of over-the-counter weight loss supplements and ketogenic diets, physicians also need to engage in dietary discussion with patients when attempting to lose weight.

1. Introduction

Obesity is an epidemic with high burden of disease. In 2016, the prevalence of obesity among adults in the United States was close to 40% [1]. Obesity is related to worse outcomes and increased physical morbidity as well as mental health disease [2]. Weight loss is a challenging journey. More than 50–60% of the American adult obese population embarks on this journey yearly [3, 4]. Obese patients try different methods and strategies to lose weight including dietary modifications, dietary restrictions, exercise, weight loss medications, or programs [3, 4]. Low carbohydrate, or ketogenic, diets have gained popularity over the past few years. Ketogenic diets and reducing carbohydrate intake will lead to weight loss through different mechanisms including appetite suppression, increased lipolysis, and changes in lipid metabolism as well as gluconeogenesis [5, 6]. Acetic acid ingestion has also been proposed to be beneficial in weight management [7]. Obese patients seek medical information and help with weight management from various sources including television, online, and social media platforms [8]. These sources may provide unreliable information [8–10]. This may translate into patients engaging in new dietary habits without consulting medical professionals. We present here a unique case of a young female patient who presented to our hospital with severe acidosis secondary to ketogenic diet and acetic acid ingestion. To our knowledge, this is the first case of combined ketogenic acid, metformin use, and acetic acid ingestion leading to severe acidemia in literature.

2. Case Presentation

A 43-year-old female with a medical history significant for diabetes mellitus type 2, hypertension, iron deficiency anemia, gastroesophageal reflux disease, and Potts syndrome presented to the emergency department with complaints of weakness and lightheadedness for two weeks. The patient started developing intermittent nausea without any abdominal pain, vomiting, or diarrhea. Symptoms started two weeks prior to presentation. The patient reported no fever, no chills, denied urinary urgency, or increased frequency but complained of dysuria. She also denied any chest pain, cough, or dyspnea. She reported recent weight loss of approximately 14 lbs after starting on ketogenic diet along with regular ingestion of apple cid vinegar. She would drink it as a stand-alone drink or add it to various foods in the last two months. Her diet included little to no carbohydrate. She did not report that she sought advice from a medical professional prior to initiation of her diet. She denied illicit drug use, significant alcohol intake, or ingestion of locally produced alcohols such as moonshine. She consumed alcohol on an infrequent basis, and her last drink was a half glass of wine a day prior to presentation. She denied any prior episodes of diabetic ketoacidosis or use of sodium-glucose cotransporter-2 (SGLT2) inhibitors. She admitted to taking ibuprofen or acetaminophen occasionally for pain. Her medications included lisinopril, hydrochlorothiazide, ferrous sulphate, omeprazole, gabapentin, and metformin. The dose of metformin was increased from 500 mg twice daily to 2000 twice daily 4–5 months before admission. On arrival to the emergency department, she was found to have hypotension and tachycardia. Physical exam was unremarkable except for labored breathing and dry mucous membranes. Her labs revealed metabolic acidosis (pH 7.15) with an increased anion gap of 27 mEq/L, lactic acid of 4.9 mmol/L, blood sugar of 108 mg/dl, serum ethanol level of 18 mg/dL, and elevated creatinine level of 2.7 mg/dL (Table 1). She received 3 L intravenous bolus of normal saline (0.9% NaCl) and was started on IV Dextrose 5% in water (D5W) @100 ml/hr for suspicion of starvation ketosis. She also received 100 mEq of sodium bicarbonate intravenously in addition to initiation of fomepizole empirically, given an elevated osmolal gap of 18 mOsm/kg. With volume expansion, bicarbonate supplementation, as well as dextrose supplementation, the patient's acidosis, acute kidney injury (AKI), and ketosis resolved. Nephrology service was consulted to assist in patient's care, and after reviewing case, they agreed that her acidosis was likely a combination of starvation ketosis, in setting of acetic acid consumption, hypovolemia, and AKI. Other etiologies like ingestion of methanol, isopropyl alcohol, salicylate, or D lactic acidosis were also ruled out. She denied frequent use of acetaminophen; hence, diagnosis of pyroglutamic aciduria was not entertained. Lactic acid level returned to normal within 4 hours and her anion gap closed in the first 14 hours after presentation. A repeat venous pH was recorded as 7.35. On urinalysis, the patient was positive for a urinary tract infection, and the patient endorsed that she had dysuria. The patient was started on IV ceftriaxone. On day 2, the patient's lab work-up was within normal limits. The patient was counseled about dietary intake and was told to abstain from use of vinegar. Metformin was discontinued. The patient was discharged with an endocrinology outpatient follow-up. Laboratory investigations at time of admission and discharge are outlined in Table 1.

3. Discussion

Ketogenic diets are popular among patients seeking weight loss. However, there is no clear consensus on the overall health benefits of these diets [11, 12]. During states of low carbohydrate intake, body will promote gluconeogenesis for endogenous glucose production. After few days of low carbohydrate intake, ketogenesis is promoted as a source of energy [5, 6]. Ketogenesis includes overproduction of acetoacetate, beta-hydroxybutyric acid, and acetone, with these processes occurring mainly in the liver. Ketogenesis associated with low carbohydrate diets or dietary ketosis is thought to be safe, which is different from pathologic cases of ketoacidosis that happens in patients with diabetes [5, 6]. During normal and controlled conditions of caloric intake and hydration, use of very low carbohydrate diet seems to produce safe levels of ketosis [13–15]. Studies have shown that restricting carbohydrate intake is safe from an electrolyte and acid base stand point, especially with adequate caloric and fluid intake as performed in such studies [13–15]. Nonetheless, there are several cases in the literature of severe acidosis associated with ketogenic diets [16–21]. Acute kidney injury, dehydration, and other complications have been also reported in the pediatric population adhering to ketogenic diets for epilepsy management [22, 23]. Ingestion of dietary forms of vinegar is usually safe. Dietary vinegar contains acetic acid [24, 25]. Normally, acetic acid is metabolized to bicarbonate in the liver and should not alter acid base balance; however, there may be a delay between the actual ingestion and buffering which could create a temporary acid base disturbance [26]. Vinegar may be ketogenic as well [27]. A link between acetic acid consumption and ketosis has been demonstrated in animal studies. [28] Reports of complications or fatalities related to vinegar or acetic acid ingestion are mostly secondary to consumption of concentrated forms of acetic acid [29–31]. We did find one fatality reported to homicidal massive ingestion of dietary vinegar in a pediatric patient [32]. The combination of metformin to carbohydrate-restricted diets has been reported to aid in management of diabetes patients [33]. None the less, metformin may exacerbate ketosis through inhibition of gluconeogenesis and stimulation of fatty acid oxidation as previously reported [34]. Our case is unique in a way that the patient engaged in aggressive carbohydrate restriction along with frequent ingestion of vinegar in the setting of an increasing dose of metformin, and all these factors worked in concert to promote unrestricted ketogenesis which led to life-threatening anion gap acidosis. She was not following with a dietician or a healthcare professional to guide her dietary changes and did not maintain appropriate fluid intake. To our knowledge, this is the first case in literature that is reported with severe acidosis in setting of ketogenic diet, vinegar ingestion, and metformin use. This should serve as a good resource for clinicians and public to educate about the risks of various, presumed to be harmless, dietary changes. In conclusion, ketogenic diets and

Table 1: Laboratory investigations at time of admission and discharge.

Laboratory variables (units)	Labs on admission	Labs on discharge	Normal values
PCO_2 (mmHg)	31	43	41–51
HCO_3 (mmol/L)	10.5	23.5	23–29
pH	7.15	7.35	7.31–7.41
WBC ($\times 10^9$/L)	10.6	2.0	4.5–10
Hemoglobin (g/dl)	11.4	7.9	12–16
Platelets ($\times 10^9$/L)	231	93	150–440
Sodium (meq/L)	131	142	135–145
Potassium (meq/L)	3.8	4.1	3.5–5.0
Chloride (meq/L)	94	104	98–108
Blood sugar (mg/dl)	108	103	74–100
HbA1C (%)	5.1	NA	<5.7
Osmolality (mOsm/kg)	298	300	281–297
Anion gap	27	6	5–14
Serum albumin	4.7	3.0	3.1–4.5
Serum acetone	3+	NA	Negative
BUN (mg/dL)	19	6.1	7–18
Creatinine (mg/dL)	2.37	0.9	0.6–1.10
Serum ethanol (mg/dL)	18	NA	Negative
Lactic acid (mmol/L)	4.19	1.89	0.7–2.10
Salicylate level (mg/dL)	<2	NA	2–20
Methanol level	Negative	NA	Negative
D-Lactate	<0.2	NA	<0.50
Isopropyl ethanol	Negative	NA	Negative
Antipancreatic islet cell Ab	Negative	NA	Negative

NA, values not available.

vinegar consumption can lead to life-threatening acidosis. It is imperative that trained healthcare providers supervise patients seeking weight loss if they want to engage in either of these options to avoid potentially serious complications. We should also work in our communities to educate the public and produce reliable media outlets to help spreading reliable medical advice.

Abbreviations

AKI: Acute kidney injury
SGLT2: Sodium-glucose cotransporter-2
D5W: Dextrose 5% in water.

References

[1] C. M. Hales, M. D. Carroll, C. D. Fryar, and C. L. Ogden, "Prevalence of obesity among adults and youth: United States, 2015–2016," *NCHS Data Brief*, vol. 288, pp. 1–8, 2017.

[2] A. Hruby and F. B. Hu, "The epidemiology of obesity: a big picture," *Pharmacoeconomics*, vol. 33, no. 7, pp. 673–689, 2015.

[3] J. Kruger, D. A. Galuska, M. K. Serdula, and D. A. Jones, "Attempting to lose weight," *American Journal of Preventive Medicine*, vol. 26, no. 5, pp. 402–406, 2004.

[4] J. M. Nicklas, K. W. Huskey, R. B. Davis, and C. C. Wee, "Successful weight loss among obese U.S. adults," *American Journal of Preventive Medicine*, vol. 42, no. 5, pp. 481–485, 2012.

[5] A. Paoli, "Ketogenic diet for obesity: friend or foe?" *International Journal of Environmental Research and Public Health*, vol. 11, no. 2, pp. 2092–2107, 2014.

[6] A. Paoli, A. Rubini, J. S. Volek, and K. A. Grimaldi, "Beyond weight loss: a review of the therapeutic uses of very-low-carbohydrate (ketogenic) diets," *European Journal of Clinical Nutrition*, vol. 67, no. 8, pp. 789–796, 2013.

[7] T. Kondo, M. Kishi, T. Fushimi, S. Ugajin, and T. Kaga, "Vinegar intake reduces body weight, body fat mass, and serum triglyceride levels in obese Japanese subjects," *Bioscience, Biotechnology, and Biochemistry*, vol. 73, no. 8, pp. 1837–1843, 2009.

[8] M. Jane, M. Hagger, J. Foster, S. Ho, and S. Pal, "Social media for health promotion and weight management: a critical debate," *BMC Public Health*, vol. 18, no. 1, p. 932, 2018.

[9] P. A. Pirraglia and R. L. Kravitz, "Social media: new opportunities, new ethical concerns," *Journal of General Internal Medicine*, vol. 28, no. 2, pp. 165-166, 2013.

[10] C. Korownyk, M. R. Kolber, J. McCormack et al., "Televised medical talk shows—what they recommend and the evidence to support their recommendations: a prospective observational study," *BMJ*, vol. 349, Article ID g7346, 2014.

[11] C. Churuangsuk, M. Kherouf, E. Combet, and M. Lean, "Low-carbohydrate diets for overweight and obesity: a systematic review of the systematic reviews," *Obesity Reviews*, vol. 19, no. 12, pp. 1700–1718, 2018.

[12] W. Masood and K. R. Uppaluri, *Ketogenic Diet*, StatPearls, Treasure Island, FL, USA, 2020.

[13] W. S. Yancy Jr., M. K. Olsen, T. Dudley, and E. C. Westman, "Acid-base analysis of individuals following two weight loss

diets," *European Journal of Clinical Nutrition*, vol. 61, no. 12, pp. 1416–1422, 2007.

[14] S. D. Phinney, B. R. Bistrian, R. R. Wolfe, and G. L. Blackburn, "The human metabolic response to chronic ketosis without caloric restriction: physical and biochemical adaptation," *Metabolism*, vol. 32, no. 8, pp. 757–768, 1983.

[15] D. Gomez-Arbelaez, A. B. Crujeiras, A. I. Castro et al., "Acid-base safety during the course of a very low-calorie-ketogenic diet," *Endocrine*, vol. 58, no. 1, pp. 81–90, 2017.

[16] T. F. Freeman, B. Willis, and D. M. Krywko, "Acute intractable vomiting and severe ketoacidosis secondary to the dukan diet," *The Journal of Emergency Medicine*, vol. 47, no. 4, pp. e109–12, 2014.

[17] S. Chalasani and J. Fischer, "South Beach Diet associated ketoacidosis: a case report," *Journal of Medical Case Reports*, vol. 2, p. 45, 2008.

[18] S. Basnet, N. Tachamo, S. Nazir, R. Dhital, A. Jehangir, and A. Donato, "Severe anion gap metabolic acidosis associated with initiation of a very low-carbohydrate diet," *Journal of Community Hospital Internal Medicine Perspectives*, vol. 9, no. 2, pp. 165–167, 2019.

[19] P. Shah and W. L. Isley, "Ketoacidosis during a low-carbohydrate diet," *New England Journal of Medicine*, vol. 354, no. 1, pp. 97-98, 2006.

[20] T.-Y. Chen, W. Smith, J. L. Rosenstock, and K.-D. Lessnau, "A life-threatening complication of Atkins diet," *The Lancet*, vol. 367, no. 9514, p. 958, 2006.

[21] L. von Geijer and M. Ekelund, "Ketoacidosis associated with low-carbohydrate diet in a non-diabetic lactating woman: a case report," *Journal of Medical Case Reports*, vol. 9, p. 224, 2015.

[22] K. H. Yoo and H. E. Yim, "Acute tubular necrosis associated with the ketogenic diet in a child with intractable epilepsy," *Childhood Kidney Diseases*, vol. 23, no. 1, pp. 48–52, 2019.

[23] H. C. Kang, D. E. Chung, D. W. Kim, and H. D. Kim, "Early- and late-onset complications of the ketogenic diet for intractable epilepsy," *Epilepsia*, vol. 45, no. 9, pp. 1116–1123, 2004.

[24] C. S. Johnston and C. A. Gaas, "Vinegar: medicinal uses and antiglycemic effect," *MedGenMed: Medscape General Medicine*, vol. 8, no. 2, p. 61, 2006.

[25] US Food and Drug Administration, *CPG Sec. 525.825 Vinegar, Definitions—Adulteration with Vinegar Eels*, US Food and Drug Administration, Silver Spring, MD, USA, 2014.

[26] K. Lhotta, G. Höfle, R. Gasser, and G. Finkenstedt, "Hypokalemia, hyperreninemia and osteoporosis in a patient ingesting large amounts of cider vinegar," *Nephron*, vol. 80, no. 2, pp. 242-243, 1998.

[27] C. J. d. C. Harvey, G. M. Schofield, and M. Williden, "The use of nutritional supplements to induce ketosis and reduce symptoms associated with keto-induction: a narrative review," *PeerJ*, vol. 6, p. e4488, 2018.

[28] M. Eaton, R. H. B. MacKay, H. O. Carne, and N. Arne, "Wick *ketogenic Activity of acetic acid*," *Journal of Biological Chemistry*, vol. 135, pp. 157–163, 1940.

[29] J. Tibballs, R. Cathie, M. Buist, K. Shimizu, K. Stokes, and J. Millar, "Upper airway obstruction caused by ingestion of concentrated acetic acid," *Anaesthesia and Intensive Care*, vol. 34, no. 3, pp. 379–381, 2006.

[30] O. Jurim, E. Gross, J. Nates, and A. Eldor, "Disseminated intravascular coagulopathy caused by acetic acid ingestion," *Acta Haematologica*, vol. 89, no. 4, pp. 204-205, 1993.

[31] A. Ratcliffe, A. Baker, and D. Smith, "Successful management of 70% acetic acid ingestion on the intensive care unit: a case report," *Journal of the Intensive Care Society*, vol. 19, no. 1, pp. 56–60, 2018.

[32] L. B. E. Shields, C. M. Rolf, and J. C. Hunsaker III, "Sudden death due to forced ingestion of vinegar," *Forensic Science International*, vol. 266, pp. e23–e26, 2016.

[33] J. E. Müller, D. Sträter-Müller, H.-J. Marks et al., "Carbohydrate restricted diet in conjunction with metformin and liraglutide is an effective treatment in patients with deteriorated type 2 diabetes mellitus: proof-of-concept study," *Nutrition & Metabolism*, vol. 8, no. 1, p. 92, 2011.

[34] V. Schwetz, F. Eisner, G. Schilcher et al., "Combined metformin-associated lactic acidosis and euglycemic ketoacidosis," *Wiener klinische Wochenschrift*, vol. 129, no. 17-18, pp. 646–649, 2017.

27

Localized Fournier's Gangrene in "End-Stage" Renal Failure: Multidisciplinary Approach and Integration of Palliative Care

M. Voordeckers,[1] J. Noels,[2] M. Brognet,[3] M. T. Salaouatchi,[3] and M. Mesquita[3]

[1]Palliative Care Unit, Centre Hospitalier Universitaire, Hospital Brugmann, Brussels, Belgium
[2]Urology Clinic, Centre Hospitalier Universitaire, Hospital Brugmann, Brussels, Belgium
[3]Department of Internal Medecine, Clinics of Nephrology and Dialysis, Hospital Brugmann, Brussels, Belgium

Correspondence should be addressed to M. Mesquita; maria.mesquita@chu-brugmann.be

Academic Editor: Anja Haase-Fielitz

Presentation of the Case. Penile gangrene is a rare entity with significant morbidity and mortality. There are only few case reports of isolated penile Fournier's gangrene in literature. Its rare occurrence, associated with complex and serious comorbidity, poses a major challenge to the attending medical personnel. A 53-year-old Caucasian patient with poorly controlled diabetes, progressive renal insufficiency, and multiple vascular complications presented with progressive necrosis of the penis (localized Fournier's gangrene). *Discussion.* Fournier's gangrene or necrotizing fasciitis refers to any synergistic necrotizing infection of the external genitalia or perineum and is a hallmark of severe systemic vascular disease. Fournier's gangrene is an absolute emergency because the time interval between diagnosis and treatment significantly influences morbidity and mortality. Despite aggressive management, the estimated mortality rates range from 57 to 71%. *Conclusions.* Improved integration of palliative care services into the care of such patients is important to improve end-of-life care even though they do not have a malignant disease. The "Palliative Care Indicator Tool" can help identifying people at risk of deteriorating health and is important to improve end-of-life care.

1. Introduction

Penile gangrene is a rare entity with significant morbidity and mortality. There are only few case reports of isolated penile Fournier's gangrene in literature [1]. Its rare occurrence associated with complex and serious comorbidity poses a major challenge to the attending medical personnel.

Penile gangrene can be due to an infection (infectious gangrene) or can occur because of traumatism or vascular problems such as atherosclerosis or arteriosclerosis (dry gangrene). Distinction between infectious and dry gangrene is essential since clinical management of these two subsets differs markedly [2].

Fournier's gangrene (FG) or necrotizing fasciitis refers to any synergistic necrotizing infection of the external genitalia or perineum. Predisposing factors such as diabetes, alcohol or intravenous drug abuse, cancer, obesity, advanced age, renal failure, immunodeficiency and HIV infection, and/or heart-and peripheral arteries disease can be identified in nearly all cases [3].

FG can be idiopathic, may result from perineal and genital skin infections, or can occur following genitourinary procedures or trauma. In approximately 95% of cases, a source of infection can be identified. The most common source of infection is urethral stricture, perianal abscesses or fissures, and fistulas [4].

The most frequent cause of ischemic penile gangrene is diabetes mellitus with end-stage renal disease leading to secondary hyperparathyroidism. This condition may cause calciphylaxis of penile arteries, leading to a decreased blood flow. It is important to exclude this diagnosis in uremic patients [5].

Fournier's gangrene is an absolute emergency because the time interval between diagnosis and treatment significantly influences morbidity and mortality. Ischemic gangrene of the male genitalia is a hallmark of severe systemic vascular disease. Because of poor blood flow leading to anoxia and inflammation, any ischemic lesion can become infected, leading to FG.

Foul, feculent odor with soft-tissue crepitation is the classical finding. Prompt surgical debridement is the norm and, if needed, suprapubic cystostomy should be performed. The definitive management is either partial or total penectomy depending upon the extent of involvement. A permanent perineal urethrostomy is needed in patients undergoing total penectomy. Diabetes with penile gangrene has a high mortality rate [6].

The treatment options for dry gangrene include surgical intervention or observation while awaiting autoamputation of the demarcated tissue. Patients with atherosclerosis, resulting from underlying diabetes mellitus and chronic renal failure, are predisposed to infection and often have extensive history of hospitalization. Weiner et al. noted 57% mortality rate in their seven patients within 6 months after initial presentation. Stein et al. noted 71% mortality rate in their series at 6 months of follow-up [7, 8].

In certain cases of FG, an early palliative care approach is required to improve the quality of life of the patient. We report a case of localized FG of the penis, which required different treatment options, and PC.

2. Case Report

2.1. Patient Information. A 53-year-old Caucasian (Syrian) patient, with poorly controlled diabetes mellitus type 2 and chronic renal insufficiency stage 3, was admitted to the nephrology department because of progressive kidney failure. His medical history was significant for left ischemic stroke with sequential right hemiparesis, arteritis of the lower limbs requiring amputation of the right leg, ischemic heart disease and coronary artery bypass grafting (CABG), long-standing arterial hypertension, and chronic obstructive pulmonary disease (COPD).

2.2. Clinical Evolution and Treatment. On the day of admission, the patient complained of pain in the penile region. A chronic indwelling urinary catheter was already in place for management of urine voiding.

A physical examination revealed a whitish liquid from the urinary meatus. The patient had a lot of pain with an estimated visual analog scale (VAS) of 8. However, because of a total language barrier, it was difficult to grasp the exact sensation. At that moment, no penile skin lesion was observed. There were no signs of inflammation or erythema. The urinary catheter seemed to provoke a painful sensation; a bladder spasm was not excluded.

Laboratory investigations at presentation were significant for serum creatinine of 4.5 mg/dL (0.7–1.2) with an estimated glomerular filtration rate of 14 ml/min/1.73 m^2 using MDRD equation, phosphate, 1.2 mmol/L (0.75–1.39); calcium, 2.26 mg/dl (2.15–2.50); albumin, 21 g/L (40–49); parathyroid hormone, 111 ng/L (>49 for end-stage renal disease (ESRD)); vitamin D, <5 μg/L (30–60); hemoglobin, 8 g/dL (13–18); HbA1c, 8.3% (4–6); and C-reactive protein (CRP), 38.5 mg/L (<5).

Urine culture grew *Staphylococcus epidermidis* (<20.000 col/ml).

The urologists suggested anticholinergics and a local antiseptic solution. Painkillers were prescribed.

One week later, a very painful, rapidly progressing lesion appeared on the anterior part of glans penis (Figure 1). The ulcer was covered with a thick layer of fibrin. The greenish coloration was suggestive for a *Pseudomonas* infection. The ulcer could be due to a traumatic wound caused by the urinary catheter, but necrosis was not excluded. The patient became agitated and developed a fever (38°C).

The laboratory examination showed elevated CRP (341 mg/L). Hemocultures were collected, and empiric antimicrobial therapy (ceftriazone) was administered parenterally.

Despite antibiotics, the patient remained febrile, and he was malnourished (BMI 18) and septic. Antimicrobial therapy was adapted by the infectiologists in order to cover a *Pseudomonas* infection, and amoxicillin + ceftazidime was prescribed.

Due to worsening of the patient's general condition, a computed tomography (CT) of the abdomen and pelvis was done and showed a global infiltration with air bubbles in the penile soft tissues reflecting gangrene. No air bubbles were visible inside the corpora cavernosa, and no infiltration of the perineum was seen (Figure 2).

The diagnosis of localized FG of the penis was primarily based on clinical findings. The common laboratory findings were nonspecific. CT scan helped in the diagnosis and evaluation of the extent of the disease to guide appropriate surgical treatment.

Because of extensive local necrosis, a chirurgical penile debridement was done, and 1/3 of the glans penis was amputated.

Histopathological examination revealed acute and chronic inflammation and extensive necrotic tissue with the presence of microorganisms (secondary infection), and no calcification of the arterial walls was seen. Diagnosis of isolated Fournier's penile gangrene was confirmed.

Hemocultures confirmed the infection with *Pseudomonas aeruginosa*. Antibiotics were adapted once again according to the results of blood cultures; a combination of Méropénéme-Colimycine-Metronidazole was prescribed.

Due to progressive necrosis of the penile shaft, the patient underwent subsequent debridations at the end a total resection of penile skin tissue, necrotized tissue, the ventral side of the glans, and resection of the necrotized part of the urethra. The patient and his family were informed of the risk of partial or total penectomy. A suprapubic catheter was placed during the second debridement (Figure 3).

Hyperbaric oxygen therapy was suggested, but because of his poor general condition (Karnofsky index 20) and frequent restlessness, this treatment could not be carried out.

Once more, the unfavorable clinical evolution was discussed with the patient and his family. They were told that, due to advanced renal insufficiency with diffuse arterial

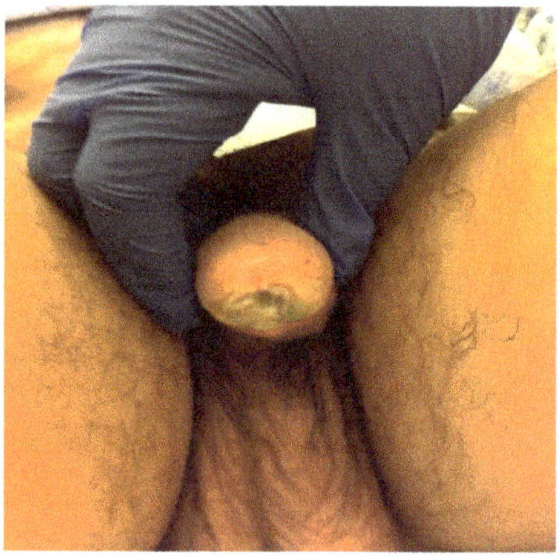

Figure 1: A rapidly progressing lesion appearing on the anterior part of the glans penis.

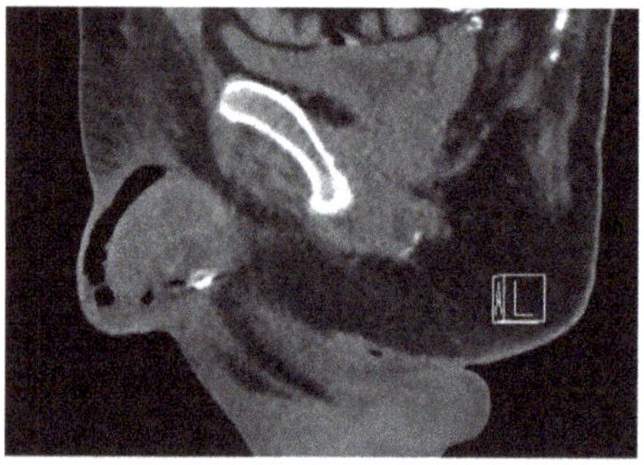

Figure 2: Computed tomography (CT) of the abdomen and pelvis: significant infiltration of the whole of the penis until its origin and its periphery at the pubic level, with many air bubbles within it. No infiltration of the perineum. Diffuse calcified atheromatous. Fournier gangrene located at the penis level.

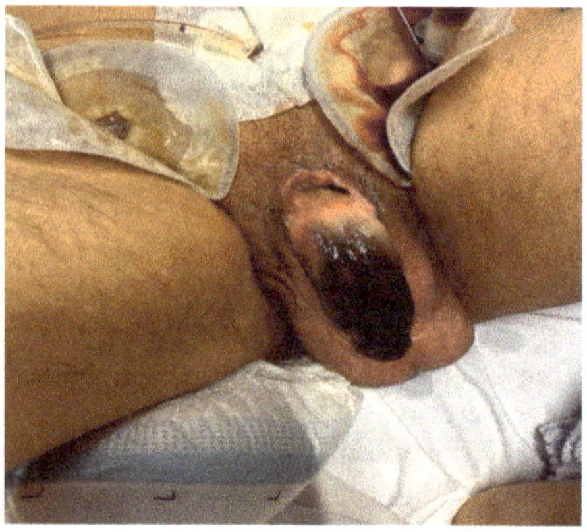

Figure 3: Due to progressive local necrosis, several debridations under narcosis were done, and a suprapubic catheter was placed.

disease and irreversible vascular penile necrosis, amputation of the penis spontaneously or surgically was inevitable.

Daily clinical worsening of the patient's condition, mental confusion with almost complete loss of contact was noted. The patient remained often in fetal position under his blanket, and he refused intake per os. Enteral or parenteral feeding/treatment became impossible because the patient tore off gastric tubes as well as perfusion catheters.

After multidisciplinary discussion, it was decided that this patient should rapidly benefit from a palliative care approach to make this patient's end-of-life comfortable. Due to language barrier, direct communication with the patient and his family was impossible. With support of an interpreter and an intercultural mediator, a meeting was organized with the family and palliative care (PC) team to discuss the patient's pernicious prognosis and the palliative setting in order to transfer the patient to the PC unit. At first, the family was reticent to this approach despite several attempts during the past two weeks to explain the difficult and serious medical condition; they found it difficult to accept the bad outcome. After several meetings, agreement between the family and the PC team was obtained; the patient was admitted to the PC unit. He died 2 days later.

3. Discussion

Following the poor clinical evolution of the penile gangrene in our patient despite treatment with antibiotics and several surgical debridements, the palliative care approach was required to improve the quality of end-of-life in our patient.

3.1. Comfort Therapy and Palliative Care. Historically, palliative care was focused on patients with incurable cancer. However, the current view is that access to palliative care should be based on need rather than diagnosis and so, many patients with nonmalignant diseases qualify as well [9, 10].

The general aim of palliative care is improving quality of life of patients and families, to help them adjusting to progressive disease and to improve care and patient-centered outcome.

One of the most important barriers for introducing palliative care is the lack of validated and practical tools to identify patients in need.

In 2002, Belgium adopted a legal framework for taking care of life's end: "The Act of 14 June 2002 on palliative care," which grants all citizens the right to palliative care in the context of support throughout the end-of-life.

Recently, a tool was developed to identify persons with palliative care needs in the population or in specific settings or conditions. This "Palliative Care Indicator Tool" (PICT) was included in "the Official Gazette" (het Belgisch staatsblad) on November 20, 2018 (M.B. 20/11/2018-A.R. du 21/10/2018).

This PICT is a guide to identifying people at risk of deteriorating health and dying. It has 6 general indicators of deteriorating health and clinical signs of advanced, progressive, underlying conditions. It helps professionals identify people for care planning. The first question is "would you be surprised if your patient died within the next 6 to 12 months?" This new index allows extending significantly the number of individuals admitted to palliative care. What will happen to each person and when is often uncertain? The PICT does not give a "prognosis" or a time frame [11].

Palliative care demands an active participation of patients, family, and team(s) in shared decision-making. Multidisciplinary and multidimensional approach is needed to identify values and preferences and to make an advance care planning. Good care for people with advanced illnesses is based on a person-centered, multidimensional (physical, emotional, social, and spiritual), and respectful care practiced by a competent interdisciplinary team.

3.2. *In Our Patient Case*

(1) This process took several days, partly influenced by cultural differences: his family could not accept the poor clinical outcome. After repeated discussion, they understood the palliative approach and accepted a transfer to a palliative care unit.

(2) His symptoms and pain were exacerbated significantly by emotional and psychological distress because of a language barrier (he only spoke Syrian). Moreover, the patient showed episodes of confusion, and direct contact with him was very difficult.

This type of complex situations emphasizes the need for multidisciplinary team involvement to address all aspects of his physical, psychological, social, and spiritual well-being [12].

Although excellent pain control was only achieved in the last days of life, a combined approach involving surgical colleagues, renal physicians, anesthetists, and palliative care physicians was essential to optimize symptom control.

Our patient's pain was exacerbated due to emotional and psychological distress because he could not communicate with us. He had been through mutilating surgery, but was not improving. It was difficult for his family to accept his condition. These situations require collaboration with interpreters and intercultural mediators.

Patients with nonmalignant diseases but life-limiting diseases, such as advanced respiratory diseases, advanced cardiac disease, advanced neurological diseases, frailty, and end-stage renal disease (ESRD), unlike patients with malignant diseases experience a low proportion of PC consultations and intense care at the end-of-life despite significant morbidity and mortality in these populations [9, 10]. This also applies to some patients with FG, whose pain is difficult to control and have poor short-time prognosis.

Family-reported quality of end-of-life care was significantly better for cancer and dementia patients than for patients with ESRD, cardiopulmonary failure, or frailty, largely due to higher rates of palliative care consultation and do-not-resuscitate orders and fewer intensive care unit (ICU) deaths among cancer and dementia patients. Increasing access to PC and goals-of-care discussion that addresses code status and preferred setting of death, particularly for patients with end-organ failure and frailty, may improve the overall quality of end-of-life care for patients dying of these illnesses [13].

Our case presentation highlights the need for improved integration of PC services into care of FG patients to improve quality of EOL care.

4. Conclusion

Isolated Fournier's penile gangrene is associated with significant morbidity and mortality. Despite prompt intervention, FG can rapidly evolve into progressive tissue destruction, sepsis and ultimately death as observed in our patient who had multiple comorbidities.

Pain control is very important in this situation and it demands a multidisciplinary team approach. Palliative care consultation should be programmed early to control symptoms and to support the family.

This case report highlights the need for improved integration of PC services into care for patients to improve quality of end of live (EOL) care.

Disclosure

This article does not contain any studies with human participants or animals performed by any of the authors.

Authors' Contributions

Each author contributed important intellectual participation during manuscript drafting or revision.

Acknowledgments

The authors thank the nursing staff of the nephrology ward of CHU-Brugmann.

References

[1] A. Obi, "Isolated Fournier's gangrene of the penis," *Nigerian Journal of Clinical Practice*, vol. 19, no. 3, pp. 426–443, 2016.

[2] M. Moussa and M. Abou Chakra, "Isolated Penile Fournier's gangrene: a case report and literature review," *International Journal of Surgery Case Reports*, vol. 62, pp. 65–68, 2019.

[3] A. Katsimantas, N. Ferakis, P. Skandalakis, and D. Filippou, "A rare case of localized isolated penile Fournier's gangrene and a short review of the literature," *Case Reports in Urology*, vol. 2018, Article ID 5135616, 2018.

[4] A. Talwar, N. Puri, and M. Singh, "Fournier's gangrene of the penis: a rare entity," *Journal of Cutaneous and Aesthetic Surgery*, vol. 3, no. 1, pp. 41–44, 2010.

[5] H. S. Jeong and A. R. Dominguez, "Calciphylaxis: controversies in pathogenesis, diagnosis and treatment," *The American Journal of the Medical Sciences*, vol. 351, no. 2, pp. 217–227, 2016.

[6] S. Vishwajeet, R. J. Sinha, and SN. Sankhwar, "Penile gangrene: a devastating and lethal entity," *Saudi Journal of Kidney Diseases and Transplantation*, vol. 22, no. 2, pp. 359–361, 2011.

[7] D. M. Weiner and F. C. Lowe, "Surgical management of ischemic penile gangrene in diabetics with end stage atherosclerosis," *Journal of Urology*, vol. 155, no. 3, pp. 926–929, 1996.

[8] M. Stein, C. Anderson, R. Ricciardi, J. W. Chamberlin, S. E. Lerner, and D. Glicklich, "Penile gangrene associated

with chronic renal failure: report of 7 cases and review of the literature," *Journal of Urology*, vol. 152, no. 6 Part 1, pp. 2014–2016, 1994.
[9] T. O'Brien, J. Welsh, and F. G. Dunn, "ABC of palliative care non-malignant conditions," *BMJ*, vol. 316, no. 24, 1998.
[10] H. P. Dharmasena and K. Forbes, "Palliative care for patients with non-malignant disease: will hospital physicians refer?" *Palliative Medicine*, vol. 15, no. 5, pp. 413–418, 2001.
[11] G. Highet, D. Crawford, S. A. Murray, and K. Boydl, "Development and evaluation of the supportive and palliative care indicators tool (SPICT): a mixed-methods study," *BMJ Supportive & Palliative Care*, vol. 0, pp. 1–6, 2013.
[12] A. Rich, A. Leach, and J. Ellershaw, "Case of difficult pain in a patient with chronic renal failure and calciphylaxis," *Journal of Pain and Symptom Management*, vol. 22, no. 1, 2001.
[13] M. W. Wachterman, C. Pilver, D. Smith, M. Ersek, S. R. Lipsitz, and N. L. Keating, "Quality of end-of-life care provided to patients with different serious illnesses," *JAMA Internal Medicine*, vol. 176, no. 8, pp. 1095–1102, 2016.

28

Accessory Renal Artery Stenosis and Secondary Hypertension

Ariel A. Chung and Patricia R. Millner

Department of Family Medicine, Tripler Army Medical Center, Honolulu, HI 96859, USA

Correspondence should be addressed to Ariel A. Chung; ariel.a.chung.mil@mail.mil

Academic Editor: Ze'ev Korzets

Background. Secondary hypertension is an uncommon cause of hypertension with extensive workup not recommended in most patients; however, further evaluation is generally recommended in young patients presenting with hypertension. *Case Presentation.* A 31-year-old female presented with history of elevated blood pressures. Secondary hypertension workup revealed no laboratory abnormalities; however, renal artery ultrasound demonstrated a left superior accessory artery and suspected bilateral renal vein congestion that was further evaluated with renal CT with contrast. Renal CT showed ostial stenosis of the left accessory renal artery. In addition, compression of the left renal vein between aorta and superior mesenteric artery was also noted, consistent with nutcracker syndrome. Hypertension was suspected to be secondary to stenosis of the accessory renal artery. Upon consultation with interventional radiology, pharmacologic treatment was recommended, and blood pressure control was ultimately achieved with a single agent. *Discussion.* Renovascular etiologies are responsible for 1% of cases of mild hypertension and up to 45% of severe hypertension. Accessory renal arteries are a normal anatomical variant in approximately 30% of the population. Secondary hypertension due to stenosis of an accessory renal artery is rare with very few cases described in case reports. *Conclusion.* Though hypertension secondary to accessory renal artery stenosis is rare and not well published in medical literature, few case reports, including this one, demonstrate that accessory renal artery stenosis can be an underlying etiology of hypertension.

1. Background

Hypertension is a common diagnosis in the United States, affecting approximately 30% of adults; however, secondary hypertension is uncommon and responsible for only 5–10% of cases [1, 2]. Hypertension due to secondary causes is more common in the younger population; however, it can occur in all ages [2]. The most common etiologies of secondary hypertension vary by age and include renal parenchymal disease, renal artery stenosis, coarctation of the aorta, thyroid dysfunction, hyperaldosteronism, obstructive sleep apnea, Cushing's syndrome, and pheochromocytoma [2]. Evaluation for secondary causes of hypertension is generally not recommended in all individuals presenting with elevated blood pressure but should be considered in patients with severe or resistant hypertension, presence of end organ damage, or onset before 30 years of age [2].

2. Case Presentation

A 31-year-old female presented for a routine clinic visit with her primary care physician and was found to have an elevated blood pressure of 150/100 that was sustained on repeat measurement. Upon further questioning, the patient reported history of elevated blood pressure readings over the past 7 years and was lost to follow up. Past medical history was significant for migraine headaches and the patient had no past surgical history. Current medications included rizatriptan and ibuprofen were used as needed for headaches, approximately 2–3 times per year, and levonorgestrel IUD for contraception. Family history was notable for maternal and paternal grandparents with hypertension and mother with hypothyroidism. The patient was a nonsmoker with occasional alcohol use. BMI was 19. Physical exam was unremarkable.

24-hour ambulatory blood pressure monitoring was performed and confirmed the diagnosis of hypertension. Due to the patient's age, a secondary hypertension workup was initiated. Laboratory evaluation included complete blood count, basic metabolic panel, and thyrotropin that showed no abnormalities; plasma aldosterone and renin were within normal limits at 2.9 and 1.069, respectively; urinalysis showed 1+ protein with protein/creatinine ratio 0.44. Renal ultrasound was performed and showed presence of left accessory renal artery and the appearance of bilateral renal vein congestion. Bilateral main renal arteries showed no signs of stenosis. Renal CT with contrast was recommended for further evaluation of renal vasculature due to appearance of renal vein congestion and showed ostial stenosis of the left accessory renal artery (Figures 1–3). In addition, compression of the left renal vein between aorta and superior mesenteric artery was also noted, consistent with nutcracker syndrome (Figures 2 and 4).

The cause of hypertension in this 31-year-old female was suspected to be due to stenosis of the left accessory renal artery that was identified on imaging. Interventional radiology was consulted and recommended trial of pharmacologic treatment before pursuing angiography or revascularization. An antihypertensive regimen was initiated with nifedipine extended release 30 mg that was discontinued due to side effects of headaches and lower extremity edema. Nifedipine was replaced with amlodipine 10 mg; however, amlodipine at maximum dose did not achieve desired blood pressure goal. Lisinopril 5 mg was added to the regimen at this time with subsequent improvement of blood pressure; however, the patient experienced several episodes of presyncope likely due to orthostatic hypotension. Amlodipine was discontinued and lisinopril dose was increased to 10 mg and desired blood pressure goal was achieved without significant side effects.

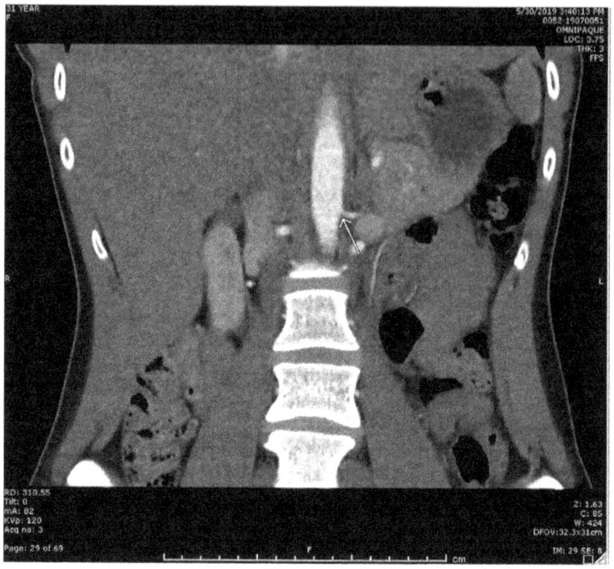

FIGURE 1: Coronal image from renal CT with contrast showing the area of ostial stenosis of left accessory renal artery.

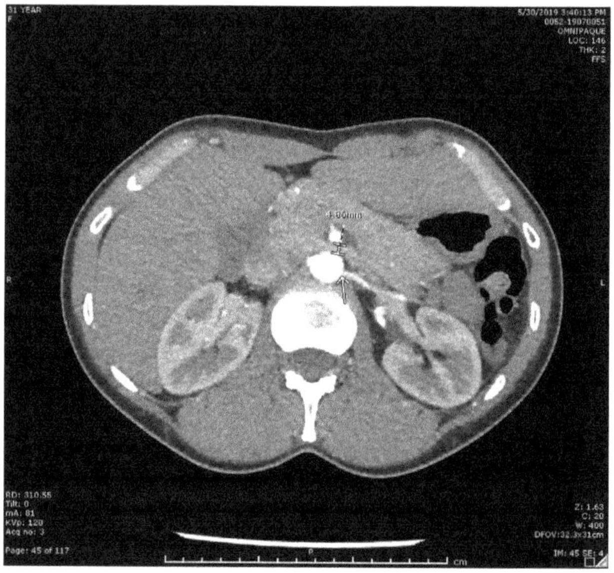

FIGURE 2: Axial image from renal CT with contrast showing the area of ostial stenosis of left accessory renal artery and compression of left renal vein between aorta and superior mesenteric artery.

3. Discussion

Renovascular hypertension is responsible for approximately 1% of cases of mild hypertension and approximately 10–45% of severe cases [3, 4]. The two main etiologies of renal artery stenosis are atherosclerosis and fibromuscular dysplasia [4]. Hypertension due to renal artery stenosis is the result of activation of the renin-angiotensin-aldosterone system due to renal ischemia [4]. The standard for diagnosis is invasive angiography; however, ultrasonography, magnetic resonance angiography (MRA), and CT angiography (CTA) are preferred as noninvasive initial studies [4]. Potential treatment options include pharmacologic as well as revascularization, with revascularization typically reserved for patients with hypertension refractory to antihypertensive medications or progressive worsening of renal function [4].

Accessory renal arteries are a normal anatomic variant in approximately 30% of the population [5]. Hypertension due to stenosis of an accessory renal artery in the absence of stenosis of the main renal arteries is exceedingly rare, with very few cases described in case reports. To the best of our knowledge, there are only two case reports that exist in published literature that describe patients with elevated blood pressure and secondary hypertension workup notable for stenosis of an accessory renal artery.

Zeina et al. describe a case of a 35-year-old female with resistant hypertension despite regimen with multiple antihypertensive agents [6]. Invasive angiography was performed and showed stenosis of an accessory renal artery with an appearance consistent with fibromuscular dysplasia [6]. Revascularization with balloon angioplasty was performed with subsequent improvement in blood pressure and the ability to achieve desired blood pressure goal with a single antihypertensive agent [6].

Akbeyaz et al. describe a case of a 13-year-old female with hypertension secondary to stenosis of an accessory

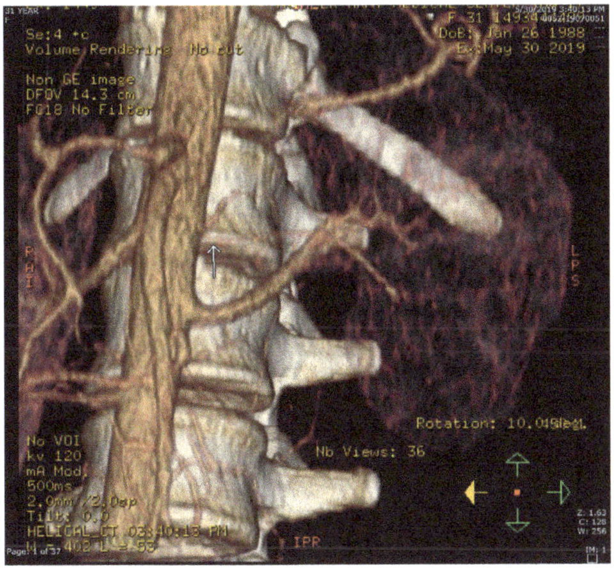

FIGURE 3: 3D image from renal CT with contrast showing the area of ostial stenosis of left accessory renal artery.

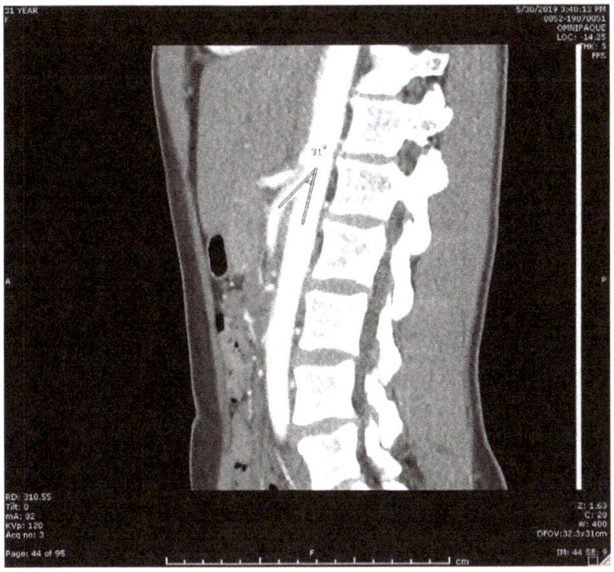

FIGURE 4: Sagittal image from renal CT with contrast showing decreased angle between aorta and superior mesenteric artery.

renal artery identified on renal ultrasound and confirmed on CT angiography [7]. The patient received antihypertensive pharmacologic treatment and blood pressure goal was achieved [7]. At routine follow-up two months later, it was discovered that the patient's blood pressure was much lower than previous measurements and antihypertensive treatment was gradually tapered and discontinued [7]. Repeat renal ultrasound was performed and the accessory artery could no longer be visualized [7]. Spontaneous collapse of the vessel was suspected [7]. The patient remained normotensive and did not require any additional treatment [7].

In our case, the patient was also a young female with hypertension suspected to be due to the accessory renal artery stenosis that was discovered on imaging. In contrast, our patient received renal CT with contrast. This imaging modality is not typically recommended to evaluate stenosis of renal arteries; however, this study was recommended to further evaluate bilateral renal vein congestion that was seen on renal ultrasound and incidentally discovered stenosis of the left accessory renal artery. Imaging also revealed compression of the left renal vein between aorta and superior mesenteric artery consistent with nutcracker syndrome. We considered nutcracker syndrome as a possible etiology of the patient's hypertension due to a small number of published case reports that suggested that hypertension may be a rare symptom of nutcracker syndrome [8–11]. However, in the vast majority of these cases, the patients presented with additional symptoms that are commonly associated with nutcracker syndrome including flank pain and hematuria [8–11]. Due to the absence of additional symptoms in our patient, we suggest that stenosis of the accessory renal artery is the most likely etiology of the patient's hypertension. Our patient's hypertension was ultimately controlled on one antihypertensive agent and did not require further invasive testing or intervention.

4. Conclusion

Though hypertension secondary to accessory renal artery stenosis is rare and not well published in medical literature, few case reports, including this one, demonstrate that accessory renal artery stenosis can be an underlying etiology of hypertension.

Disclosure

The views expressed in this article are those of the authors and do not reflect the official policy or position of the Department of the Army, Department of Defense, or the U.S. Government.

References

[1] C. D. Fryar, Y. Ostchega, C. M. Hales, G. Zhang, and D. Kruszon-Moran, "Hypertension prevalence and control among adults: united states, 2015–2016," *NCHS Data Brief*, vol. 289, pp. 1–8, 2017.

[2] S. F. Rimoldi, U. Scherrer, and F. H. Messerli, "Secondary arterial hypertension: when, who, and how to screen?" *European Heart Journal*, vol. 35, no. 19, pp. 1245–1254, 2014.

[3] A. Lewin, M. D. Blaufox, H. Castle, G. Entwisle, and H. Langford, "Apparent prevalence of curable hypertension in the hypertension detection and follow-up program," *Archives of Internal Medicine*, vol. 145, no. 3, pp. 424–427, 1985.

[4] S. C. Textor and L. Lerman, "Renovascular hypertension and ischemic nephropathy," *American Journal of Hypertension*, vol. 23, no. 11, pp. 1159–1169, 2010.
[5] E. Gulas, G. Wysiadecki, T. Cecot et al., "Accessory (multiple) renal arteries - differences in frequency according to population, visualizing techniques and stage of morphological development," *Vascular*, vol. 24, no. 5, pp. 531–537, 2016.
[6] A. Zeina, W. Vladimir, and E. Barmeir, "Fibromuscular dysplasia in an accessory renal artery causing renovascular hypertension: a case report," *Journal of Medical Care Reports*, vol. 1, no. 58, 2007.
[7] I. H. Akbeyaz, A. Tirosh, C. Robinson et al., "Spontaneously resolving hyperreninemic hypertension caused by accessory renal artery stenosis in a 13-year-old girl: a case report," *The Journal of Clinical Hypertension*, vol. 19, no. 1, pp. 100–102, 2017.
[8] Y. Hosotani, H. Kiyomoto, H. Fujioka, N. Takahashi, and M. Kohno, "The nutcracker phenomenon accompanied by renin-dependent hypertension," *The American Journal of Medicine*, vol. 114, no. 7, pp. 617-618, 2003.
[9] A. Mazarakis, G. Almpanis, N. Tragotsalou, D. Karnabatidis, and C. Fourtounas, "Is hypertension a manifestation of the nutcracker phenomenon/syndrome? Case report and brief review of the literature," *Hippokratia*, vol. 16, pp. 187–189, 2012.
[10] N. Narkhede, A. Deokar, K. Mehta, and N. Kamat, "Nutcracker syndrome with hypertension as an unusual initial presentation," *Indian Journal of Nephrology*, vol. 27, no. 6, p. 472, 2017.
[11] A. Azhar, N. Zeb, S. Shah, and A. Khalid, "Nutcracker syndrome with hypertension: a case report," *Cureus*, vol. 11, no. 5, e4781 pages, 2019.

29

Focal Segmental Glomerulosclerosis and Scheduled Pretransplant Plasmapheresis: A Timely Diagnosis of Nail-Patella Syndrome Avoided More Futile Immunosuppression

H. Trimarchi

Nephrology Service, Hospital Británico de Buenos Aires, Buenos Aires, Argentina

Correspondence should be addressed to H. Trimarchi; htrimarchi@hotmail.com

Academic Editor: Salih Kavukcu

Focal and segmental glomerulosclerosis (FSGS) is a histopathological pattern of injury. As such, it encompasses a wide variety of dissimilar entities with different pathophysiologic mechanisms. Although ultrastructural morphological characteristics can specifically diagnose certain diseases and genetic mutations can also be unravelled, this ideal situation is generally not available worldwide. In this respect, when proteinuria with or without nephrotic syndrome is encountered and FSGS is the histological lesion, patients start to be prescribed different regimes of immunosuppression, which should only be indicated in cases of primary FSGS, a rare entity that is elusive to response and can hardly be precisely diagnosed. We present a 35-year-old female patient with a life-long diagnosis of FSGS and a heavy burden of immunosuppressants, which had been unable to manage the persistent proteinuria that eventually led to end-stage kidney disease. She was referred to us to organize the kidney transplant. Plasmapheresis had been previously suggested to her to prevent the relapse of primary FSGS. A genetic test disclosed that the patient was heterozygous for LMX1B, and the diagnosis of nail-patella syndrome was made. In this entity, immunosuppression is not indicated, and there is no recurrence of the disease in the transplanted allograft.

1. Introduction

Focal and segmental glomerulosclerosis (FSGS) is not a disease. It is a histologic pattern of injury with several morphological variants that reflects the repairing mechanisms employed in response to past and/or present insults received by the kidney. It has been classically classified as primary or secondary [1, 2]. The origin of these insults is quite diverse. In the case of primary FSGS, it includes circulating factors mainly secreted by neutrophils or mononuclear cells that affect the podocyte. In secondary FSGS, it encompasses mutations of genes that codify podocyte proteins, hyperfiltration settings such as obesity, reduced nephron mass, vesical-ureteral reflux, drepanocytosis, certain drugs as biphosphonates and cocaine, and HIV, among others [3]. The clinical picture is generally more aggressive in primary FSGS, where nephrotic syndrome is prevalent and a progressive decline in glomerular filtration rate is faster than in secondary FSGS, where proteinuria is generally lower than the nephrotic range. Nephroprotection is indicated in both primary and secondary FSGS. However, management of primary FSGS is mainly based on immunosuppression, with a discrete rate of successful response, while the secondary forms approach is mainly based on treating the primary cause [4]. Finally, approximately 30–55% of primary FSGS cases recur in the transplant with a high rate of graft loss, while most of secondary causes do not recur [5].

Genetic causes of FSGS due to mutations in podocyte proteins are frequently not diagnosed due to the lack of access to these genetic studies, and subdiagnosis exists. While some cases appear clinically soon after birth with severe nephrotic syndrome and renal failure, as it occurs with mutations in nephrin, other cases must be suspected early in childhood, as is the case of mutations in podocin, CD2-associated protein (CD2AP), and actinin-IV [6]. Finally, others manifest in later adolescence or early adulthood, as transient receptor potential cation channel subfamily C member 6 (TRPC6) and Wilms' tumor 1 (WT-1) [6]. The amount of proteinuria varies, generally increasing with age and reaching high levels, but nephrotic syndrome is not as frequent as in primary FSGS. In general, there are no pathognomonic features that determine the cause of FSGS in optic microscopy, while immunofluorescence is not contributory. Electron microscopy may be diagnostic in some cases and is not always available. Thus, the precise diagnosis of FSGS is mandatory, particularly to distinguish primary from genetic causes. In this work, we present a case that was assumed as primary FSGS for over 30 years of age, and the patient had been treated with different and aggressive immunosuppressive regimes with poor results. In fact, plasmapheresis was scheduled for the forthcoming peritransplant period. The patient was referred to our unit. A genetic study was asked, and the diagnosis of nail-patella syndrome was made due to a mutation in *LMX1B*. Immunosuppression has no place in the treatment of this cause of secondary FSGS.

2. Case Presentation

A 35-year-old female with a history of chronic proteinuria since early childhood was assessed due to end-stage kidney disease. She lacked a family history of chronic renal disease. At the age of 5 years, with a 2.9 g/day of proteinuria, she was empirically prescribed meprednisone 1 mg/kg/day for 12 weeks and, then, tapered down, without response. She was first biopsied at the age of 9 due to 3.9 g/day of proteinuria and normal kidney function without nephrotic syndrome. She was started on a low-protein and low sodium diet and enalapril at a dose of 5 mg twice daily. The kidney biopsy disclosed focal and segmental glomerulosclerosis and minimal interstitial fibrosis and tubular atrophy. Secondary causes were discarded, and since then, she had been prescribed different immunosuppression regimes that included steroids, cyclophosphamide, cyclosporine, and tacrolimus along her life. All the treatments failed to reduce proteinuria, which on the contrary, progressively increased until adulthood. Her glomerulosclerosis was filiated as primary. She was biopsied again at the age of 29 with a glomerular filtration rate of 55 mL/min and 6 g/day of proteinuria. The biopsy revealed 8 obliterated glomeruli plus focal and segmental glomerulosclerosis with segmental hyalinosis of the glomerular tuft in the remaining 9 glomeruli, plus a 40% of interstitial fibrosis. She was referred to our clinic at the age of 34 for a second opinion, as a kidney transplant had been counselled in another hospital, where plasmapheresis was to be performed as part of the induction therapy, with her father as the potential donor. We first indicated a genetic assessment of the glomerulosclerotic pattern, as the diagnosis of primary glomerulosclerosis appeared doubtful. The genetic study, performed with sequence analysis and copy number variation analysis of a panel of podocyte genes informed that the patient was heterozygous for *LMX1B* c.737G > A, p. (Arg246Gln), which was classified as pathogenic (Blueprint Genetics Oy, Keilaranta 16 A-B, 02150 Espoo, Finland). The molecular diagnosis of nail-patella syndrome was made. Knee and elbow X-Rays were normal, ophthalmologic evaluation discarded glaucoma, and nail features were unremarkable. The patient has recently been started on hemodialysis. She has recently received a kidney transplant from her father, in whom the genetic assessment had been previously made and the mutation was not encountered. The initial prescription of plasmapheresis as part of the induction approach to the transplant therapy was obviously discarded.

3. Discussion

In the present report, it is underscored that FSGS is a morphological pattern of injury that does not necessarily implie the necessity to employ immunosuppression despite elevated proteinuria, as commonly observed. The diagnosis of secondary causes of FSGS as genetic mutations is mandatory to undertake specific therapeutic indications and genetic counselling.

Focal and segmental glomerulosclerosis describes a distortion of the normal glomerular architecture characterized by a certain number of glomeruli with different degrees of sclerosis while others remain normal. The histological Columbia classification of FSGS identified five morphological variants of primary and secondary forms with dissimilar frequencies of diagnosis: (a) not otherwise specified form (NOS) or "classic FSGS" (68%of cases); (b) tip variant or tip lesion, with the sclerotic lesion next to the proximal tubule (10% of cases); (c) cellular variant with segmental endocapillary hypercellularity (3%); (d) perihilar variant, with perihilar hyalinosis and sclerosis in >50% of the glomeruli with segmental lesions (7%); and (e) collapsing variant, which requires at least a single glomerulus with a collapsing lesion, defined as segmental or global collapse of the tuft with overlying visceral epithelial cell hyperplasia (12%) [1, 2].

Segmental sclerosis lesions are consequently heterogeneous, and the different morphological variants may shed some light onto the many different pathogenetic pathways that share the unspecific morphology of FSGS. In this respect, the broad-based scars suggest previous healed necrotizing lesions; perihilar segmental sclerosis and hyalinosis are hallmarks of adaptive haemodynamic changes; visceral epithelial hyperplasia and hypertrophy and tip lesions are markers of podocyte injury, known as podocytopathies [2, 7].

Podocyte mutations can lead to FSGS and to alterations in the normal glomerular filtration barrier, clinically characterized by varying degrees of proteinuria and a progressive decrease in renal function [3, 6]. A rare cause of FSGS is the nail-patella syndrome.

The nail-patella syndrome or osteo-onychodysplasia that the reported patient presents is a rare autosomal dominant disorder with full gene penetrance but variability of expression within families, characterized by limb and pelvic skeletal abnormalities as hypoplastic or absent patella, dysplasia of elbows, iliac horns, nail and distal digital abnormalities, sensorineural hearing loss, ophthalmological abnormalities including glaucoma, gastrointestinal dysmotility, and kidney disease. The estimated incidence of nail-patella syndrome is estimated to be 1 per 50,000 [8–11].

Approximately 85 percent of families with nail-patella syndrome present with mutations of the *LMX1B* gene located at the distal end of the long arm of chromosome 9 [12]. LMX1B is a transcription factor of the LIM-homeodomain type that plays an important role for limb and renal development in vertebrates; however, it is expressed lifelong within the podocyte, and it is essential for the maintenance of the structured actin cytoskeleton in podocytes [13]. The identification of complete *LMX1B* deletions confirms that haploinsufficiency is the principal pathogenetic mechanism of nail-patella syndrome. Studies in homozygous knock-out mice and *in vitro* assays demonstrated that *LMX1B* protein expressed in glomerular podocytes helps control the transcription of multiple genes integral for proper glomerular basement membrane formation and/or glomerular podocyte differentiation and function during the early stages of renal development [12]. Putative target genes include *COL4A3* and *COLA4*, genes for alpha-4 chains of collagen type IV, and *NPHS2* and *CD2AP* genes, which encode podocyte proteins podocin and CD2-associated protein (CD2AP), respectively [14, 15].

In addition, there are case reports of *LMX1B* mutation (R246 or R249 missense mutations) associated with familial focal segmental glomerulosclerosis (FSGS), but without any other clinical features of nail-patella syndrome [16–18]. As in our patient, the kidney appears to be the only clinically affected organ, but her biological parents lacked the mutation, suggesting a spontaneous or *de novo* mutation. Renal biopsy is not necessary if the diagnosis is confirmed by genetic testing. However, if electron microscopy is performed, besides podocyte foot-process effacement, unique or pathognomonic changes in the kidney comprise focal or diffuse thickening of the glomerular basement membrane, with electron-lucent areas containing bundles of type III collagen alternating with areas of fibrillar inclusions in the glomerular basement membrane, giving a "moth-eaten appearance" [6]. In mice, the splitting of the glomerular basement membrane and the reduced number of endothelial fenestrations have been observed because podocytes synthesize proteins of the glomerular basement membrane and control differentiation of glomerular endothelial cells, as the vascular endothelial growth factor (VEGF) [6]. There is no clear relationship between the clinical course and renal histopathology [19], and findings on renal biopsy appear not to alter the clinical management [20, 21].

Renal involvement in nail-patella syndrome can be a significant threat to the quality of life in patients. Urinary abnormalities often manifest as asymptomatic proteinuria (20–30% of cases) or hematuria, but it can progress to end-stage renal disease, even during early childhood [10, 19]. Most affected individuals manifest only an accelerated age-related loss of filtration function, and development of symptomatic kidney failure is rare [19, 21]. However, a small minority (5–10%) of individuals with NPS develop nephrotic-range proteinuria as early as childhood or young adulthood and progress to end-stage kidney failure over variable periods of time [19, 21]. The severity of the nephropathy is extremely variable both within and between families, suggesting that genetic, epigenetic or environmental factors might modulate the severity of the nephropathy [19]. The prevalence of nephropathy has been reported to vary widely between 10–40% of individuals with nail-patella syndrome [10, 11, 19], depending maybe on the phenotypic selection of the cohort.

In nail-patella syndrome, the prognosis is determined by the nephropathy. Comparable with the human syndrome, homozygous *LMX1B* knock-out mice lack patellae and suffer from severe podocyte damage. In contrast, however, podocin and the $\alpha3$ and $\alpha4$ chains of collagen IV are absent in the glomeruli of *LMX1B* knock-out mice. Further studies with podocyte-specific *LMX1B* knockout mice have confirmed the importance of *LMX1B* in podocytes, as these mice apparently develop foot processes initially but lose them later on [6]. Thus, *LMX1B* is essential for the development of metanephric precursor cells into podocytes and possibly also for maintaining the differentiation of podocytes [6].

Nail-patella nephropathy includes renin-angiotensin system blockade to manage proteinuria, based on data that angiotensin antagonism reduces protein excretion through hemodynamic mechanisms and podocyte protection, slowing renal disease progression [20]. However, this therapy is palliative and is not always successful, as different mutations in LMB1X may determine the response to renin-angiotensin system blockade [21]. For patients with end-stage renal disease, as our patient, renal transplantation is the preferred renal replacement therapy, as nail-patella nephropathy does not relapse after transplantation.

In summary, the pursue of genetic causes in patients with proteinuria and a histological diagnosis of FSGS, particularly the young, are mandatory in many aspects. Not only it offers a precise cause of chronic kidney disease and potential genetic counseling but also avoids the prescription of unnecessary immunosuppression, often employed as an attempt to reduce proteinuria. In cases of proteinuria due to podocyte genetic mutations, the use of immunosuppressants has no place. Since early childhood, our patient received an unnecessary burden of toxic immunosuppression, with potential consequences for her future, added to the recently prescribed ones to manage the transplanted allograft.

References

[1] V. D. D'Agati, A. B. Fogo, J. A. Bruijn, and J. C. Jennette, "Pathologic classification of focal segmental glomerulosclerosis: a working proposal," *American Journal of Kidney Diseases*, vol. 43, no. 2, pp. 368–382, 2004.

[2] V. D. D'Agati, J. M. Alster, J. C. Jennette et al., "Association of histologic variants in FSGS clinical trial with presenting features and outcomes," *Clinical Journal of the American Society of Nephrology*, vol. 8, no. 3, pp. 399–406, 2013.

[3] H. Trimarchi, "Primary focal and segmental glomerulosclerosis: Why are pieces of this puzzle still missing?"

European Medical Journal Nephrology, vol. 3, no. 1, pp. 104–110, 2015.

[4] B. H. Rovin, D. J. Caster, D. C. Cattran et al., "Management and treatment of glomerular diseases (Part 2): conclusions from a kidney disease: improving global outcomes (KDIGO) controversies conference," *Kidney International*, vol. 95, no. 2, pp. 281–295, 2019.

[5] R. Trachtman, S. S. Sran, and H. Trachtman, "Recurrent focal segmental glomerulosclerosis after kidney transplantation," *Pediatric Nephrology*, vol. 30, no. 10, pp. 1793–1802, 2015.

[6] E. Machuca, G. Benoit, and C. Antignac, "Genetics of nephrotic syndrome: connecting molecular genetics to podocyte physiology," *Human Molecular Genetics*, vol. 18, no. 2, pp. R185–R194, 2009.

[7] W. Kriz, "Maintenance and breakdown of glomerular tuft architecture," *Journal of the American Society of Nephrology*, vol. 29, no. 4, pp. 1075–1077, 2018.

[8] N. Dombros and A. Katz, "Nail-patella-like renal lesions in the absence of skeletal abnormalities," *American Journal of Kidney Diseases*, vol. 1, no. 4, pp. 237-240, 1982.

[9] M. Levy and J. Feingold, "Estimating prevalence in single-gene kidney diseases progressing to renal failure," *Kidney International*, vol. 58, no. 3, pp. 925–943, 2000.

[10] E. M. H. F. Bongers, F. T. Huysmans, E. Levtchenko et al., "Genotype-phenotype studies in nail-patella syndrome show that LMX1B mutation location is involved in the risk of developing nephropathy," *European Journal of Human Genetics*, vol. 13, no. 8, pp. 935–946, 2005.

[11] E. Sweeney, A. Fryer, R. Mountford et al., "Nail-patella syndrome: a review of the phenotype aided by developmental biology," *Journal of Medical Genetics*, vol. 40, no. 3, pp. 153–162, 2003.

[12] H. Chen, Y. Lun, D. Ovchinmikov et al., "Limb and kidney defects in LMX1B mutant mice suggest an involvement of LMX1B in human nail patella syndrome," *Nature Genetics*, vol. 19, no. 1, pp. 51–55, 1998.

[13] T. Burghardt, J. Kastner, H. Suleiman et al., "LMX1B is essential for the maintenance of differentiated podocytes in adult kidneys," *Journal of the American Society of Nephrology*, vol. 24, no. 11, pp. 1830–1848, 2013.

[14] J. H. Miner, R. Morello, K. L. Andrews et al., "Transcriptional induction of slit diaphragm genes by LMX1B is required in podocyte differentiation," *Journal of Clinical Investigation*, vol. 109, no. 8, pp. 1065–1072, 2002.

[15] C. Rohr, J. Prestel, L. Heidet et al., "The LIM-homeodomain transcription factor LMX1B plays a crucial role in podocytes," *Journal of Clinical Investigation*, vol. 109, no. 8, pp. 1073–1082, 2002.

[16] O. Boyer, S. Woermer, F. Yang et al., "LMX1B mutations cause hereditary FSGS without extrarenal involvement," *Journal of the American Society of Nephrology*, vol. 24, no. 8, pp. 1216–1222, 2013.

[17] T. Isojima, Y. Harita, M. Furuyama et al., "LMX1B mutation with residual transcriptional activity as a cause of isolated glomerulopathy," *Nephrology Dialysis Transplantation*, vol. 29, no. 1, pp. 81–88, 2014.

[18] N. Edwards, S. J. Rice, S. Raman et al., "A novel LMX1B mutation in a family with end-stage renal disease of "unknown cause"" *Clinical Kidney Journal*, vol. 8, no. 1, pp. 113–119, 2015.

[19] K. V. Lemley, "Kidney disease in nail-patella syndrome," *Pediatric Nephrology*, vol. 24, no. 12, pp. 2345–2354, 2009.

[20] H. Trimarchi, "Primary focal and segmental glomerulosclerosis and suPAR: where do we stand and where are we heading to?" *World Journal of Nephrology*, vol. 2, no. 4, pp. 103–110, 2013.

[21] Y. Harita, S. Kitanaka, T. Isojima, A. Ashida, and M. Hattori, "Spectrum of LMX1B mutations: from nail-patella syndrome to isolated nephropathy," *Pediatric Nephrology*, vol. 32, no. 10, pp. 1845–1850, 2017.

Leptospirosis Presenting with Features of Thrombotic Microangiopathy

Chaudhry Adeel Ebad,[1] **Nabeehah Moollan**,[1] **Adeel Rafi Ahmed**,[1] **Anthony Dorman**,[2,3] **and Colm Magee**[1]

[1]*Department of Nephrology, Beaumont Hospital, Dublin, Ireland*
[2]*Department of Pathology, Beaumont Hospital, Dublin, Ireland*
[3]*Royal College of Surgeons Ireland (RCSI), Dublin, Ireland*

Correspondence should be addressed to Chaudhry Adeel Ebad; adeelebad@hotmail.com

Academic Editor: Yoshihide Fujigaki

Leptospirosis is an exceptionally rare infectious disease in the Republic of Ireland. Leptospirosis can present with or mimic thrombotic microangiopathies (TTP/HUS). A 48-year-old male presented to a peripheral hospital with a short history of diarrhoea, anaemia, hyperbilirubinemia, raised lactate dehydrogenase, thrombocytopenia, and severe acute kidney injury and was transferred to our tertiary care kidney centre. A form of acute thrombotic microangiopathy (TMA) was suspected. However, no schistocytes were seen on the blood film, and the reticulocyte count was depressed. A kidney biopsy was performed before initiating any potential treatment which revealed acute interstitial nephritis (AIN). Leptospirosis was considered and subsequently serologically confirmed. The patient was managed with antimicrobials and supportive therapy. Acute kidney injury is common in leptospirosis and is often due to AIN. Initial presentation can mimic TMA; however, a differential diagnosis of leptospirosis should be considered even in nonendemic areas due to re-emergence of the disease.

1. Background

Systemic infections can mimic the features of thrombotic microangiopathies (TMAs) [1]. Leptospirosis is a common tropical zoonotic infection, but its incidence in the Republic of Ireland (ROI) is less than 0.4/100,000 population. In its fulminant form, leptospirosis can present with multiorgan failure, pulmonary haemorrhage, acute liver injury, acute kidney injury (AKI), and haematological abnormalities being a prominent feature which may overlap with other disorders such as TTP [2]. The reported kidney biopsy findings in leptospirosis-associated AKI suggest acute interstitial nephritis (AIN) with acute tubular injury as being the most common histopathological lesion [3]. We report a rare case of leptospirosis with a clinical presentation of features consistent with TMA and an acute kidney injury with a kidney biopsy showing features of AIN.

2. Case Presentation

A 48-year-old Caucasian man presented to the emergency department with lethargy, malaise, myalgias, nausea, calf pain, loss of appetite, and decreased urine output. This was preceded by 1 episode of nonbloody diarrhoea and fever following consumption of chicken at a barbeque 10 days beforehand.

He had no significant past medical or surgical history. He was not on any regular medication but had used an antibiotic metronidazole prior to hospital admission. He denied the use of any over-the-counter, herbal, or illicit drug use. He had no history of known allergies. He smoked 5–10 cigarettes per day for the last 10 years and consumed 20–30 units of alcohol per week. He worked in information technology and had no recent history of travels or contact with pets or animals.

He had a blood pressure check while seated 131/85, heart rate 88 beats per minute, respiratory rate 16 per minute, temperature 36.7 celsius, and oxygen saturation 98% on ambient room air. His further physical examination showed pallor and jaundice with no evidence of conjunctivitis or neurological manifestations. He had no other remarkable findings on systemic examination. His initial investigation results are shown in Table 1.

His laboratory features showed AKI KDIGO stage 3, thrombocytopenia, anaemia, hyperbilirubinemia, raised lactate dehydrogenase (LDH), and active urinary sediments suggesting an acute TMA. He was transferred to our hospital for further investigations and treatment with a working diagnosis of an acute TMA and a possible requirement for haemodialysis and plasmapheresis.

On arrival to the tertiary care hospital, his haemodynamic status was stable. He had relatively preserved urine output without any urgent indication for the initiation of renal replacement therapy. With a recovering kidney function and no schistocytes on a blood film (schistocytes on blood film are usually seen in TMA), it was decided not to commence plasmapheresis. A kidney biopsy was performed to clarify the underlying diagnosis. He was commenced on antibiotics for a presumed abdominal or urinary source of infection.

The kidney biopsy showed no features of TMA but severe AIN. The inflammation included eosinophils; Grocott's methenamine silver stain was negative for leptospira organisms (Figures 1, 2(a), and 2(b)). Eosinophilic-rich AIN is typically seen due to a drug reaction; however, clinical and laboratory features suggested a systemic cause, particularly leptospirosis. Despite being extremely rare in ROI, diagnostic tests for leptospirosis were sent.

Our patient did not recall a history of exposure to any animals. He had a fall in a small lake about 2 weeks prior to symptoms onset. The lake water was likely the source of his leptospira infection.

He had a serological test IgM positive for leptospirosis, and his microscopic agglutination test (MAT) result confirmed leptospirosis (Table 2).

3. Management

In this case, patient's acute kidney injury improved without renal replacement therapy or plasmapheresis. He was commenced on intravenous fluid and empirical penicillin antibiotic treatment for presumed abdominal or urinary source of infection. His creatinine, bilirubin, and platelet trends are presented in Figure 3.

Our patient's kidney biopsy showed AIN with no significant medication exposure prior to kidney biopsy. In view of improvement in kidney functions, a decision was made not to commence steroids treatment and to await leptospirosis results.

Once his diagnosis of leptospirosis was confirmed, the antibiotic regimen was switched to doxycycline 100 mg twice a day for a duration of one week. The patient had a follow-up in a clinic after two weeks with resolution of all his symptoms and normal blood results.

Table 1: Investigation results.

Test	Results (reference range)
Creatinine	623 (59–104 μmol/L)
Urea	22 (2.8–8.1 mmol/L)
Sodium	125 (133–146 mmol/L)
Potassium	3 (3.5–5.3 mmol/L)
Hb	8.8 (13–17.5 gm/dL)
WBC	8.42 (4–11·10^9/L)
Platelets	73 (140–400·10^9/L)
Neutrophils	6.59 (2–7.5·10^9/L)
Lymphocytes	1.02 (1–4·10^9/L)
CRP	80 (0–5 mg/L)
ALT	48 (0–41 I.U./L)
AST	44 (0–40 U./L)
Alkaline phosphatase	75 (40–130 I.U./L)
GGT	41 (0–59 I.U./L)
Bilirubin	134 (0–21 μmol/L)
LDH	355 (135–225 I.U./L)
Reticulocyte count	8 (10–80 10^9/L)
Fibrinogen	4.5 (1.9–3.5 g/L)

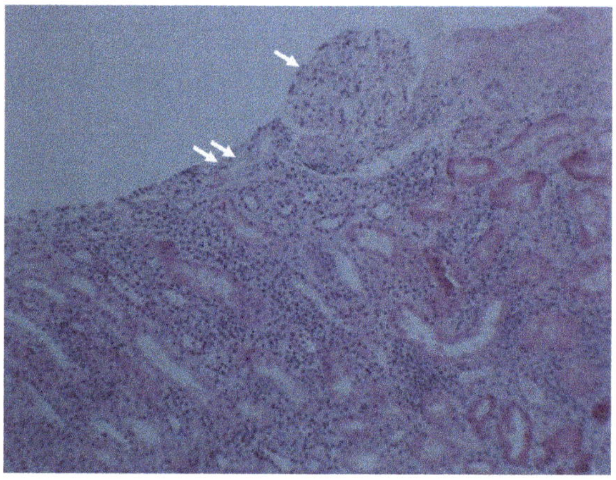

Figure 1: Hematoxylin and eosin staining (H&E)* with 100 magnification. The image shows a normal glomerulus (single arrow) and arteriole (double arrow) moderate tubulointerstitial inflammation and oedema.

4. Discussion

Leptospirosis is a zoonotic disease caused by a spirochete of the genus *Leptospira interrogans* [4]. Rodents and other animals (pigs, goats, cattle, horses, and dogs) are the natural reservoirs of this disease. The transmission of this infection results from contact with contaminated water, soil, or direct contact with animal urine or blood. An outbreak of leptospirosis was reported in triathlon athletes who were infected from the lake water [5]. In our case, the patient probably got infected when he accidentally fell into the lake.

The spirochetes cause infection by entering through skin abrasions, conjunctiva, and oral mucosal route as they cannot penetrate through intact skin [4]. The disease is commonly prevalent in the tropical region but does have a worldwide distribution. The domestic animal vaccination and eradication of rodents are important control measures which prevent the spread of infection. There is no current vaccine available for human use.

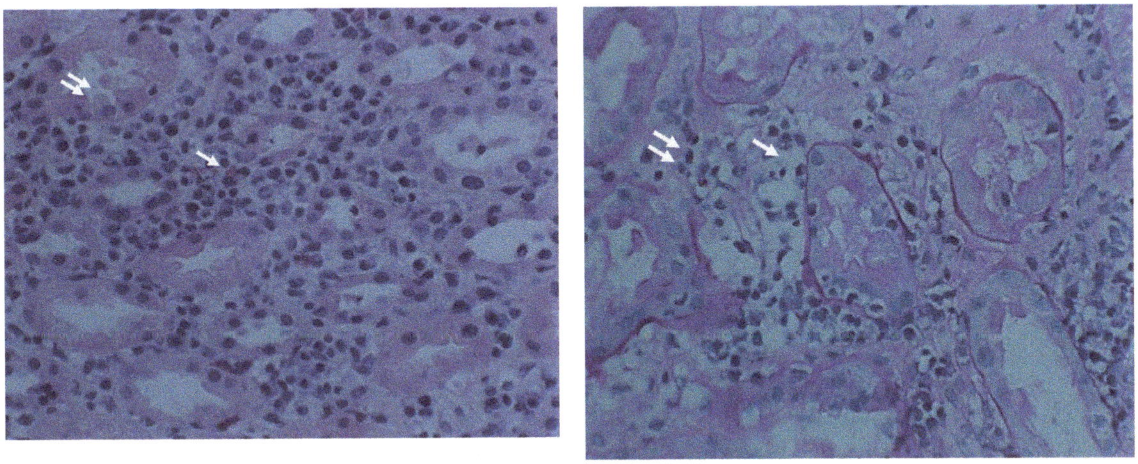

(a) (b)

FIGURE 2: (a) Hematoxylin and eosin staining (H&E)* with 400 magnification. The image shows tubulointerstitial inflammation with lymphocytes, plasma cells, and some eosinophils (single arrow) interstitial oedema with wide spacing of the tubule (double arrow). (b) Periodic acid Schiff (PAS)* with 600 magnification. The image shows moderate tubulitis with lymphocytes in the wall of the tubule (single arrow) and tubule destruction (double arrow) with fragmented tubular basement membrane.

TABLE 2: Investigation results.

Investigations	Result
Blood film	Target cells, hypersegmented neutrophils, and hypochromasia without schistocytes or spherocytes
Hep A, Hep B, Hep C, HIV, CMV	Negative
Vasculitis screen (ANCA, C3, C4, and CTD)	Negative
Urine analysis	Blood+ and protein+
Midstream urine (MSU)	No growth
Chest X-ray	Nil acute
Ultrasound kidneys	No evidence of obstruction or any other abnormality
Echocardiogram	No valvular or other abnormalities including evidence of infiltrative diseases
CT TAP	No mass, lymphadenopathy, or organomegaly incidental finding of liver haemangioma
Bone marrow biopsy	Maturation of all cell lines was unremarkable
Kidney biopsy	Acute eosinophil-rich tubulointerstitial nephritis
Microscopic agglutination test	Positive for leptospirosis
Serum protein electrophoresis	No abnormal bands

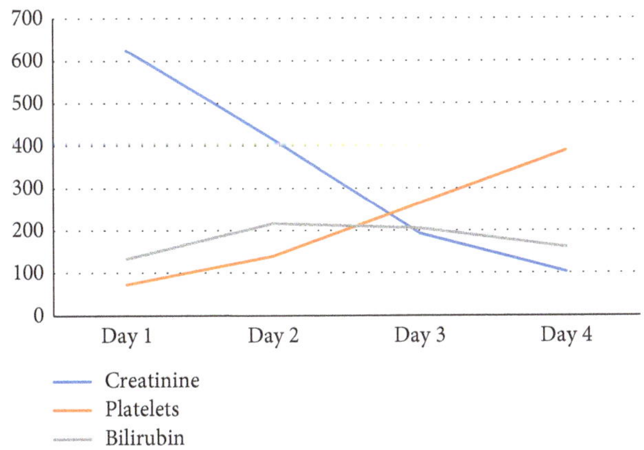

FIGURE 3: Trends of creatinine, platelets, and bilirubin.

The presentation of this disease is very variable with the spectrum of disease ranging from a mild self-limiting infection to a severe life-threatening infection with acute kidney injury, pulmonary haemorrhage, and haematological abnormalities (Weil's disease) which is associated with a mortality rate of over 20% [6].

Systemic infections can show similar features as acute thrombotic microangiopathy (TMA) with some reports of leptospirosis-induced TMA [1, 2]. A TMA (TTP/HUS) registry showed 7% of patients presented with features of TMA were subsequently diagnosed with a systematic infection [1]. A suggested approach to unmask an underlying aetiology for AKI with jaundice includes consideration of differential diagnosis, as shown in Table 3.

The kidney manifestations of leptospirosis mostly include microscopic haematuria, proteinuria, and

Table 3: Differential diagnosis of acute kidney injury with jaundice.

Acute thrombotic microangiopathy (TMA) includes TTP and HUS
Thrombotic thrombocytopenic purpura (TTP)
Haemolytic uremic syndrome (HUS)
Atypical haemolytic uremic syndrome (aHUS)
Hepatorenal syndrome
Rhabdomyolysis
Leptospirosis/Weil's disease
Malaria

nonoliguric AKI [7]. The electrolyte abnormalities of hyponatremia, hypomagnesaemia, and hypokalaemia are also seen in this disease attributed to kidney tubular damage associated with the disease [8]. The kidney injury usually has multifactorial aetiologies secondary to critical illness, AIN, direct nephrotoxic damage to tubule by leptospira organism or toxin, hyperbilirubinemia, and rhabdomyolysis [3, 8]. Few cases result in chronic kidney disease but rarely end up in dialysis-dependent chronic kidney disease [9].The common histologic changes in kidney biopsy include AIN, bile acid cast nephropathy, and acute tubular necrosis [10].

The treatment of this infection includes supportive care and antibiotic therapy. The antibiotics used for the treatment include penicillin, cephalosporin, doxycycline, and azithromycin [11]. Doxycycline is usually the preferred antibiotic unless contraindicated due to allergies or pregnancy [11].

5. Conclusion

Leptospirosis is an important consideration in patients presenting with suspected features of acute TMA (TTP/HUS). In nonendemic regions, the re-emergence of the disease results in new cases. The management is primarily antibiotics and supportive therapy. AKI commonly has nonoliguric association with hypokalaemia, and kidney biopsy shows AIN and acute tubular injury.

Additional Points

Learning Points. 1. Leptospirosis can mimic thrombotic microangiopathies and should be part of differential diagnosis even in a nonendemic area. 2. The most common histological finding on kidney biopsy is acute interstitial nephritis and acute tubular necrosis. 3. Acute kidney injury has often nonoliguric association with hypokalaemia and hyponatraemia. Active urinary sediment with blood and protein is commonly seen on urinalysis.

Consent

Written informed consent for the paper to be published (including images) was obtained from the patient. He understood that the information should be published without his name attached, but that full anonymity could not be guaranteed. He understood that the text and any pictures published in the article would be freely available on the Internet and may be seen by the general public. The pictures and text may also appear on other websites or in print and may be translated into other languages or used for commercial purposes.

References

[1] K. K. Booth, D. R. Terrell, S. K. Vesely, and J. N. George, "Systemic infections mimicking thrombotic thrombocytopenic purpura," *American Journal of Hematology*, vol. 86, no. 9, pp. 743–751, 2011.

[2] M. Małecki, E. Gołembiewska, A. M. Muraszko et al., "Atypical renal presentation in severe leptospirosis," *Kidney International Reports*, vol. 4, no. 1, pp. 168–170, 2019.

[3] F. Daher Ede, K. L. de Abreu, and G. B. da Silva Junior, "Leptospirosis-associated acute kidney injury," *Jornal Brasileiro de Nefrologia*, vol. 32, no. 4, pp. 400–407, 2010.

[4] P. N. Levett, "Leptospirosis," *Clinical Microbiology Reviews*, vol. 14, no. 2, pp. 296–326, 2001.

[5] J. Morgan, S. L. Bornstein, A. M. Karpati et al., "Outbreak of leptospirosis among triathlon participants and community residents in Springfield, Illinois, 1998," *Clinical Infectious Diseases: An Official Publication of the Infectious Diseases Society of America*, vol. 34, no. 12, pp. 1593–1599, 2002.

[6] K. B. Karpagam and B. Ganesh, "Leptospirosis: a neglected tropical zoonotic infection of public health importance-an updated review," *European Journal of Clinical Microbiology & Infectious Diseases*, vol. 39, no. 5, pp. 835–846, 2020.

[7] L. Andrade, E. de Francesco Daher, and A. C. Seguro, "Leptospiral nephropathy," *Seminars in Nephrology*, vol. 28, no. 4, pp. 383–394, 2008.

[8] A. C. Seguro and L. Andrade, "Pathophysiology of leptospirosis," *Shock*, vol. 39, no. 1, pp. 17–23, 2013.

[9] R. Ghasemian, M. Shokri, A. Makhlough, and M. A. Suraki-Azad, "The course and outcome of renal failure due to human leptospirosis referred to a hospital in North of Iran; a follow-up study," *Caspian Journal of Internal Medicine*, vol. 7, no. 1, pp. 7-12, 2016.

[10] K. V. Evangelista and J. Coburn, "Leptospiraas an emerging pathogen: a review of its biology, pathogenesis and host immune responses," *Future Microbiology*, vol. 5, no. 9, pp. 1413–1425, 2010.

[11] D. M. Brett-Major and R. Coldren, "Antibiotics for leptospirosis," *Cochrane Database of Systematic Reviews*, no. 2, Article ID CD008264, 2012, doi: 10.1002/14651858.CD008264.pub2.

Focal Segmental Glomerulosclerosis in Waldenström's Macroglobulinemia

Akshee Batra, Shatha Herz Allah, and Bijin Thajudeen

Department of Nephrology, Banner University of Arizona Medical Center, 1501 North Campbell Ave, Tucson, AZ, USA

Correspondence should be addressed to Bijin Thajudeen; bijint@gmail.com

Academic Editor: Bernard G. Jaar

Renal involvement in Waldenström's macroglobulinemia is a rare manifestation. Although most renal involvement is due to monoclonal immune deposits, pathology can also be unrelated to it. Here, we describe a 68-year-old female with a history of Waldenström's macroglobulinemia who presented with generalized edema and nephrotic range proteinuria. A renal biopsy showed findings consistent with focal segmental glomerulosclerosis. Treatment with oral prednisone leads to the resolution of proteinuria. This case highlights the importance of identifying pathology that might not be directly related to monoclonal gammopathy, which could have implications on the management.

1. Introduction

Waldenström's macroglobulinemia (WM) is a lymphoproliferative disorder involving B cells characterized by an IgM monoclonal protein >1 g/dl and 10% lymphoplasmacytic infiltrate in the bone marrow [1]. Kidney disease is a common presentation of WM usually characterized by IgM deposits along the glomerular basement membrane (GBM), infiltration of the interstitium, or amyloidosis [1, 2]. However, occasionally the pathology could be unrelated to the immunoglobulin deposition (Tables 1 and 2). Here, we report a case of focal segmental glomerulosclerosis (FSGS) in a patient with WM. According to our knowledge, there is only one other reported case of FSGS in WM [1].

2. Case Report

A 68-year-old female presented to the outpatient clinic with complaints of lower extremity edema for four weeks. Her past medical history was significant for lymphoplasmacytic lymphoma with IgM monoclonal gammopathy or WM. Since the criteria for treatment were not met, she did not receive any treatment for WM. Her home medications included omeprazole and ferrous sulfate. Her vitals showed a temperature of 98°F, blood pressure of 136/78 mmHg, pulse rate of 84/minute, respiratory rate of 16/min, and body mass index of 22.35 kg/m^2. The rest of the physical examination was unremarkable except for 2+ edema of the lower extremities. Laboratory studies yielded the following values: hemoglobin 8.3 g/dl, white blood cell count 14400/mm^3, platelet count 496000/mm^3, blood urea nitrogen 13 mg/dl, creatinine 0.6 mg/dl, calcium 8.5 gm/dl, erythrocyte sedimentation rate (ESR) 94 mm/1st hour, LDH 340 IU/I, and total protein 7.5 g/dl with albumin 3.9 g/dl. Urine sediments contained few erythrocytes and hyaline casts. The spot protein/creatinine ratio was 16.2 gm/gm creatinine, and the albumin-to-creatinine ratio was 9.9 gm/gm creatinine. Serum immunoelectrophoresis showed IgM 1693 mg/dl, IgG 453 mg/dl, and IgA 23 mg/dl. Serum immunofixation revealed monoclonal IgM kappa light chains. The concentration of serum kappa and lambda light was 73.74 mg/L and 2.38 mg/L, respectively. The ratio of kappa to lambda was 30.98. Peripheral blood flow cytometry revealed a monocytic kappa light-chain-restricted B-cell population. Cryoglobulins were absent. All serologies, including complements, ANA, anti-dsDNA, ANCA, HIV, and hepatitis panel, were negative. A renal biopsy was performed. Light microscopy showed glomeruli with thin and delicate capillary loops,

Table 1: Clinical studies, types of renal disease, and treatment in Waldenström's macroglobulinemia.

Study	Number of patients	Pathology seen	Treatment
Morel-Maroger et al. [2]	16 patients	3 amyloidosis 6 nonamyloid glomerular disease (3 cryoglobulinemia) 7 had no detectable lesions	Not available
Higgins et al. [1]	44 patients	17 amyloidosis 9 nonamyloid glomerular disease 7 tubulointerstitial nephritis 9 non-monoclonal gammopathy-related glomerular disease (1FSGS)	Amyloid glomerulopathy: Rituximab R Ituximab Chemotherapy Bortezomib Nonamyloid glomerulopathy: Steroid Rituximab Rituxima Bendamustine Bortezomib Chemotherapy
Vos et al. [3]	44 patients	Amyloidosis 11 Cryoglobulinemia 10 Light-chain deposition disease 4 Cast nephropathy 4 TMA 3 Minimal change disease 2 Membranous nephropathy 1 LPL infiltration 8 Light-chain tubulopathy 1	Proteosome inhibitor + rituximab Alkylator + rituximab Nucleoside analogue + rituximab Bendamustine Single-agent rituximab

LPL: lymphoplasmacytic lymphoma infiltration; TMA: thrombotic microangiopathy.

Table 2: Renal diseases associated with Waldenström's macroglobulinemia.

Amyloid glomerulopathy	Nonamyloid glomerulopathy	Tubulointerstitial lesions	Non-paraprotein-related lesions
Monoclonal light-chain amyloidosis	Cryoglobulinemic GN	Light-chain cast nephropathy	Minimal change disease
Monoclonal heavy-chain amyloidosis	Non-cryoglobulinemic GN	Lymphoma infiltration	Thrombotic microangiopathy
Monoclonal light- and heavy-chain amyloidosis	Light- and/or heavy-chain deposition disease Proliferative glomerular diseases Immunotactoid glomerulopathy	Lymphoma infiltration with light-chain cast nephropathy	Membranous GN Acute tubular necrosis Diabetic nephropathy FSGS

GN: glomerulonephritis; FSGS: focal segmental glomerulosclerosis.

three glomeruli showed segmental sclerosis, and two glomeruli demonstrated mild attachment to Bowman's capsule without significant tubulointerstitial inflammation (Figure 1). Immunofluorescence showed a tubular cast that stained for IgG, IgM, and kappa. Electron microscopy revealed more than 90%-foot process effacement without any evidence of immune deposits (Figure 2). The final diagnosis was primary glomerulosclerosis. Treatment with oral prednisone was started at 60 mg daily, and the dose of prednisone was tapered and stopped over eight months. Additional treatment included losartan for proteinuria and Bactrim as well as fluconazole for infection prophylaxis (stopped after six months). Protein/creatinine ratio improved to 330 mg/gm creatinine at the end of eight months. There was a complete disappearance

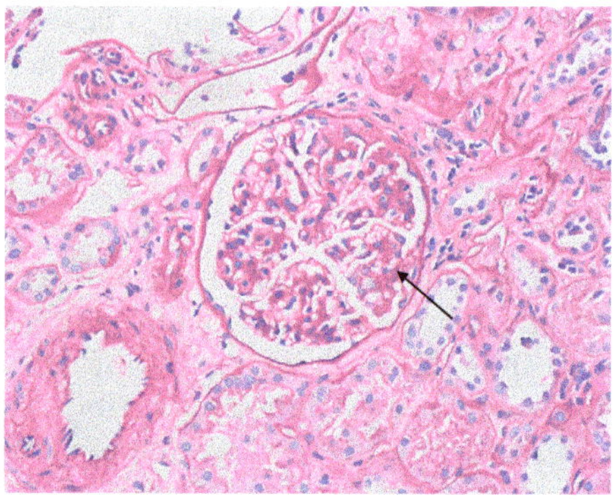

Figure 1: Light microscopy showing glomeruli with segmental sclerosis and attachment of the glomerular tuft to Bowman's capsule (arrow) (H&E stain).

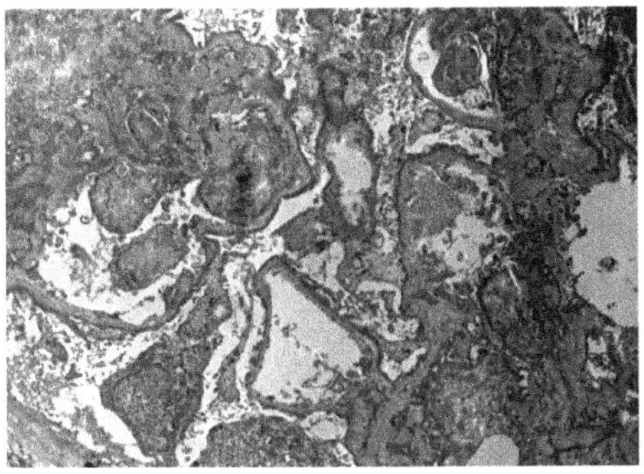

FIGURE 2: Electron microscopy showing more than 90%-foot process effacement.

of edema of extremities. The plan is to continue monitoring without any maintenance treatment.

3. Discussion

Pathogenesis of renal involvement in WM can range from direct infiltration of the lymphoplasmacytic cells, glomerular or tubular deposition of paraprotein, or an immune-mediated reaction [1–3]. Glomerular involvement due to paraprotein includes amyloid related and nonamyloid related, of which amyloid light-chain- (AL-) related glomerulopathy is the most common [1–3]. Among the nonamyloid glomerulopathies, cryoglobulinemia is the most reported renal pathology [1, 2]. Non-paraprotein-mediated kidney pathologies have also been reported, including minimal change disease, focal segmental glomerulosclerosis, membranous glomerulopathy, and thrombotic microangiopathy [1, 3]. Table 2 shows a diverse array of kidney diseases reported in WM patients.

This case highlights an unusual presentation of FSGS in kidney biopsy of a patient with prediagnosed WM. FSGS pathogenesis involves a sequel of glomerular podocyte damage and dysfunction [4]. However, at the same time, the pathogenesis of FSGS in WM is not well defined in the literature. The three possible explanations for the presence of FSGS in this patient include idiopathic FSGS unrelated to WM, paraprotein-induced podocyte injury, and paraneoplastic phenomenon affecting the genes associated with cytoskeleton organization and podocyte signaling [1–3, 5]. In the largest published study on IgM-producing B-cell lymphoproliferative disorders, Higgins et al. revealed the presence of one FSGS from the kidney biopsies of 44 patients [1]. In another cohort where 44 patients had pathology related to WM, two of the patients had minimal change, and one had membranous nephropathy [3]. Due to limited literature and failure to establish a direct causal relationship with WM, we ascertained the diagnosis as primary FSGS unrelated to WM.

Treatment for renal manifestations in WM consists of supportive therapy with hydration, plasmapheresis, and combination chemotherapy for underlying hematologic malignancy [6]. Novel therapeutics like bortezomib, lenalidomide, and ibrutinib can be considered [7]. An intervention like autologous stem cell transplantation has also been found to be effective on a case-to-case basis [8]. Table 1 shows the medications used in the treatment of WM. Since there was no histopathological finding relating the pathogenesis to paraprotein, we decided to treat this as a primary FSGS. The presence of immune deposits in immunofluorescence or electron microscopy could have favored the treatment of WM rather than primary FSGS. This case highlights the importance of individualizing therapy according to clinical presentation and kidney biopsy results.

Consent

Consent was obtained for publication of the case report.

References

[1] L. Higgins, S. H. Nasr, S. M. Said et al., "Kidney involvement of patients with Waldenström macroglobulinemia and other IgM-producing B cell lymphoproliferative disorders," *Clinical Journal of the American Society of Nephrology*, vol. 13, no. 7, pp. 1037–1046, 2018.

[2] L. Morel-Maroger, A. Basch, F. Danon, P. Verroust, and G. Richet, "Pathology of the kidney in Waldenström's macroglobulinemia," *New England Journal of Medicine*, vol. 283, no. 3, pp. 123–129, 1970.

[3] J. M. Vos, J. Gustine, H. G. Rennke et al., "Renal disease related to Waldenström macroglobulinaemia: incidence, pathology and clinical outcomes," *British Journal of Haematology*, vol. 175, no. 4, pp. 623–630, 2016.

[4] J. A. Jefferson and S. J. Shankland, "The pathogenesis of focal segmental glomerulosclerosis," *Advances in Chronic Kidney Disease*, vol. 21, no. 5, pp. 408–416, 2014.

[5] Y.-H. H. Lien and L.-W. Lai, "Pathogenesis, diagnosis and management of paraneoplastic glomerulonephritis," *Nature Reviews Nephrology*, vol. 7, no. 2, pp. 85–95, 2011.

[6] V. Leblond, E. Kastritis, R. Advani et al., "Treatment recommendations from the Eighth International Workshop on Waldenström's Macroglobulinemia," *Blood*, vol. 128, no. 10, pp. 1321–1328, 2016.

[7] P. Advani, A. Paulus, and S. Ailawadhi, "Updates in prognostication and treatment of Waldenström's macroglobulinemia," *Hematology/Oncology and Stem Cell Therapy*, vol. 12, no. 4, pp. 179–188, 2019.

[8] R. Chakraborty, E. Muchtar, and M. A. Gertz, "The role of stem cell transplantation in Waldenstrom's macroglobulinemia," *Best Practice & Research Clinical Haematology*, vol. 29, no. 2, pp. 229–240, 2016.

32

Renal Cell Carcinoma Associated with Mycosis Fungoides: A Paraneoplastic Syndrome

Jessica Tran,[1,2] Auris Huen,[1] and Madeleine Duvic[1]

[1]*Department of Dermatology, The University of Texas MD Anderson Cancer Center, Houston, TX, USA*
[2]*Baylor College of Medicine, Houston, TX, USA*

Correspondence should be addressed to Jessica Tran; jessica.tran@bcm.edu

Academic Editor: Phuong Chi Pham

Patients with mycosis fungoides have an increased risk for additional malignancies, particularly hematologic malignancies. Of the malignancies that have been associated with mycosis fungoides, renal cell carcinoma and other solid tumor malignancies have not been studied extensively. In this case series, we describe three mycosis fungoides patients who were diagnosed with clear cell renal cell carcinoma and discuss the potential pathophysiology underlying this association.

1. Introduction

Patients with mycosis fungoides (MF) have an increased risk for additional malignancies, particularly hematologic malignancies [1–3]. MF patients are also at an increased risk for solid tumor malignancies, but this association is less frequent and not well-characterized [2]. In 2019, Goyal et al. detailed a link between MF and solid tumor malignancies such as RCC. The study found elevated standardized incidence ratios (SIRs) for kidney and renal pelvis cancer in patients with MF [2]. SIR for kidney and renal pelvis cancer within a year of diagnosis of MF was 12.05. In our study of 672 patients with cutaneous T-cell lymphoma (CTCL) in 2008, 112 patients (17%) had at least one additional malignancy. Overall, patients with CTCL had a 1.79-fold risk for developing an additional malignancy [4]. In this case series, we describe three MF patients who were diagnosed with clear cell RCC and discuss the potential pathophysiology underlying this association.

2. Case Presentation

2.1. Case 1: Patient A. A 54-year-old male presented to MD Anderson Cancer Center (MDACC) in October 2003 for the management of newly diagnosed stage IA MF. The patient first noted a small brown macule on his left waist in May 2003. Over the next few months, several additional lesions erupted on his left lower abdomen, back, and neck. He also experienced abdominal bloating. His local dermatologist performed a biopsy of the left lower abdomen, revealing a diagnosis of MF. At MDACC, triamcinolone 0.1% cream was prescribed for the patient, and he received UVB light therapy three times a week with noticeable improvement of the lesions. A full-body computed tomography (CT) scan was performed, which revealed an 8 centimeter (cm) x 5.6 cm mass in the upper pole of the right kidney. Urinary testing was positive for hematuria. The patient denied any urinary symptoms. Flow cytometry was negative for atypical T cells in peripheral blood. A biopsy of the mass revealed clear cell RCC. The patient underwent a laparoscopic right radical nephrectomy in October 2003 to remove the mass. Follow-up CT scan in March 2004 demonstrated no RCC recurrence and complete remission of MF. The patient still remains disease-free from RCC and MF.

2.2. Case 2: Patient B. A 52-year-old female presented to MDACC in October 2019 for the management of MF with large cell transformation. In June 2019, she noticed a lesion on her left thigh resembling a spider bite and multiple “eczema-like” patches on the forearms and feet. Her local dermatologist performed a punch biopsy on the left lateral back and left posterior thigh, revealing MF with large cell transformation. Flow cytometry was negative for atypical T cells in peripheral blood. Triamcinolone 0.1% cream was prescribed for the patient. At MDACC, full-body skin exam revealed a 10.5 cm × 6.5 cm tumor on the left inner thigh (Figure 1) and a 3 cm × 4 cm tumor on the right posterior thigh. A positron emission tomography/computed tomography (PET/CT) scan revealed enlarged FDG-avid bilateral inguinal and right external iliac lymph nodes and an 8.5 cm × 7.7 cm exophytic right renal mass with extension into the renal sinus. Lymph node biopsy of the left inguinal lymph node demonstrated evidence of CD4-positive T-cell lymphoma. A biopsy of the mass revealed clear cell RCC. The patient underwent an open right radical nephrectomy and regional lymphadenectomy in December 2019. She received local radiation therapy to the lesions and one cycle of romidepsin. Follow-up CT scan demonstrated complete response of her lymph nodes and near complete response of her skin lesions. She remains stable on observation.

2.3. Case 3: Patient C. A 66-year-old male presented to MDACC in July 1996 for the management of stage IA MF. The patient first noticed a lesion on his right thigh approximately 10 years prior. He was diagnosed as having "dry skin" and treated with an unknown ointment with no improvement. The lesion continued to expand, becoming raised and indurated. In June 1996, a skin biopsy was performed by the patient's local dermatologist, which was consistent with MF. On presentation at MDACC, full-body skin exam revealed an 18 cm × 13 cm dusky red plaque on the right upper thigh with a net-like pattern. The plaque was rebiopsied at MDACC, which confirmed MF. The patient's MF lesion was treated with tazarotene 0.05% gel and mometasone 0.1% cream with minimal improvement. In February 1998, the patient was hospitalized for atrial fibrillation. During hospitalization, he was found to have a 3.3 cm × 2.5 cm solid mass on the left lower pole of the kidney. A biopsy of the mass revealed clear cell RCC. The patient denied any urinary symptoms. A left partial nephrectomy was performed. Within months of removal of the renal mass, the patient began to notice significant flattening and decreased hyperpigmentation of his MF lesion without changes to his treatment regimen (Figure 2). His skin lesion has since remained stable.

3. Discussion

Decreased cellular immunity and immune surveillance in MF patients may be a driving factor for secondary malignancies [2]. While the occurrence of RCC in our patients may have been incidental, the expanded number of CD4+ lymphocytes present in existing MF may have triggered the development of RCC. Using both in vitro and in vivo studies of mice RCC tissue, Wang et al. found that RCC cells have a better ability to recruit CD4+ lymphocytes than normal renal cells [5]. The recruited CD4+ lymphocytes stimulate RCC cell proliferation, promoting RCC [5].

The senior authors of this manuscript report that, in their clinical experience, nearly all MF patients have a tendency to

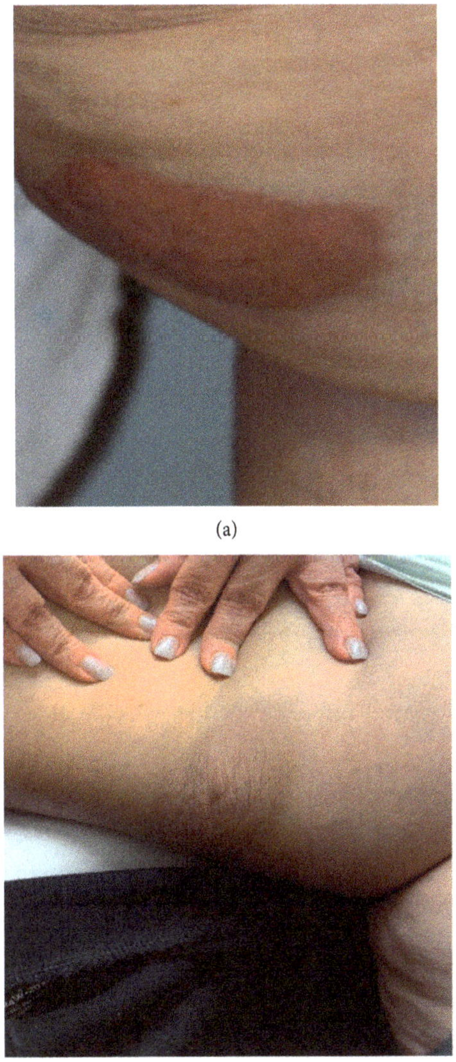

(a)

(b)

Figure 1: Patient B: clinical images of MF tumor before (a) and 1 month after (b) the removal of RCC and local radiation therapy.

relapse despite adequate treatment, and periodic flares are expected throughout their lifetime. In our patients, the absence of MF flares in over 16 years following removal of their RCC increases suspicion of a paraneoplastic syndrome. Paraneoplastic syndrome refers to specific clinical manifestations that are triggered by an altered immune system in response to a malignancy; the symptoms may not be directly attributable to invasion of the primary tumor, metastasis, or direct compression [6]. The stimulation of lymphocytes in response to RCC may have triggered the development of MF, and subsequent removal of the RCC resulted in return to normal lymphocyte levels, halting progression of MF.

While RCC was found after the diagnosis of MF in each of these patients, it remains unknown how long the RCC was present. Due to the lack of widely accepted guidelines regarding screening for renal cancer, more stringent screening guidelines may be required. Routine screening for underlying solid organ malignancies in patients with MF may be

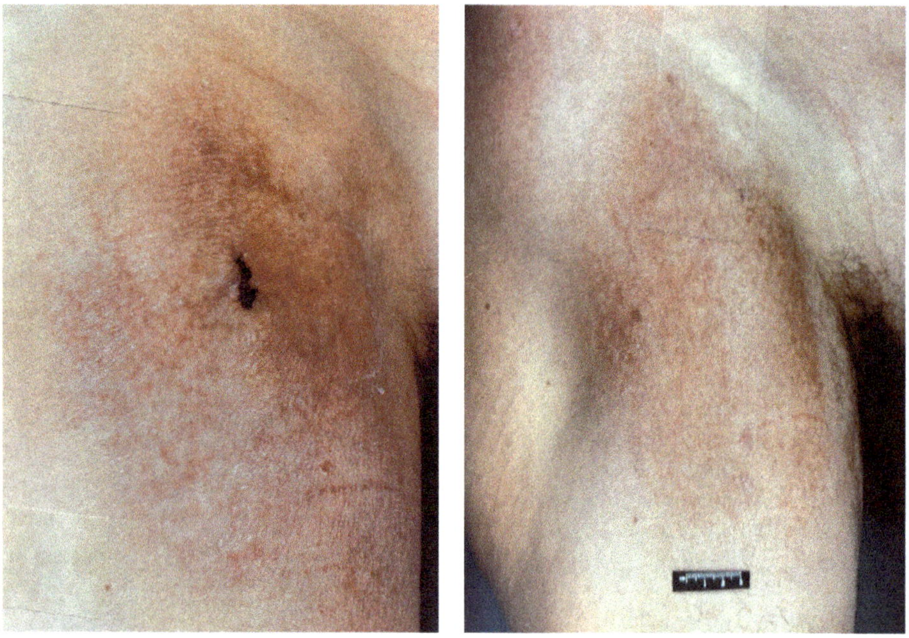

(a) (b)

FIGURE 2: Patient C: clinical images of MF lesion before removal of RCC (a) and 2 years following removal of RCC (b).

costly and impractical. However, screening is warranted in patients presenting with symptoms that may indicate an underlying malignancy, and greater emphasis should be placed on age-appropriate cancer screenings in MF patients. Refractory or rapidly progressing disease may require CT scan.

4. Conclusion

Patients with MF are at higher risk for second malignancies [4]. Of the malignancies that have been associated with MF, renal cell carcinoma (RCC) and other solid tumor malignancies have not been studied extensively [2]. The presence of a second malignancy, such as RCC, in MF patients may be a result of a paraneoplastic syndrome. Further research is needed to characterize the association between MF and RCC.

References

[1] K. T. Amber, R. Bloom, and K. Nouri, "Second primary malignancies in CTCL patients from 1992 to 2011: a SEER-based, population-based study evaluating time from CTCL diagnosis, age, sex, stage, and CD30+ subtype," *American Journal of Clinical Dermatology*, vol. 17, no. 1, pp. 71–77, 2016.

[2] A. Goyal, D. O'Leary, K. Goyal et al., "Increased risk of second primary hematologic and solid malignancies in patients with mycosis fungoides: a Surveillance, Epidemiology, and End Results analysis," *Journal of the American Academy of Dermatology*, vol. 83, no. 4, pp. 404–411, 2020.

[3] Y. J. Kim, H. J. Shin, C. H. Won et al., "The incidence of other primary cancers in patients with cutaneous lymphoma," *Annals of Dermatology*, vol. 30, no. 3, pp. 335–341, 2018.

[4] I. Brownell, C. J. Etzel, D. J. Yang, S. H. Taylor, and M. Duvic, "Increased malignancy risk in the cutaneous T-cell lymphoma patient population," *Clinical Lymphoma and Myeloma*, vol. 8, no. 2, pp. 100–105, 2008.

[5] Y. Wang, Y. Wang, L. Xu et al., "CD4+ T cells promote renal cell carcinoma proliferation via modulating YBX1," *Experimental Cell Research*, vol. 363, no. 1, pp. 95–101, 2018.

[6] G. K. Dimitriadis, A. Angelousi, M. O. Weickert, H. S. Randeva, G. Kaltsas, and A. Grossman, "Paraneoplastic endocrine syndromes," *Endocrine-Related Cancer*, vol. 24, no. 6, pp. R173–R190, 2017.

33

Previously Unidentified Gene Variation Associated with Fabry Disease: The Impact on One Family

Amaresh R. Vanga[1] **Samantha A. Schrier Vergano,**[2,3] **Jolanta Kowalewska,**[4] **and Thomas R. McCune**[1,5]

[1]*Division of Nephrology, Department of Internal Medicine, Eastern Virginia Medical School, Norfolk, VA, USA*
[2]*Division of Medical Genetics and Metabolism, Children's Hospital of the King's Daughters, Norfolk, VA, USA*
[3]*Department of Pediatrics, Eastern Virginia Medical School, Norfolk, VA, USA*
[4]*Department of Pathology and Anatomy, Eastern Virginia Medical School, Norfolk, VA, USA*
[5]*Center for Congenital Kidney Diseases, Eastern Virginia Medical School, Norfolk, VA, USA*

Correspondence should be addressed to Amaresh R. Vanga; amareshvanga@yahoo.com

Academic Editor: Ze'ev Korzets

Fabry disease is an X-linked lysosomal storage genetic disorder associated with over 1000 mutations in the *alpha-galactosidase-A* gene region. We report here a 69-year-old male who underwent a kidney biopsy to evaluate progressive renal failure. He was found to have zebra bodies in visceral epithelial cells on biopsy, with electron microscopy showing inclusions within the cytoplasm of multiple podocytes consistent with Fabry disease. An alpha-galactosidase level was found to be 21 nm/hr/mg (normal range 50–150 nm/hr/mg). Genetic studies revealed a missense variant in the *GLA* gene with alanine replaced by cysteine at position 682 (c.682 A > C, p.N228H) that had not been previously associated with Fabry disease. The same variant was detected in two additional family members. The pathologic findings, clinical features, and low alpha-galactosidase level suggest that the c.682 A > C variant is associated with Fabry disease.

1. Introduction

Fabry disease is an X-linked lysosomal storage disease caused by a deficiency in the alpha-galactosidase enzyme, which affects both males and females. The signs and symptoms of Fabry disease include skin angiokeratomas, neuropathic limb pain, abdominal complaints, corneal opacities, transient ischemic events/strokes, left ventricular hypertrophy, and renal impairment. These can be manifestations and complications of other diseases such as diabetes and hypertension; therefore, Fabry disease may not be considered. Screening of populations at risk for Fabry disease based on ESRD [1–4], cryptogenic strokes [5], and left ventricular hypertrophy [6] found an instance of 1.0% or less. There are over 1,000 known mutations associated with the region that codes for the alpha-galactosidase enzyme [7]. Because of the large number of gene variations, there is a great deal of heterogeneity in the presentation of this multiorgan disease. This article presents a case of Fabry disease due to the *GLA* pathogenic variant not previously associated with the disease.

2. Case Report

A 69-year-old male with a past medical history of hypertension, diabetes, morbid obesity requiring gastric bypass, and metastatic prostate cancer presented for evaluation of progressive kidney disease with subnephrotic-range proteinuria. His glomerular filtration declined by greater than 5 ml per minute per 1.73 m^2 per year. His diabetes mellitus was diet controlled. Medications included atorvastatin, amlodipine, aspirin, calcium carbonate, and leuprolide injection every three months. There were no known drug allergies. The family history was positive for renal failure of undetermined etiology in a brother in his forties. His review of systems was remarkable for peripheral neuropathy with unstable balance, but he denied any symptoms of hypohidrosis, extremity pain, GI complaints, rashes, or cardiac issues. He denied any skin issues. Physical exam revealed a blood pressure of 160/78 mmHg, pulse of 72, and BMI of 24.5. There were no abnormal physical findings of his lungs, heart, abdomen, extremities, or skin. The serum laboratory revealed a creatinine of 4.3 mg/dl and BUN of 47 mg/dl and CO_2 of 19 mg/dl. The remainder of the electrolytes was within normal limits. On CBC, there was hemoglobin of 10.9 but normal platelets and WBC. Urinalysis was remarkable for mild proteinuria. The urine protein/creatinine ratio was 2.2. Initial evaluation of SPEP, UPEP, and free light chains failed to demonstrate any abnormalities. Ultrasound of kidneys showed slightly atrophic kidneys with echogenic parenchyma. A kidney biopsy was performed to complete the evaluation. Light Microscopic evaluation showed normocellular glomeruli with uniform capillary walls and prominent visceral epithelial cells (podocytes) with foamy cytoplasm (Figure 1) and myelin/zebra bodies in visceral epithelial cells (Figure 2) suggesting Fabry disease. Ultrastructural examination revealed osmophilic lamellated inclusions within the cytoplasm of multiple podocytes with concentric of striped appearance (zebra bodies) suggestive of defective lysosomal metabolism of glycolipids, as seen in Fabry disease.

After the biopsy report has been explained to the patient, his brother confirmed that he had been told he had Fabry disease. Lysosomal GL-3 was not drawn as biopsy findings and clinical symptomology were consistent with this diagnosis. The family history is limited as his brother is estranged. He had not had any genetic testing.

The alpha-galactosidase level was 21 nm/hr/mg protein (50–150 nm/hr/mg protein). Genetic studies were sent to EGL fenetics for evaluation. They detected a missense variant in the *GLA* gene sequence in which the nucleotide alanine is replaced by cysteine at position 682 in (c.682 A > C). The variation c.682 A > C in the GLA sequence was a known variant but previously had not been associated with clinical Fabry disease. Genetic testing performed on his daughter and his grandson confirmed that they were positive for this same variant. The testing of other family members is ongoing. Testing of this mutation by Cambridge Biomedical determined that Migalastat chaperon therapy would be appropriate.

3. Discussion

This case suggests that the c.682 A > C variant is associated with Fabry disease based on low alpha-galactosidase levels and pathologic lesions on kidney biopsy. The late age at onset of renal disease and only a 50% decrease in alpha-galactosidase level suggest an atypical variant. However, the fact that the patient's brother developed ESRD in his forties suggests a more classic form of the disease. Another Fabry disease mutation, p.R301Q, which is not related to this mutation, is also associated with both classic and atypical presentations [8]. This suggests that both classic and atypical presentations can be observed in multiple Fabry disease mutations.

The diagnosis of Fabry disease requires a high index of suspicion as many symptoms, such as hypohidrosis, go unrecognized. Other Fabry disease symptoms related to the gastrointestinal, cardiac, and neurologic systems may be attributed to other common conditions such as diabetes mellitus and hypertension. This patient had multiple indicators of Fabry disease, such as a male relative with ESRD at an early age and neuropathy not in proportion to his diet-controlled diabetes yet went undiagnosed. Measuring serum alpha-galactosidase enzyme levels can be a useful screening study in male patients but can yield false-positive results, particularly in patients who are malnourished and with chronic inflammation [9]. Genetic testing for mutations and deletions in the GLA segment of the X chromosome is vital to obtaining the correct diagnosis in females and is required in males to rule out false-positive low alpha-galactosidase levels. Genetic testing is also necessary to assess if a mutation is amenable to oral chaperone therapy as an alternative to enzyme replacement therapy. This patient's genetic variation is an N228H mutation. We found this mutation responsive to migalastat based on (GLP-validated) HEK assay. Unfortunately, this mutation was not included in either the ATTRACT [8] or FACETS [10] studies of migalastat, so monitoring of serum GL-3 levels, kidney function, and left ventricular mass will be vital. Enzyme replacement is available for all patients with Fabry disease mutations but is required for patients with mutations that are not amenable to migalastat chaperone therapy.

The low incidence of diagnosing Fabry disease through screenings programs in patients at high risk such as ESRD, early-onset ischemic strokes, and left ventricular hypertrophy suggests that this form of screening may not be warranted. The incidence of Fabry disease in ESRD patients is upwards of 1% (one in a hundred). It suggests that nephrologists should not ignore the possibility of the disease and maintain a healthy index of suspicion.

More importantly, identifying Fabry disease in the ESRD population benefits the patient's family. A Spanish review of 3,650 dialysis patients identified only 11 new cases of Fabry disease but diagnosed 23 family members out of 66 tested [3]. A Turkish study of 1136 ESRD patients only found one new case of Fabry disease but identified six additional affected family members [4]. A French survey of 106 patients with ESRD found one new case of Fabry disease with seven new family members diagnosed [11]. Having a high index of suspicion for Fabry disease benefits both the patient and their family in avoiding the complications of this disease.

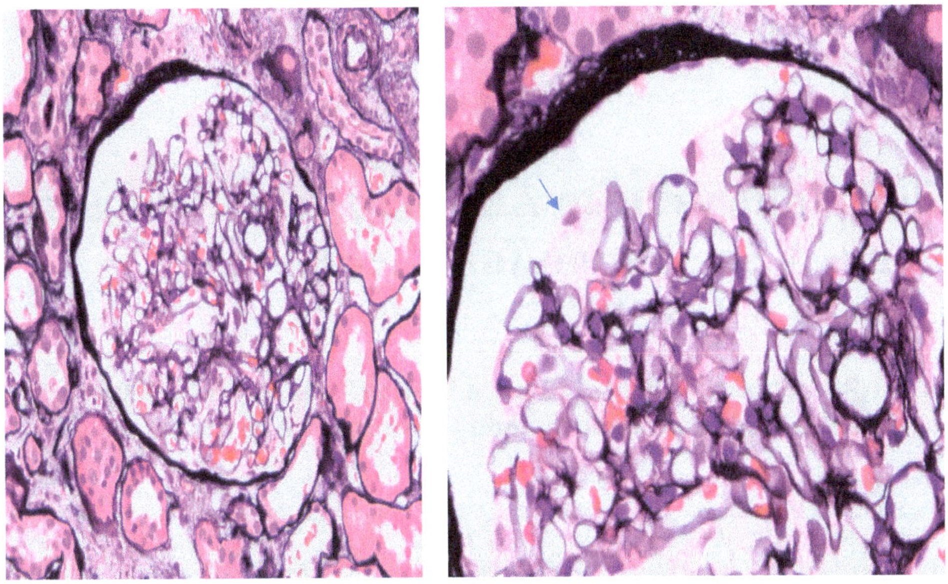

(a) (b)

FIGURE 1: Normocellular glomerulus showing podocytes with foamy cytoplasm (blue arrow). Hematoxylin eosin stain; original magnification 200x (a) and 400x (b).

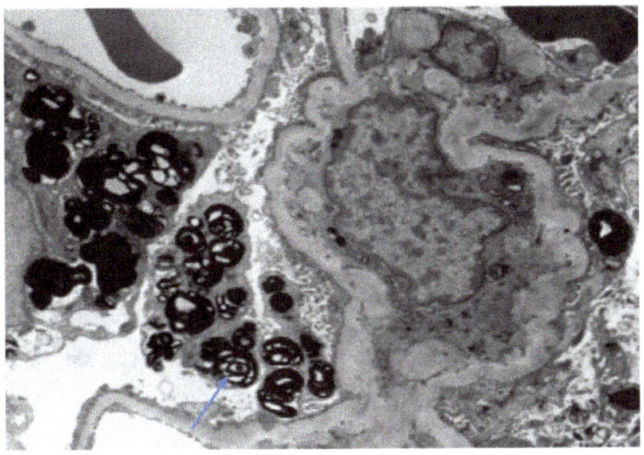

FIGURE 2: Electron microscopy showing podocytes containing dark lamellated osmophilic inclusions, some with appearance of zebra bodies (blue arrow). Transmission electron microscopy; original magnification 3000x.

References

[1] G. E. Linthorst, C. E. Hollak, J. C. Korevaar, J. G. Van Manen, and J. M. Aerts, E. W. Boeschoten, "Alpha-galactosidase A deficiency in Dutch patients on dialysis: a critical appraisal of screening for Fabry disease," *Nephrology Dialysis Transplantation*, vol. 18, no. 8, pp. 1581–1584, 2003.

[2] S. Nakao, C. Kodama, T. Takenaka et al., "Fabry disease: detection of undiagnosed hemodialysis patients and identification of a "renal variant" phenotype," *Kidney International*, vol. 64, no. 3, pp. 801–807, 2003.

[3] J. Herrera and C. S. Miranda, "Prevalence of Fabry's disease within hemodialysis patients in Spain," *Clinical Nephrology*, vol. 81, no. 2, pp. 112–120, 2014.

[4] I. Okur, F. Ezgu, G. Biberoglu et al., "Screening for Fabry disease in patients undergoing dialysis for chronic renal failure in Turkey: identification of new case with a novel mutation," *Gene*, vol. 527, no. 1, pp. 42–47, 2013.

[5] A. Rolfs, T. Böttcher, M. Zschiesche et al., "Prevalence of Fabry disease in patients with cryptogenic stroke: a prospective study," *The Lancet*, vol. 366, no. 9499, pp. 1794–1796, 2005.

[6] W. S. Kim, H. S. Kim, J. Shin et al., "Prevalence of Fabry disease in Korean men with left ventricular hypertrophy," *Journal of Korean Medical Science*, vol. 34, no. 7, p. e62, 2019.

[7] A. Tuttolomondo, I. Simonetta, G. Duro et al., "Inter-familial and intra-familial phenotypic variability in three Sicilian families with Anderson-Fabry disease," *Oncotarget*, vol. 8, no. 37, pp. 61415–61424, 2017.

[8] D. P. Germain, D. A. Hughes, K. Nicholls et al., "Treatment of Fabry's disease with the pharmacologic chaperone migalastat," *New England Journal of Medicine*, vol. 375, no. 6, pp. 545–555, 2016.

[9] S. Jahan, S. Sarathchandran, S. Akthar et al., "Prevalence of Fabry disease in dialysis patients: western Australia Fabry disease study—the forward study," *Orphanet Journal of Rare Diseases*, vol. 15, no. 1, p. 10, 2020.

[10] D. A. Hughes, K. Nicholls, S. P. Shankar et al., "Oral pharmacological chaperone migalastat compared with enzyme replacement therapy in Fabry disease: 18-month results from the randomized phase III attract study," *Journal of Medical Genetics*, vol. 54, no. 4, pp. 288–296, 2017.

[11] S. Bekri, A. Enica, T. Ghafari et al., "Fabry disease in patients with end-stage renal failure: the potential benefits of screening," *Nephron Clinical Practice*, vol. 101, no. 1, pp. c33–c38, 2005.

34

Acute Kidney Injury due to Anticoagulant-Related Nephropathy: A Suggestion for Therapy

Letizia Zeni, [1,2] **Chiara Manenti**, [3] **Simona Fisogni**, [4] **Vincenzo Terlizzi**, [3,4] **Federica Verzeletti**, [3] **Mario Gaggiotti**, [3] **and Giovanni Cancarini** [3,4]

[1] *University of Campania Luigi Vanvitelli, Naples, Italy*
[2] *Fondazione Policlinico Universitario A. Gemelli IRCCS, O. U. of Nephrology, Rome, Italy*
[3] *O. U. of Nephrology, ASST Spedali Civili Brescia, Brescia, Italy*
[4] *Nephrology, Department of Medical and Surgical Specialties, Radiological Science and Public Health, University of Brescia, Brescia, Italy*

Correspondence should be addressed to Letizia Zeni; letizia.zeni@policlinicogemelli.it

Academic Editor: Anja Haase-Fielitz

The relationship between kidneys and anticoagulation is complex, especially after introduction of the direct oral anticoagulants (DOAC). It is recently growing evidence of an anticoagulant-related nephropathy (ARN), a form of acute kidney injury caused by excessive anticoagulation. The pathogenesis of kidney damage in this setting is multifactorial, and nowadays, there is no established treatment. We describe a case of ARN, admitted to our Nephrology Unit with a strong suspicion of ANCA-associated vasculitis due to gross haematuria and haemoptysis; the patient was being given dabigatran. Renal biopsy excluded ANCA-associated vasculitis and diagnosed a red blood cell cast nephropathy superimposed to an underlying IgA nephropathy. Several mechanisms are possibly responsible for kidney injury in ARN: tubular obstruction, cytotoxicity of heme-containing molecules and free iron, and activation of proinflammatory/profibrotic cytokines. Therefore, the patient was given a multilevel strategy of treatment. A combination of reversal of coagulopathy (i.e., withdrawal of dabigatran and infusion of its specific antidote) along with administration of fluids, sodium bicarbonate, steroids, and mannitol resulted in conservative management of AKI and fast recovery of renal function. This observation could suggest a prospective study aiming to find the best therapy of ARN.

1. Introduction

Despite initial scepticism, anticoagulant-related nephropathy is now considered in the lexicon of nephrologists. If suggestions for diagnostic pathway are available [1], a standardised strategy of treatment is still lacking. This report is intended to describe a case of biopsy-proven dabigatran-related nephropathy superimposed to undiagnosed IgA nephropathy and discuss a possible therapy.

2. Case Presentation

A 71-year-old Caucasian male was admitted to our hospital with severe acute kidney injury (AKI) and multiple overt bleedings. His medical history included hypertension, chronic obstructive pulmonary disease, obesity, heavy smoking, obstructive sleep apnoea, and hypercholesterolemia. In May 2017, the patient underwent pacemaker implant due to atrioventricular block; one month later, prolonged episodes of parossistic atrial fibrillation were recorded. Since the renal function was normal, serum creatinine (sCr) 0.97 mg/dL and estimated glomerular filtration rate (eGFR) 78 ml/min/1.73 m^2, a direct oral anticoagulant (DOAC), i.e., dabigatran 150 mg twice a day, was started.

In March 2018, the patient reported persistent fatigue after a flu-like syndrome and occasional episodes of haematuria, haemoptysis, and epistaxis. The blood tests performed on 26th of March showed anaemia with haemoglobin (Hb) of 9.4 g/dL and severe renal failure with sCr 5.12 mg/dL; therefore, the patient was urgently referred to emergency service. In the emergency room on 29th of March, sCr was 6.4 mg/dL, activated partial thromboplastin time was 70 seconds, international normalized ratio was 2.3, and Hb was 8 g/dL. Idarucizumab, the antidote to dabigatran, was readily administered. Chest CT-scan showed bilateral localized ground glass lesions partly with pseudonodular pattern, while no significant abnormalities were seen at abdominal sonography. Rapidly progressive glomerulonephritis with a lung-kidney syndrome was suspected, and tests for anti-neutrophil cytoplasmic antibodies (ANCA) and anti-glomerular membrane antibodies (anti-GBMAb) were urgently performed. Shortly after ELISA confirmation of antimyeloperoxidase antibodies positivity (anti-MPO titre of 61.4 RU/mL), the patient was transferred, on 30th of March, to our Nephrology Unit with a hypothesis of new onset ANCA-associated vasculitis (AAV). Based on this hypothesis, an i.v. bolus of methylprednisolone 100 mg was empirically given on 5th of April and the day after. Renal ultrasound showed normal-sized kidneys, increased cortical echogenicity, and slight reduction in corticomedullary differentiation. Given the chest images are not entirely suggestive for haemorrhagic alveolitis, the absence of systemic signs and symptoms, the negativity of anti-GBMAb and the low levels of inflammatory markers (protein reactive C was 9 mg/L, normal range < 5 mg/L), and the hypothesis of AAV were revised. The morphology of urine red blood cells (RBC) confirmed glomerular haematuria. A renal biopsy was performed on 6th of April when sCr reached its peak of 7.9 mg/dL, and coagulopathy was safely reversed. Few hours later, the patient developed loin pain and a large self-limiting perirenal haematoma. Renal biopsy showed complex features: mesangial matrix expansion and hypercellularity at glomerulus; prominent acute tubular injury with several obstructive RBC casts; interstitium with blood extravasation and moderate inflammation; arteriosclerosis; and arteriolar hyalinosis. Immunofluorescence studies showed 4 + positivity for IgA (Figure 2). Therefore, AAV was excluded, and IgA nephropathy (Oxford score M1, E1, S1, T0, and C0) with possibly iatrogenic acute tubular-interstitial damage was diagnosed.

To promote a "flushing" effect within tubules, mannitol was given from the 9th of April onwards, with rapid and progressive decrease in sCr (Figure 1). Twenty-four hours urinary output was persistently above 1.5–1.8 litres, since the admission to hospital. Given the absence of plasma hyperosmolality and hyperosmolar hyponatremia and presuming mannitol effectiveness in maintaining osmotic diuresis, we decided to slightly increase mannitol dose from two to three times daily. Sodium bicarbonate was initially started for metabolic acidosis (arterial blood gas analysis showed a pH 7.34, pCO_2 38 mmHg, pO_2 85 mmHg, HCO_3- 20 mmol/L, and BE −4 mmol/L), and subsequently maintained to force alkaline diuresis (urinary pH was increased from 5.0 and to 8.0 before discharge) and prevent occurrence of protein (haemoglobin) casts. Then, oral prednisone, 50 mg/day was associated and slowly tapered to 25 mg/day. The patients showed neither significant electrolyte disturbances nor symptoms/signs of uraemia and fluid overload. Balancing the potential risks of bleeding and infection related to central line placement and the benefits of intermittent haemodialysis in the lack of clinically relevant uraemia, renal replacement therapy (RTT) was not performed. The patient was discharged with sCr of 3.3 mg/dL, glomerular proteinuria 3.1 g/24 hours, and plenty of erythrocytes per high power field (HPF) at urine sediment.

Dabigatran was no longer restarted, and 4000 units/day of enoxaparin were introduced, until the patient underwent successful percutaneous closure of left atrial appendage in June. Renal function has progressively improved over time, and proteinuria and haematuria remarkably decreased. Prednisone was withdrawn in September 2018 when sCr was 1.2 mg/dL, proteinuria was 0.9 g/24h, and 1–5 RBC per HPF were detectable.

3. Discussion

After the introduction of direct oral anticoagulants OAC), few papers have reported AKI associated to their use, so the term "Anticoagulant-related nephropathy" (ARN) was coined to describe AKI caused by overanticoagulation [2].

Interestingly, it is suggested that overanticoagulation alone cannot provoke kidney damage. The main risk factors are glomerular overperfusion in the presence of reduced number of functioning nephrons and an underlying inflammatory glomerular disease [3]. In our patient, vascular and inflammatory factors together with advanced age could be the susceptible conditions for AKI, eventually triggered by overanticoagulation. We could not determine whether there was a preexisting kidney disease recognizable at the time of initiation of anticoagulation, as only sCr was available. The estimation of kidney function does not provide an exhaustive renal risk; urinalyses are useful to identify patients that deserve close attention during anticoagulation follow-up [4].

Generally, glomerular macrohematuria is considered a marker of glomerular basement membrane damage and inflammation [5] but, it can be also associated to AKI [6]; in fact, haematuria results in tubular injury in pigment-induced nephropathy (PIN), IgA nephropathy (IgAN), thin basement membrane nephropathy, and ARN [6, 7]. In vitro tubular cytotoxicity after RBC administration encouraged reevaluation of the predominant role of tubular obstruction in haematuria-associated renal damage. In fact, RBC is subjected to intratubular degradation and release heme-containing molecules and free iron [8], that have a direct oxidative cytotoxic effect on tubular cells. Overall, the pathogenesis of ARN is complex and multifactorial: significant erythrocytes filtration through an altered glomerular barrier is triggered by overanticoagulation and results in tubular obstruction and necrosis, inflammation, vasoconstriction-ischemia damage, proapoptosis, and oxidative stress [6]. This interplay between glomerulus and tubule in haematuria-associated renal damage recalls their interaction in many proteinuric glomerulonephritis. Consequently, the first question is whether the induction of inflammation and fibrosis by haematuria promotes chronic kidney disease (CKD), likewise proteinuria. No prospective studies are available probably because ARN is still underestimated.

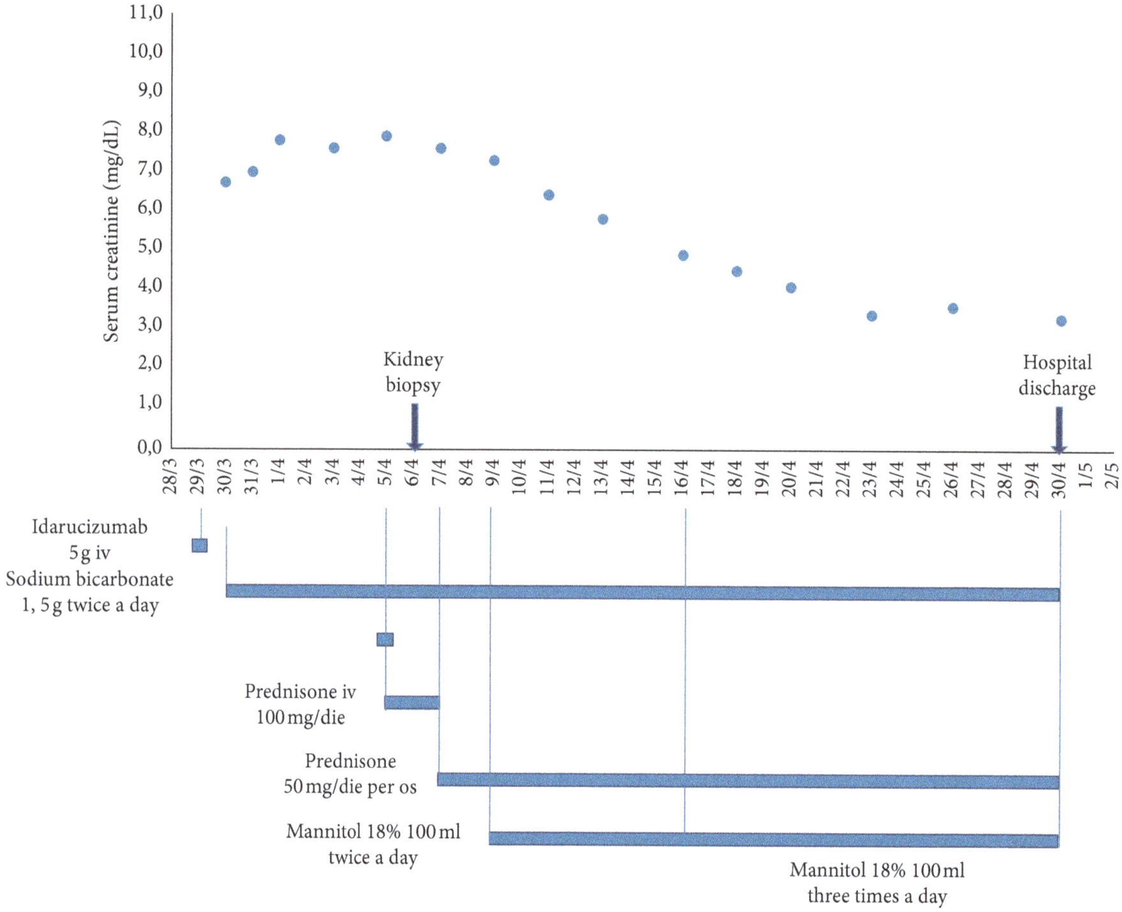

Figure 1: Kidney function trends and therapeutic strategies' timeline during hospitalization.

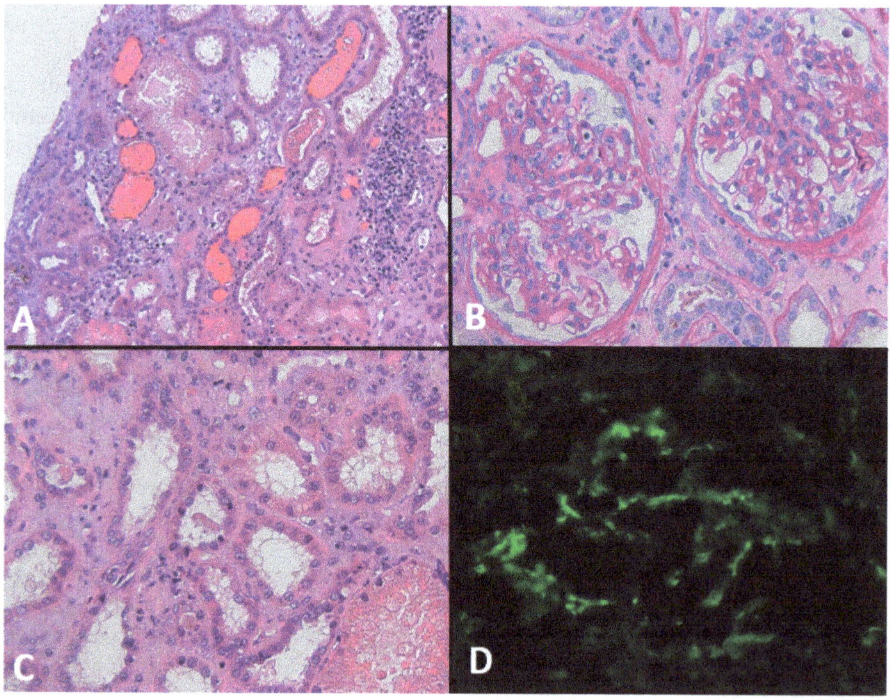

Figure 2: (A) Extensive tubular injury, partially haemolyzed and/or fragmented red blood cells within tubular lumen (H&E 10x). (B) In light microscopy, 10 glomeruli were identified; two glomeruli with mild expansion of mesangial matrix, minimal segmental endocapillary proliferation, flocculo-capsular adhesion with irregularities of Bowman's capsule, and activation of parietal epithelium; tubular injury (PAS 20x). (C) Tubular injury (H&E 20x). (D) IF stain for IgA with mesangial, vessels walls, and endotubular material staining pattern (20x).

However, given the growing evidence of progression of kidney disease in many haematuric conditions, the risk of CKD due to ARN remains a possibility [6]. A second issue is the importance of kidney biopsy in ARN. Considering the association between presumptive ARN with an increase in acute mortality rate [9], a rapid biopsy-proven diagnosis can be helpful [3]. Due to overanticoagulation and severe impairment of kidney function and coexisting comorbidities, renal biopsy is not always feasible. Although the coagulopathy was apparently reversed and the biopsy was performed by an expert physician, a clinically relevant bleeding occurred in our patient after procedure. Notably, this is not the only case of biopsy complicated by bleeding in the contest of dabigatran-induced nephropathy [10]. However, thanks to a biopsy-proven diagnosis, the management dramatically changed, RTT was avoided, and renal function rapidly improved.

To date, no guidelines for ARN treatment are available, and suggestions are gathered from case reports. Correction of coagulopathy (i.e., discontinuation of anticoagulant and administration of antidote) and general supportive care are the mainstays [11].The latter should include fluids administration and urine alkalinisation to prevent RBC precipitation in acidic environment. Early use of steroids to promote renal function recovery and minimize the risk for CKD is suggested by observational studies. Steroids were useful in our patient probably because of underlying IgAN; however, promoting an anti-inflammatory response could be beneficial also for haematuria-associated renal damage. Anti-inflammatory pathway induced by CD163 may decrease haemoglobin cytotoxicity and repair damaged tissues [12].

ARN and PIN share some pathogenetic features. Few evidence [7, 13] suggest that mannitol together with bicarbonate have no advantage over fluid resuscitation in managing AKI due to rhabdomyolysis, and its use remains controversial. However, randomized controlled trials are lacking, and its beneficial effect cannot be excluded [14]. The rationale to use mannitol consists first in a washout effect, that flushes out intratubular necrotic debris [2]; second, in scavenger ability of hydroxyl and other free radicals [13], minimizing cells' injury through an antioxidant effect, and last, in vasodilatation and improvement of renal blood flow [15]. Although it is a long-standing drug, its benefits in haematuria-associated renal damage have not been established yet.

To the best of our knowledge, there are 8 published case reports describing biopsy-proven dabigatran-induced RBC cast nephropathy. Three patients needed RRT, with only two patients with eventually full recovery of renal function. Among patients conservatively treated, sCr returned to the baseline value in three patients only [10, 11, 16–21]. In the contest of overanticoagulation in a subject on NOAC, haematuria suggests that ARN should be taken into account in differential diagnosis; renal biopsy plays a crucial role in this field. None of these patients was treated with mannitol and bicarbonate; in our patient, the sharp and progressive decrease of sCr shortly after their initiation suggests that they could be an option.

Although warfarin has a stronger association with renal events compared to NOAC, several cases have highlighted safety issues for kidney related to NOAC use. In patients on anticoagulants presenting with AKI and haematuria, ARN should be always considered. Once coagulopathy is reversed, performing a kidney biopsy is important to identify any form of renal disease. Mannitol together with sodium bicarbonate and steroids was associated with rapid improvement in renal function. Although only a multicentric prospective study could establish the best strategy for ARN, the combination therapy described in the present case could be informative.

Authors' Contributions

LZ and CM gave the research idea and study design. LZ, CM, SF FV, VT, and MG conducted data acquisition. MG and GC supervised or mentored the study. Each author contributed important intellectual content during manuscript drafting or revision.

References

[1] R. J. Glassock, "Anticoagulant-related nephropathy: it's the real McCoy," *Clinical Journal of the American Society of Nephrology*, vol. 14, no. 6, 2019.

[2] D. S. Wheeler, R. P. Giugliano, and J. Rangaswami, "Anticoagulation-related nephropathy," *Journal of Thrombosis and Haemostasis*, vol. 14, no. 3, pp. 461–467, 2016.

[3] S. Brodsky, J. Eikelboom, and L. A. Hebert, "Anticoagulant-related nephropathy," *Journal of the American Society of Nephrology*, vol. 29, no. 12, pp. 2787–2793, 2018.

[4] C. Cavanaugh and M. A. Perazella, "Urine sediment examination in the diagnosis and management of kidney disease: core curriculum 2019," *American Journal of Kidney Diseases*, vol. 73, no. 2, 2018.

[5] S. M. Jalalah, I. H. Alzahrani, and P. N. Furness, "Glomerular changes in microscopic haematuria, studied by quantitative immunoelectron microscopy and in situ zymography," *Nephrology Dialysis Transplantation*, vol. 17, no. 9, pp. 1586–1593, 2002.

[6] J. A. Moreno, C. Yuste, E. Gutiérrez et al., "Haematuria as a risk factor for chronic kidney disease progression in glomerular diseases: a review," *Pediatric Nephrology*, vol. 31, no. 4, pp. 523–533, 2016.

[7] R. Sakthirajan, J. Dhanapriya, A. Varghese et al., "Clinical profile and outcome of pigment-induced nephropathy," *Clinical Kidney Journal*, vol. 11, no. 3, pp. 348–352, 2017.

[8] J. A. Moreno, C. Martín-Cleary, E. Gutiérrez et al., "AKI associated with macroscopic glomerular hematuria: clinical and pathophysiologic consequences," *Clinical Journal of the American Society of Nephrology*, vol. 7, no. 1, pp. 175–184, 2012.

[9] S. V. Brodsky, T. Nadasdy, B. H. Rovin et al., "Warfarin-related nephropathy occurs in patients with and without chronic kidney disease and is associated with an increased mortality rate," *Kidney International*, vol. 80, no. 2, pp. 181–189, 2011.

[10] R. Escoli, P. Santos, S. Andrade, and F. Carvalho, "Dabigatran-related nephropathy in a patient with undiagnosed IgA nephropathy," *Case Reports in Nephrology*, vol. 2015, Article ID 298261, 4 pages, 2015.

[11] J. Awesat, I. Sagy, Y. S. Haviv et al., "Dabigatran-induced nephropathy and its successful treatment with Idarucizumab-case report and literature review," *Thrombosis Research*, vol. 169, pp. 120–122, 2018.

[12] J. Ballarín, Y. Arce, R. Torra Balcells et al., "Acute renal failure associated to paroxysmal nocturnal haemoglobinuria leads to intratubular haemosiderin accumulation and CD163 expression," *Nephrology Dialysis Transplantation*, vol. 26, no. 10, pp. 3408–3411, 2011.

[13] H. Shawkat, M.-M. Westwood, and A. Mortimer, "Mannitol: a review of its clinical uses," *Continuing Education in Anaesthesia Critical Care & Pain*, vol. 12, no. 2, pp. 82–85, 2012.

[14] J. S. Nielsen, M. Sally, R. J. Mullins et al., "Bicarbonate and mannitol treatment for traumatic rhabdomyolysis revisited," *The American Journal of Surgery*, vol. 213, no. 1, pp. 73–79, 2017.

[15] G. Bragadottir, B. Redfors, and S.-E. Ricksten, "Mannitol increases renal blood flow and maintains filtration fraction and oxygenation in postoperative acute kidney injury: a prospective interventional study," *Critical Care*, vol. 16, no. 4, p. R159, 2012.

[16] R. G. Kalaitzidis, A. Duni, G. Liapis et al., "Anticoagulant-related nephropathy: a case report and review of the literature of an increasingly recognized entity," *International Urology and Nephrology*, vol. 49, no. 8, pp. 1401–1407, 2017.

[17] L. Jansky, P. Mukkamala, D. Jebakumar, A. Rao, T. M. Goldson, and S. N. Forjuoh, "Acute Kidney Injury and Undiagnosed Immunoglobulin A Nephropathy after Dabigatran Therapy," *Proceedings (Baylor University. Medical Center)*, vol. 31, no. 3, pp. 321–323, 2018.

[18] N. Sharfuddin, M. Nourbakhsh, A. Box, H. Benediktsson, and D. A. Muruve, "Anticoagulant related nephropathy induced by dabigatran," *Case Reports in Nephrology*, vol. 2018, Article ID 7381505, 7 pages, 2018.

[19] X. Li and C. Y. Cheung, "Dabigatran causing severe acute kidney injury in a patient with liver cirrhosis," *CEN Case Reports*, vol. 8, no. 2, pp. 1–3, 2019.

[20] G. W. Moeckel, R. L. Luciano, and U. C. Brewster, "Warfarin-related nephropathy in a patient with mild IgA nephropathy on dabigatran and aspirin," *Clinical Kidney Journal*, vol. 6, no. 5, pp. 507–509, 2013.

[21] M. Ikeda, M. Tanaka, S. Shimoda et al., "Dabigatran-induced anticoagulant-related nephropathy with undiagnosed IgA nephropathy in a patient with normal baseline renal function," *CEN Case Reports*, vol. 8, no. 4, pp. 292–296, 2019.

35

Silicone-Induced Granulomatous Reaction Causing Severe Hypercalcemia: Case Report and Literature Review

Gulshan Man Singh Dangol[1,2] and Hilmer Negrete[1,2]

[1]*Department of Internal Medicine, St. Elizabeth Health Center, Youngstown, Ohio, USA*
[2]*Department of Internal Medicine, Northeastern Ohio Medical University, Rootstown, Ohio, USA*

Correspondence should be addressed to Gulshan Man Singh Dangol; gulshanms@gmail.com

Academic Editor: Raoul Bergner

A 67-year-old woman presented to the hospital with complaints of abdominal pain. Physical exam was significant for signs of severe dehydration, mild epigastric tenderness and multiple non-tender hard nodules over her arms and thighs. Incidental finding of severe hypercalcemia led to negative workups for hyperparathyroidism, vitamin D intoxication, and malignancy. However, elevated levels of 1,25-hydroxy vitamin D raised the possibility of granulomatous diseases. Imaging and patient report revealed silicone-induced foreign body granulomatous reaction as the cause of hypercalcemia. Use of silicone for cosmetic enhancement of body contours can result in siliconomas, severe hypercalcemia, and complications. Treatment is unestablished for this condition. Increasing prevalence of cosmetic enhancement should prompt vigilance for this rare disease entity. Providers should counsel and educate individuals undergoing such procedures.

1. Introduction

Hypercalcemia is a common electrolyte abnormality with multiple etiologies, including hyperparathyroidism and malignancy [1]. Rare causes, accounting for less than 10% of cases, should be entertained when more prevalent etiologies have been eliminated. One such cause is extra-renal production of 1,25-hydroxy (OH) vitamin D (calcitriol) produced by silicone-induced foreign body granulomas, siliconomas [2–13].

Silicone, chemically inert, has been used for cosmetic enhancement either in the form of liquid silicone injections (LSI) or as silicone filled breast implants (SBI) [14]. In this article, we report a case of silicone-induced hypercalcemia, and review the literature, highlighting the pathophysiology and discuss therapeutic approaches for this exceedingly rare phenomenon.

2. Case

A 67-year-old woman presented to the hospital with complaint of burning epigastric pain over the past two months. Pain was intermittent, non-radiating, and associated with nausea and vomiting. She admitted to unintentional weight loss, approximately 30 pounds, during the past three months. She denied diarrhea, hematemesis, or melena. Significant past surgical history included bilateral silicone breast implants, exploratory laparotomy following gunshot wound with partial bowel resection, Billroth I gastrectomy following peptic ulcer disease, and partial thyroidectomy for a follicular adenoma.

On examination, she appeared pale and severely dehydrated. Vital signs were 141 beats/minute, blood pressure 143/72 mm of Hg, temperature 97.4°F (36.3°C), and respiratory rate 18 breaths/minute. Current weight was 44 kg with a body mass index of 18.3 kg/m^2. A right-sided thyroid lump was palpable, firm in consistency with regular margins, and moved with swallowing. Breast implants were "rock hard" in consistency with loss of distinct margin over the lower part of the right implant. Heart and lungs were clear to auscultation. Abdomen was soft with multiple surgical scars from previous surgeries. There was mild tenderness over the epigastric region without any guarding or rigidity. There was

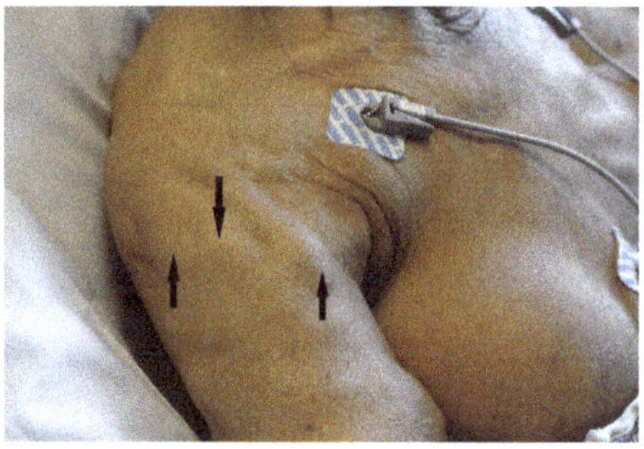

FIGURE 1: Palpable nodules (arrows) over the right arm.

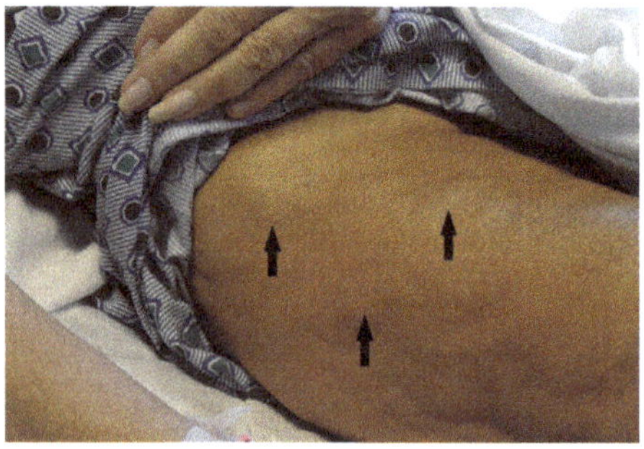

FIGURE 2: Palpable nodules (arrows) over the right thigh.

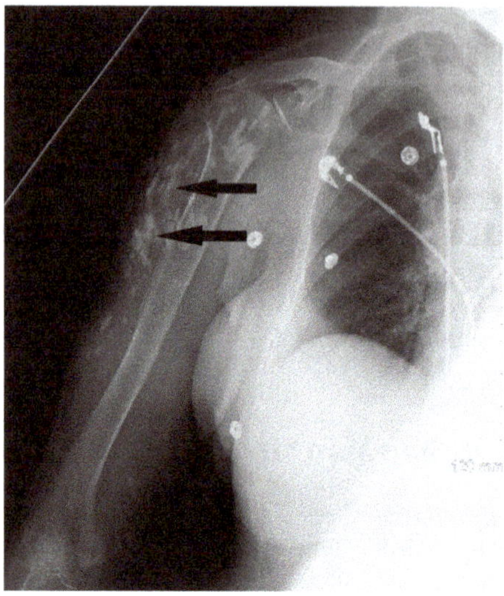

FIGURE 3: X-ray of the right arm showing soft tissue calcifications.

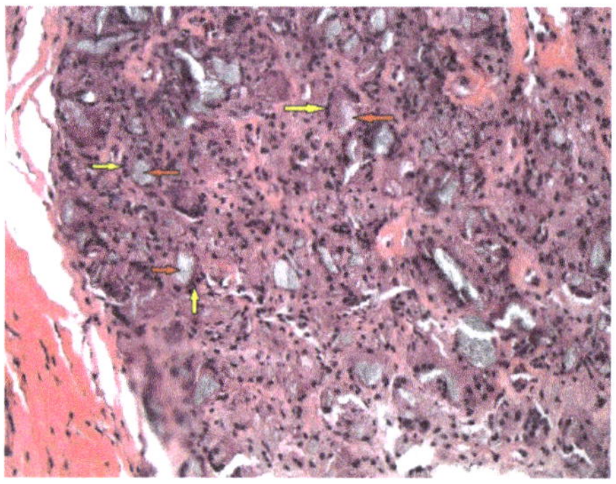

FIGURE 4: Microscopy of the biopsied mass from the left arm showing foreign body granulomatous reaction (high power view, 200 X). Foreign bodies (silicone materials) are shown by black arrows. These are surrounded by multi-nucleated giant cells (white arrows).

no rebound tenderness. Stool guaiac was weakly positive. Multiple fixed hard masses were palpable over both arms and thighs, but not painful, tender, or erythematous (Figures 1 and 2). On further questioning, she described right breast implant rupture diagnosed several years previous, but did not seek any medical advice because of financial issues.

Admission blood work revealed severe hypercalcemia, Ca 18.4 mg/dL (normal: 8.6-10.2 mg/dl), and hyperphosphatemia, Phosphorus 6.8 mg/dL (normal: 2.5-4.5 mg/dl). Initial differential diagnosis for hypercalcemia included excessive antacid use, hyperparathyroidism, malignancy, and vitamin D intoxication. She denied any antacid use, but reported vitamin D 5000 U supplementation twice daily for the past five years. Parathyroid hormone was low, 13 pg/mL (normal 15-65 pg/ml); parathyroid hormone-related peptide,, was normal, <2 pmol/L (normal 0.0 – 3.4 pmol/L); serum and urine protein electrophoresis were both normal; and 25-hydroxy (OH) vitamin D was 40 ng/mL (normal 30-100 ng/mL). Esophagogastroduodenoscopy (EGD) and computed tomography (CT) of the chest and abdomen were negative for malignancy. EGD revealed moderate chronic gastritis; biopsies returned negative for *Helicobacter pylori* or intestinal metaplasia. Chest CT showed clear lung fields with stable bilateral pulmonary nodules, 3-5 mm, in the lower lobes. X-rays of the arms (Figure 3) and thighs revealed extensive soft tissue calcifications. Biopsy of the thyroid mass demonstrated benign-appearing follicular cells with abundant colloid, negative for malignancy. Abdominal CT was negative for any acute intra-abdominal pathology but showed universal calcinosis bilaterally affecting the musculature of the upper thighs. Colonoscopy demonstrated a hyperplastic polyp with evidence of melanosis coli; no malignant cells were seen.

Serum 1,25-OH vitamin D was very elevated 290.7 pg/mL (normal 19.9-79.3 pg/mL), raising the suspicion of an underlying granulomatous disease. Angiotensinogen converting enzyme was mildly elevated, 137 U/L (Normal 9-67 U/L). Tissue biopsy of soft tissue calcifications was discussed; however, the patient refused. She was managed symptomatically and discharged home. Approximately three months later, the patient was re-admitted with hypercalcemia, 17.4 mg/dL. Abdominal CT scan revealed a 7 mm right sided ureteral calculus with mild hydronephrosis. Need for tissue biopsy was re-discussed with the patient and she agreed. Biopsy of the calcified mass on the left arm demonstrated dystrophic calcifications and foreign body granulomatous reaction (Figure 4).

During initial admission, the patient was managed with intravenous normal saline, subcutaneous calcitonin (4 units/kg) every 12 hours for three doses, and a dose of

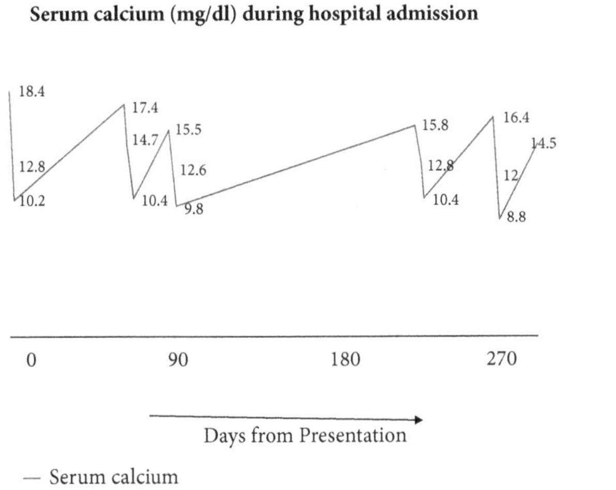

FIGURE 5: Graph showing serum calcium of patient during presentations.

pamidronate (60 mg) intravenously. Despite treatment, the patient remained hypercalcemic, 12.8 mg/dL on hospital day 2. An additional dose of intravenous pamidronate (60 mg) was administered, and calcium level improved to 10.8 mg/dL. After hypercalcemia improved, the patient was discharged with consideration for low dose prednisone on an outpatient basis. However, she failed to follow-up.

On her second admission, three months later, she underwent right ureteral lithotripsy with placement of a ureteral stent, in addition to intravenous hydration, calcitonin, and bisphosphonates. After biopsy confirmed foreign body granulomatous reaction, plastic surgery was consulted for removal of breast implants and calcified granulomas. Given extensive extremity distribution of granulomas, surgical excisions were unfeasible. Removal of breast implants was considered but not done because of her financial constraints. The patient was started and maintained on prednisone 20 mg daily. Despite steroid initiation, the patient remained hypercalcemic and was readmitted after one month, a third time, with a serum calcium of 15 mg/dL.

For the past year, she has had multiple admissions with hypercalcemia and its complications (Figure 5). However, after steroid initiation, her hypercalcemic events were less severe.

3. Discussion

Silicone breast implants consist of a silicone gel enclosed within an outer shell, also known as an elastomer, which provides protection against contracture and rupture [15]. However, breast implant rupture may occur following trauma or during mammography. Once ruptured, silicone materials may disperse to distant sites, either through lymphatic or vascular systems.

The immune system can induce a foreign body reaction in response to administration of organic or inorganic materials, leading to chronic granulomatous inflammation. Epidemiological data has suggested higher rates of sarcoidosis in women receiving silicone breast implants [16]. Such reaction has a latent phase, usually following an acute inflammatory phase, and can last several years, prompting delayed clinical presentation. Typical presentation includes hardening of the skin and tissues, formation of lumps and nodules, and occasional ulcerations [17]. Silicone, either in the form of LSI or following SBI rupture, induces granulomatous reaction leading to the formation of foreign body tumors or siliconomas. Formation of siliconomas following silicone use was first described by Winer et al. in 1964 [18]. However, siliconomas causing hypercalcemia are extremely rare; only a handful of cases have been reported in the literature. Kozeny et al., in 1984, published the first incident of this rare condition [2]. Subsequently, thirteen cases have been reported (Table 1) [2–13]. Most of the cases reported were female; four were transgender. LSI were used in most cases with or without the implantation of SBI. In only one case, SBI was identified as the sole cause of hypercalcemia [10]. Also reported was the use of silicone with the help of transdermal ultrasound to remove wrinkles from the face and neck in one of the cases [5]. Hydration and steroids, with or without bisphosphonates, were the mainstay of treatment, but with improvement in only five cases [3, 5, 6, 12, 13]. Surgical excision of silicone granulomas helped normalize serum calcium in two of the reported cases, [9] and removal of breast implants resulted in improvement in one case [10]. The current case is the second case involving hypercalcemia solely secondary to SBI rupture. While our patient denied any LSI use, including on follow-up, silicone from implant rupture alone may be insufficient in quantity to cause the clinical and radiological findings. Typically, SBI ruptures contribute to local inflammation, and blood or lymphatic silicone transport is microscopic. However, distant multiple siliconomas in lower extremities following breast implant rupture have been described [19]. Among the cases reported, the current case has the highest serum calcium level reported. Use of steroid resulted in temporary improvement, and removal of granulomas and SBI were not pursued in our case.

The exact mechanism of silicone induced hypercalcemia is unknown. Formation of foreign-body granulomas by silicone may play a role in producing hypercalcemia. Granulomatous diseases, especially sarcoidosis, are known to cause calcitriol-related hypercalcemia. In these disorders, macrophages are known to produce 1-alpha-hydroxylase, responsible for the conversion of inactive vitamin D to its active form. Postulated pathophysiology includes the immunomodulatory effect of calcitriol, which decreases T cell activity at the site of inflammation, probably by inhibiting interleukin-2 and γ-interferon [20]. In addition, immunohistochemical studies in vitro have demonstrated 1-alpha-hydroxylase activity in macrophages of sarcoid and foreign-body granulomas [20, 21].

Normally, the enzyme 1-alpha-hydroxylase is present in renal tubular cells, regulating the production of calcitriol. High serum levels of calcitriol cause negative feedback, leading to inhibition of 1-alpha-hydroxylase enzyme. However, these regulatory mechanisms are deficient in macrophages, resulting in unregulated 1,25-OH vitamin D production [18]. This unregulated extra-renal production of calcitriol causes

TABLE 1: Literature reported hypercalcemia cases following use of cosmetic silicone.

Authors (year)	Age (years)	sex	Site of silicone administration	Serum Calcium (mg/dL)**	1,25-OH vitaminD (pg/mL)***	Treatment received	Overall outcome
Kozeny, et al. (1984)	33	Transgender	Silicone injections to face, breasts and both hips	14.7	85.0	Hydration and steroids	Serum calcium improved while on steroid, but increased after it was stopped
Singapuri, et al. (2010)	49	Female	silicone injections to gluteal region	14.6	NA*	Hydration, bisphosphonates and steroids	Serum calcium stabilized
Ogbuagu, et al. (2010)	38	Female	Silicone breast implants; silicone injections to lips, hip and breasts	14.0	51.0	NA*	NA*
Ogbuagu, et al. (2010)	48	Transgender	Silicone injections to hips, face and breasts	11.8	63.0	NA*	NA*
Schanz, et al. (2012)	72	Female	Topical silicone applied over face and neck with transdermal ultrasound for wrinkles removal	12.1	39.0	Steroids	Serum calcium normalized
Agrawal, et al. (2013)	45	Transgender	Bilateral breast implants and silicone injections to buttocks	13.1	147.0	Hydration and steroids	Serum calcium normalized
Camuzard, et al. (2014)	63	Female	Silicone injections to buttocks and hips	13.0	65.0	Hydration, bisphosphonates and steroids	No improvement in serum calcium, patient refused surgical treatment
Visnyei, et al. (2014)	40	Transgender	Silicone injections to thigh and gluteal region	12.3	47.0	Hydration, bisphosphonates and steroids	Initial improvement in serum calcium, but noncompliance resulted in elevation of serum calcium

TABLE 1: Continued.

Authors (year)	Age (years)	sex	Site of silicone administration	Serum Calcium (mg/dL)**	1,25-OH vitaminD (pg/mL)***	Treatment received	Overall outcome
Edwards, et al (2015)	50	Female	Silicone injections to gluteal region	17.3	71.0	Steroid and pentoxiphylline; surgical removal of granulomas	Steroid and pentoxiphylline did not help; surgical removal of granulomas normalized serum calcium
Edwards, et al. (2015)	NA	Female	Silicone injections to gluteal region	11.5	89.0	Steroids and surgical excision of silicone granulomas	Surgical excision improved serum calcium levels
Melnick et al. (2016)	41	Female	Silicone injections to buttocks	13.5	84.0	IV hydration, pamidronate	Serum calcium improved at one year followup
Rodriguez, et al. (2017)	74	Female	Silicone breast implants	14.0	NA*	Hydration, calcitonin and removal of breast implants	Improvement in serum calcium
Noreña, et al. (2017)	40	Female	Silicone injections to gluteal region	13.0	69.1	Hydration, calcitonin, bisphosphonates, sevelamer, chloroquine, and steroids	No improvement in serum calcium, patient died from complications of hypercalcemia
Hamadeh, et al. (2018)	35	Male	Silicone injections to shoulder, arms and forearms	13.1	19.3	Mass excision; hydration, and tapering course of steroids (40 mg daily for three weeks, tapered by 5 mg weekly thereafter)	Improvement in serum calcium
Dangol, et al. (current case) (2018)	67	Female	Silicone breast implants	18.4	290.7	Hydration, calcitonin, bisphosphonate and steroids	No improvement in serum calcium; multiple admissions with hypercalcemia and its complications

*NA = not available.
**Across the series, normal range for serum calcium was 8.2 – 10.3mg/dl.
***Across the series, normal range for 1, 25-OH vitamin D was 15.0 – 86.5 pg/ml.

increased intestinal absorption and calcium mobilization from bones, resulting in hypercalcemia.

Definitive treatment of silicone-induced hypercalcemia is unknown. The benefit of targeted monoclonal antibody treatment for molecular pathways, especially in interleukin production, is unknown, but may be beneficial in the fibrotic phase of silicone induced reactions [22]. Unlike sarcoidosis, where corticosteroids markedly improve production of 1,25-OH vitamin D, treatment with steroids is of limited value in silicone-induced hypercalcemia. While the addition of steroids and removal of foreign body granulomas and implants were helpful in some cases, no treatment modalities or response was noted in other cases. In our patient, steroids were of minimal benefit; removal of granulomas was unfeasible, given extensive dissemination. While steroids may decrease hypercalcemia severity, the adverse profile of steroids over long periods raises the question of possible risk versus benefit. Silicone-induced foreign-body granulomatous reaction should be considered in patients who have undergone cosmetic enhancement and developed hypercalcemia. Treating physicians should be aware of limited treatment modalities available for silicone hypercalcemia and educate individuals of the risk of silicone cosmesis.

Acknowledgments

The authors wish to thank David Gemmel, Ph.D. for critique, manuscript review, and editing.

References

[1] F. W. Lafferty, "Differential diagnosis of hypercalcemia," *Journal of Bone and Mineral Research*, vol. 6, pp. S51–S59, 1991.

[2] G. A. Kozeny, A. L. Barbato, V. K. Bansal, L. L. Vertuno, and J. E. Hano, "Hypercalcemia associated with silicone-induced granulomas," *The New England Journal of Medicine*, vol. 311, no. 17, pp. 1103–1105, 1984.

[3] S. Singapuri, D. Patel, and F. Rahbari-Oskoui, "285: Hypercalcemia Associated With Gluteal Silicone Injections: A Case Report," *American Journal of Kidney Diseases*, vol. 55, article B103, 2010.

[4] O. Ogbuagu, P. Soltani, K. Lawrence, and A. Stern, "216: Unique Etiology of Hypercalcemia in Male to Female Transgender Patients," *American Journal of Kidney Diseases*, vol. 55, no. 4, p. B85, 2010.

[5] J. Schanz, K. Flux, C. Kircher et al., "Mirror, mirror on the wall: Hypercalcemia as a consequence of modern cosmetic treatment with liquid silicone," *Medical Science Monitor*, vol. 18, pp. CS5–CS7, 2012.

[6] N. Agrawal, S. Altiner, N. H. E. Mezitis, and S. Helbig, "Silicone-induced granuloma after injection for cosmetic purposes: A rare entity of calcitriol-mediated hypercalcemia," *Case Reports in Medicine*, vol. 2013, pp. 1–3, 2013.

[7] O. Camuzard, P. Dumas, R. Foissac et al., "Severe granulomatous reaction associated with hypercalcemia occurring after silicone soft tissue augmentation of the buttocks: A case report," *Aesthetic Plastic Surgery*, vol. 38, no. 1, pp. 95–99, 2014.

[8] K. Visnyei, M. Samuel, L. Heacock, and J. A. Cortes, "Hypercalcemia in a male-to-female transgender patient after body contouring injections: A case report," *Journal of Medical Case Reports*, vol. 8, article 71, 2014.

[9] B. J. Edwards, S. Saraykar, M. Sun, W. A. Murphy, P. Lin, and R. Gagel, "Resection of granulomatous tissue resolves silicone induced hypercalcemia," *Bone Reports*, vol. 5, pp. 163–167, 2016.

[10] I. E. Rodriguez and F. W. Deleyiannis, "Hypercalcemia secondary to silicone breast implant rupture," *Plastic and Reconstructive Surgery - Global Open*, vol. 5, article e1416, 2017.

[11] J. A. Noreña, C. D. Niño, S. Gallego et al., "Calcitriol-mediated hypercalcemia secondary to granulomatous disease caused by soft-tissue filler injection: A case report," *Clinical Cases in Mineral and Bone Metabolism*, vol. 14, pp. 340–346, 2017.

[12] M. Hamadeh, J. Fares, K. Maatouk et al., "Hypercalcemia in a bodybuilder with cosmetic silicone injections," *The New Zealand Medical Journal*, vol. 131, pp. 78–81, 2018.

[13] S. Melnick, A. Abaroa-Salvatierra, M. Deshmukh, and A. Patel, "Calcitriol mediated hypercalcaemia with silicone granulomas due to cosmetic injection," *BMJ Case Reports*, 2016, online accessed 12/15/2018.

[14] P. E. Chasan, "The history of injectable silicone fluids for soft-tissue augmentation," *Plastic and Reconstructive Surgery*, vol. 120, no. 7, pp. 2034–2040, 2007.

[15] M. Grigg, S. Bondurant, V. L. Ernster et al., *Information for Women about the Safety of Silicone Breast Implants*, National Academies Press, Washington, DC, USA, 2000.

[16] A. Watad, V. Rosenberg, S. Tiosano et al., "Silicone breast implants and the risk of autoimmune/rheumatic disorders: a real-world analysis," *International Journal of Epidemiology*, vol. 47, no. 6, pp. 1846–1854, 2018.

[17] M. J. Rapaport, C. Vinnik, and H. Zarem, "Injectable silicone: Cause of facial nodules, cellulitis, ulceration, and migration," *Aesthetic Plastic Surgery*, vol. 20, pp. 267–276, 1996.

[18] L. H. Winer, T. H. Sternberg, R. Lehman, and F. L. Ashley, "Tissue reactions to injected silicone liquids," *Arch Dermatol*, vol. 90, pp. 588–592, 1964.

[19] J. H. Oh, S. Y. Song, D. H. Lew, and D. W. Lee, "Distant migration of multiple siliconomas in lower extremities following breast implant rupture," *Plastic and Reconstructive Surgery - Global Open*, vol. 4, pp. 1–3, 2016.

[20] M. Conron, C. Young, and H. L. C. Beynon, "Calcium metabolism in sarcoidosis and its clinical implications," *Rheumatology*, vol. 39, pp. 707–713, 2000.

[21] A. G. Moraitis, M. Hewison, M. Collins, C. Anaya, and M. F. Holick, "Hypercalcemia associated with mineral oil-induced sclerosing paraffinomas," *Endocrine Practice*, vol. 19, pp. 50–56, 2013.

[22] A. M. Desai, J. Browning, and T. Rosen, "Etanercept therapy for silicone granuloma," *Journal of Drugs in Dermatology*, vol. 5, pp. 894–896, 2006.

36

An Exceptional Case of Light Chain Only Variant of Proliferative Glomerulonephritis with Monoclonal Immunoglobulin Deposits Secondary to Chronic Lymphocytic Leukemia: A Case Report and Review of the Literature

José C. De La Flor,[1] Jacqueline Apaza,[2] Francisco Díaz,[3] Edna Sandoval,[4] Tania Linares,[1] Alexander Marschall,[5] Patricia Núñez,[3] Andrea Cecilia Rivas-Nieto,[6] and Elisa Ruiz[1]

[1]*Department of Nephrology, Hospital Central Defense Gomez Ulla, Madrid, Spain*
[2]*Department of Nephrology, Hospital Fuenlabrada, Madrid, Spain*
[3]*Department of Anatomic Pathology, Hospital Gregorio Marañon, Madrid, Spain*
[4]*Department of Hematology, Hospital Central Defense Gomez Ulla, Madrid, Spain*
[5]*Department of Cardiology, Hospital Central Defense Gomez Ulla, Madrid, Spain*
[6]*Department of Nephrology, Hospital Cayetano Heredia, Lima, Peru*

Correspondence should be addressed to José C. De La Flor; josedelaflor81@yahoo.com

Academic Editor: Kouichi Hirayama

We present the case of an 86-year-old Caucasian male with an 11-year history of low-grade chronic lymphocytic leukemia (CLL) presenting with nephrotic syndrome (NS). Renal biopsy findings showed a diffuse mesangial and endocapillary proliferative glomerulonephritis (GN) lesion with fine granular deposits, consistent with a rare morphologic variant of proliferative glomerulonephritis with monoclonal immunoglobulin deposits (PGNMID)-lambda light chain (LC) only. Monthly combination therapy of rituximab (500 mg/m^2 on day 1), fludarabine (30 mg/m^2 on days 1–3), and cyclophosphamide (750 mg/m^2 on days 1–3) was administered. Five courses of this regimen resulted in hematological remission, as well as a partial renal response with a reduction in the spot urine protein-to-creatinine ratio (UPCR) of 815.3 mg/g (reduction > 50% proteinuria without improvement in kidney function). This condition is a rare morphological variant of PGNMID, poorly described in CLL patients. We review the literature and suggest that this case provides sheds light on the unknown pathophysiological mechanisms of monoclonal immunoglobulins (MIg)-mediated glomerular damage in CLL patients, and may be helpful for the investigation of a more effective treatment.

1. Introduction

Chronic lymphocytic leukemia (CLL) is one of the most common chronic lymphoproliferative disorders, accounting for 30% of all leukemias, with an incidence of 4–5 cases per 100,000 habitants per year, and an average age at the time of diagnosis of 60 years [1], making it the most common leukemia in the elderly. CLL is a disease of neoplastic clonal B cells, primarily involving bone marrow, peripheral blood, lymph nodes, liver, and spleen. Extranodal manifestations of CLL are rare and renal involvement is relatively uncommon. The spectrum of kidney pathology includes immune-mediated glomerulonephritis (GN), interstitial infiltration, tubular obstruction, and drug toxicity.

The association between glomerular disease and CLL is apparently rare despite the relative frequency of this type of leukemia [2]. In CLL, the proliferation of the *B*-cell clone does not lead to plasma-cell terminal differentiation. The incidence of GN in CLL is low and the physiopathology links with the hematologic malignancy appear most often hypothetical [3]. The most frequently reported glomerular lesions are membranoproliferative glomerulonephritis (MPGN) and membranous nephropathy. Less commonly, minimal change disease (MCD), focal segmental glomerulosclerosis, amyloidosis, cryoglobulinemic glomerulonephritis, and immunotactoid/microtubular glomerulopathies, have been described [4]. Cases where the monoclonal immunoglobulins (MIg) secreted by the clone of *B* cells may be directly and indirectly involved in the pathogenesis of the glomerular lesions, would be categorized as monoclonal gammopathy lesions of renal significance (MGRS), according to the recent classification [5]. The lesions are governed by the physicochemical properties of the pathogenic MIg rather than the proliferation rate or tumor burden of the *B*-lymphocyte that produces them. MGRS-related kidney lesions are classified according to the characteristics of the MIg deposits on electron microscopy as follows: organized, nonorganized, or absent deposits. The proliferative glomerulonephritis with monoclonal immunoglobulin deposits (PGNMID) is a form of MGRS-associated lesion showing nonorganized MIg granular electron-dense deposits in absence of cryoglobulins [6]. This entity, described by Nasr et al. [7], was characterized by diffuse proliferative (mesangial and endocapillary), membranoproliferative or membranous features with fine granular deposits, mimicking immune complex-type deposits on electron microscopy. In most PGNMID cases, the pathogenic deposited MIg is IgG, but in rare cases, it can be IgA or IgM [8]. However, cases of PGNMID with deposition of nonorganized MIg light chains (LC) only (PGNMID-LC), particularly associated with pathogenic plasma cell clones, are exceptional [9]. Herein, we describe a rare case of CLL with a *B*-cell clonal disorder showing PGNMID-lambda light chain on renal biopsy.

2. Case Report

Our patient is an 86-year-old Caucasian male with an 11-year history of low-grade CLL being followed conservatively by a hematologist. Over 3 months, he developed progressive edema in his lower legs, asthenia, fatigue, and uncontrolled arterial hypertension (AHT). His medication included angiotensin II receptor blockers (ARBs), furosemide, and statin.

On admission, physical examination revealed a blood pressure of 180/87 mmHg, a respiratory rate of 24 breaths/min, oxygen saturation of 96% while breathing ambient air, pulmonary rales, and peripheral edema. His laboratory values indicated a creatinine (Cr) level of 1.67 mg/dl, estimated GFR (eGFR) 36.5 mL/min/1.73 m^2 by chronic kidney disease epidemiology (CKD-EPI) formula, and hypoalbuminemia without hypercholesterolemia. His urine showed 15–25 red blood cells per high-power field (RBC/HPF) with dysmorphic cells. The 24-hour urine protein excretion was 7.72 g with a significant disproportion of spot urine protein-to-creatinine ratio (UPCR) and urine albumin-to-creatinine ratio (UACR) of 7614.94 and 2635.39 mg/g, respectively. Serum protein immunofixation/electrophoresis (IFE) revealed a trace band positive for IgG-kappa and IgG-lambda *M*-protein. Urine IFE also showed only a weak band of IgG-lambda. Other laboratory findings revealed the following: leukocyte count, 6.92×10^3/uL with 35.4% lymphocyte; erythrocyte count, 3.56×10^6/uL with his other hematologic cell lines being normal. The rest of his investigations were normal (cryoglobulins, hepatitis B and C, antinuclear antibody (ANA), antineutrophil cytoplasmic antibody (ANCA), rheumatoid factor, serum complement-3 (C3), and complement-4 (C4). The patient's creatinine rose to 2.3 mg/dl during the in-hospital stay after starting depletive treatment, probably associated with hemodynamic changes due to antiproteinuric medication. Other laboratory test results are shown in Table 1.

A renal biopsy was performed and 38 glomeruli were examined under light microscopy (LM), 17 of which (44%) were globally sclerotic. All of the remaining glomeruli exhibited a global and diffuse expansion of the mesangial matrix, with a focally (<50% of glomeruli) increase of mesangial cells. A variable degree of pericapsular fibrosis was observed. The capillary loops were slightly thickened and no double contours, endocapillary proliferation, or intravascular thrombi were observed. In addition, three glomeruli showed extracapillary epithelial cell proliferation, two of them cell lesions and one fibrocellular. A mild degree of interstitial scarring (30%) and tubular atrophy were also noted. A mild infiltration of lymphocytes, histologically nonspecific, occupying less than 5% of the cortical surface was observed. Mild arteriolosclerosis was seen. No intravascular thrombi or vasculitis was observed. Congo red and thioflavin staining were negative (Figures 1(a)–1(c)). Marked intensity for the lambda light chain (2+) and weak intensity for the kappa light chain (1+) in both the mesangium and peripheral capillary loops were demonstrated by frozen tissue immunofluorescence (IF-F). In contrast, the IF was negative for IgG, IgM, IgA, C1q, and C3. On the other hand, the IF on pronase-digested paraffin-embedded (IF-P) sections showed no subendothelial or mesangial deposits of IgG, IgM, or IgA (Figure 1(d)). Electron microscopy (EM) revealed large electron-dense nonorganized deposits in mesangial and subendothelial areas (Figures 1(e) and 1(f)). The immunohistochemistry technique for DNAJB9 was performed with a negative result.

The bone marrow (BM) aspiration showed increased cellularity. The immunophenotypic study showed that 45.4% of the total cellularity was lymphocytes. Of this population, 27.7% were mature lymphocytes of monoclonal origin with moderate intensity lambda light chain restriction, with an immunophenotype compatible with CLL (CD19+, CD45+, CD5++, CD200+++, and weakly positive for CD20). The few plasma cells revealed a phenotype without abnormalities or restriction of intracytoplasmic light chains. A fluorescence in situ hybridization (FISH) cytogenetic study was performed in bone marrow, being negative for BCL-2 and *t* (11; 14). A positron emission tomography-computed tomography scan (PET/CT) did not suggest lymphoproliferative syndrome, solitary plasmacytoma, or other extramedullary affectations.

Table 1: Laboratory findings on admission.

		Reference range/Unit
WBC	6920	U/L
Hemoglobin (Hb)	11	12–16 g/dL
Platelet count (PLt)	131	10^3/uL
Reticulocytes count	2.77	2–4%
Erythrocyte count	3.56	4.2–5.8 10^6/uL
Lactate dehydrogenase (LDH)	180	135–214 IU/L
Coombs test	Negative	NA
Total bilirubin	0.5	0.1–1 mg/dL
Total protein (TP)	5.5	6.4–8.7 g/dL
Serum albumin (Alb)	2.56	3–5.5 g/dL
GOT	21	5–32 IU/L
GPT	12	5–33 IU/L
Urea	98	17–60 mg/dL
Creatinine	1.67	0.6–1.2 mg/dL
Na	138	135–145 mmol/L
K	5.2	3.5–5.5 mmol/L
Cl	99	95–110 mmol/L
CRP	1.5	0.1–0.5 mg/dL
Hbs-Ag	Negative	NA
HCV-Ab	Negative	NA
HIV	Negative	NA
CH50	50	40–90 U/ml
CFH	250	225–760 μg/mL
Autoantibodies CFH	Negative	<18 AU/L
C3 nephritic factor (C3NF)	Negative	Ratio >1.022
C3	116	90–180 mg/dL
C4	22.5	10–40 mg/dL
RF	Negative	<15 IU/ml
ANA, anti-dsDNA, ANCA, and cryoglobulin	Negative	NA
Anti-GBM	Negative	<1 AI
Anti-PLA2R Ab (ELISA)	Negative	NA
Beta 2 microglobulin	1.09	<0–20 mg/dL
IgG	1200	800–1600 mg/dL
IgA	151	70–400 mg/dL
IgM	67.7	90–180 mg/dL
UPCR	7614.94	<20 mg/g
UACR	2635.39	<30 mg/g
Urine red blood cells	15–25	/HPF
24 h urine total protein excretion	7.72	<0.15 g/24 h
SPEP M-protein concentration	2 M-protein: 1.5 and 2.9%	NA
SIF	IgG κ, IgG λ	NA
Urine immunofixation electrophoresis	IgG λ	NA mg/dL
Urine IgG	52.70	NA mg/dL
FLC κ	30.1	4.90–13.70 mg/L
FLC λ	53	7.60–19.50 mg/L
FLC κ/λ	0.57	0.27–1.67

AI: activity index; AU: arbitrary units; NA: not applicable; WBC: white blood cells; GOT: glutamate-oxaloacetate transaminase; GPT: glutamate pyruvate transaminase; Na: sodium serum; K: potassium serum; Cl: chloride serum; CRP: C—reactive protein; CH50: complement hemolytic activity-50; CFH: complement factor H; C3NF: complement-3 nephritic factor; C3: complement-3; C4: complement-4; RF: rheumatoid factor; ANA: antinuclear antibody; anti-dsDNA: anti-double stranded DNA antibody; ANCA: anti-neutrophil cytoplasmic autoantibody; anti-GBM: anti-glomerular basement membrane; anti-PLA2R Ab: anti-phospholipase a2 receptor antibody; Ig: immunoglobulin; UPCR: spot urine protein-to-creatinine ratio; UACR: spot urine albumin-to-creatinine ratio; ELISA: enzyme-linked immunosorbent assay; SPEP: serum protein electrophoresis; SIF: serum immunofixation; FLC: free light chain; κ: kappa; λ: lambda; HPF: high-power field.

Therefore, the present case was diagnosed as lesions PGNMID-Lambda LC only associated with CLL. Monthly combination therapy of rituximab (500 mg/m^2 on day 1), fludarabine (30 mg/m^2 on days 1–3), and cyclophosphamide (750 mg/m^2 on days 1–3) was administered. Five courses of this regimen resulted in hematological remission, as well as a partial renal response with a reduction in the UPCR of 815.3 mg/g (reduction >50% proteinuria without improvement in kidney function).

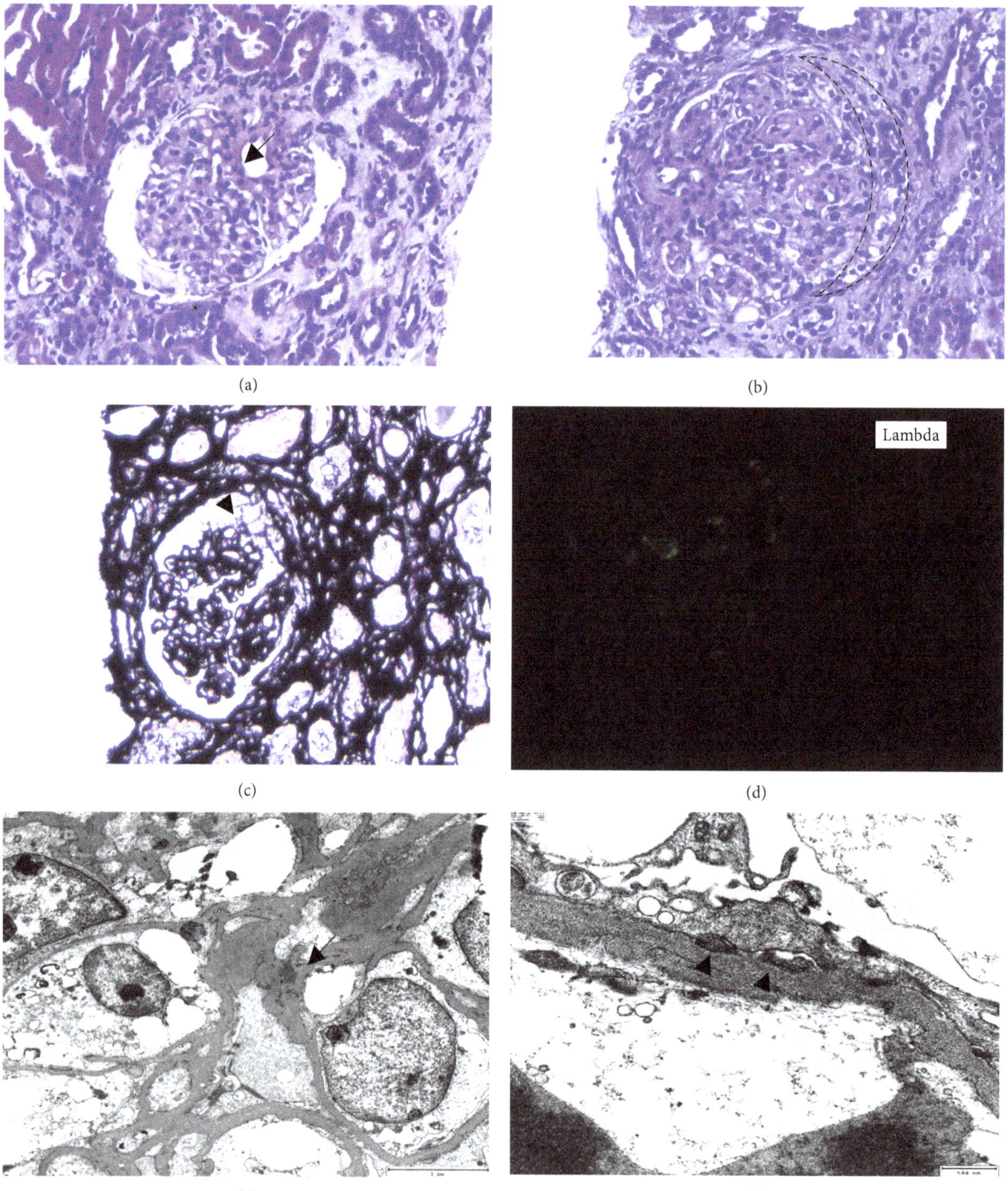

(a) (b) (c) (d) (e) (f)

Figure 1: Light microscopy shows a global increase of mesangial matrix, with focally mesangial hypercellularity (arrow). (a) Hyalinosis of the afferent arteriole was observed (asterisk) (*H-E*, 200*x*). (b) The glomerulus shows irregular capillary wall thickening and a cellular crescent (dashed crescent) (*H-E*, 200*x*). (c) Methanamine-silver stain (200x) shows a glomerulus with a cellular crescent (arrowhead). (d) Direct immunofluorescence showing bright granular staining of glomerular mesangium for lambda light chain (lambda++/kappa+, 200*x*). (e) Electron microscopy revealed large electron-dense nonorganized deposits in mesangial areas (arrow) (10000*x*). (f) Electron microscopy showing segmental subendothelial mesangial deposits (arrow-head) (10000*x*).

3. Discussion

In this report, we describe a case of CLL presenting with NS. Renal biopsy findings showed a diffuse mesangial and endocapillary proliferative GN lesion with fine granular deposits, consistent with a rare morphologic variant of PGNMID-Lambda LC only. The LM, IF and EM findings of our patient described MGRS-related renal lesions with deposit Ig nonorganized. These findings were completely different from those of monoclonal immunoglobulin deposition disease (MIDD). MIDD comprises a group of diseases characterized by the deposition of light chains (LCDD), heavy chains (HCDD), or both light and heavy chains deposits (LHCDD) are seen along both the glomerular basement membrane (GBM) and the tubular basement membrane (TBM). In addition, LCDD is characterized by nodular mesangial glomerulosclerosis resembling Kimmelstiel–Wilson nodules and the continuous deposition of fine, electron-dense granular materials along the inner aspect of the glomerulus [10].

The incidence of NS in patients with CLL is approximately 1% to 2% [11]. While the renal complications of plasma cell dyscrasia have been well described, most information on patients with CLL is derived from case reports. There are two large case series published in the literature [2, 4]. The larger of the two was that of Strati et al. [4], who completed a retrospective analysis of patients with CLL or monoclonal *B*-cell lymphocytosis that underwent kidney biopsy for renal insufficiency and/or NS. Between January 1995 and June 2014, 49 of 4,024 (1.2%) patients with CLL ($n = 44$) or monoclonal *B*-cell lymphocytosis ($n = 5$) had a renal biopsy: 34 (69%) for renal insufficiency and 15 (31%) for nephrotic syndrome. The most common findings were MPGN ($n = 10$, 20%), chronic lymphocytic leukemia interstitial infiltration as primary etiology ($n = 6$, 12%), thrombotic microangiopathy ($n = 6$, 12%), and minimal change disease ($n = 5$, 10%). MPGN is one of the most frequent kidney diseases described in association with CLL, which is caused by cryoglobulinemia, predominantly type II [12], or may be associated with deposition of a MIg secreted by leukemia *B* cells [3, 11], recently included in a new diagnostic term denominated MGRS [6]. The MGRS is pathogenically characterized by the proliferation of B-lymphocyte clones or plasma cell clones that synthesize and secrete a MIg or its components (light or heavy chains), with the ability to cause damage at the tubular, glomerular, vascular, and interstitial compartments through direct (deposition) or indirect (alterations of the alternative complement pathway) mechanisms, constituting a heterogeneous group of entities [13, 14].

In 2004, Nasr et al. [15] described for the first time a new type of glomerular injury related to MIg deposition without involving TBM, which they classified as PGNMID. PGNMID are characterized by deposits typically composed of intact MIg with both Ig heavy and light chains, particularly by IgG (PGNMID-IgG) or exceptionally by deposits of nonorganized MIg light chains (LC) only (PGNMID-LC). According to Nasr et al. [9] in a series of 17 cases with PGNMID-LC, based on the pathologic findings by LM and EM, they described several notable pathological and immune-hematologic differences between PGNMID-LC and the considerably more common variant-PGNMID-IgG primarily, the deposits on IF in PGNMID-LC stain only for Ig-LC without staining for IgG neither other Ig type (IgA or IgM). These observations are consistent with our findings, as we confirmed the absence of IgG, IgA, or IgM by IF-P and EM. Secondly, both in PGNMID-IgG and PGNMID-LC, the codeposit of C3 is nearly always described, while the deposits of C1q are more frequent in PGNMID-IgG than PGNMID-LC [9]. In contrast, the present case did not show C3 or C1q codeposits on IF or IF-P. At this point, the liquid chromatography-mass spectrometry (LC-MS) study would have been very useful. Leung et al., in the expert consensus document of the International Kidney and Monoclonal Gammopathy Research Group, recommend the usefulness of LC-MS for the diagnosis of MGSR lesions when IF studies have negative findings [5], as in our case. However, this technique is not available in our center. Thirdly, the subendothelial deposits in most cases of PGNMID-IgG are small and best seen by EM, while that in PGNMID-LC are frequently large and easily identified by LM [9], these findings are in line with the biopsy of our case, except for the presence of diffuse proliferative mesangial and endocapillary lesions. Nasr et al. [9] hypothesized that this could be due to the higher concentration of circulating MIg levels in PGNMID-LC than in PGNMID-IgG and this may also reflect differences in the mechanisms of complement activation induced by the deposition of monoclonal LCs. Lastly, clonal identification is most difficult in patients who have PGNMID-IgG, in more than 80%, pathological clones of B cells and plasma cells are not detected in BM at diagnosis or on follow-up [8, 9, 15]. Nasr et al. [9] reported that the underlying clone in all PGNMID-LC cases was a plasma cell clone, these nephropathic clone was detected in the BM in 88% (14 of 16), coinciding with other case reports [16–20]. Unlike in our case, proliferative glomerulonephritis was caused by the secretion and deposition of lambda LC in a patient with CLL, in which the pathological clone was a *B*-lymphocyte. Therefore, to the best of our knowledge, this case could be one of the first to describe PGNMID-LC associated with CLL.

Regarding the hematological characteristics of PGNMID-LC, the serum free light chain (FLC) ratio was abnormally elevated in almost 83% (10 of 12 patients tested) of PGNMID-LC cases reported by Nasr et al. [9], including 3 patients with a serum FLC ratio > 100, and normal in 2 (17%) patients. On the other hand, in a study by Buthani et al. [8], only 20% of patients with PGNMID-IgG presented abnormal FLC. In our patient, we found two serum bands of monoclonal IgG-kappa and IgG-lambda, urine IFE with a faint band of IgG-lambda, and renal deposits of lambda LCs in mesangial and capillary loops. In addition, the serum FLC kappa and lambda were slightly elevated with a normal serum FLC ratio. On the other hand, our patient did not present hypocomplementemia or alterations in the study of the alternative pathway of complement (APC). In the cohort of PGNMID-LC reported by Nasr et al. [9], they detected hypocomplementemia (low C3 with normal C4) in 6 (50%) of 12 patients. Four of these patients had complement factor B (CFB), factor H (CFH), and factor I (CFI) levels within normal limits and none had detectable C3 nephritic factor (C3FN) or antifactor H IgG autoantibody.

The pathogenesis of PGNMID-LC remains uncertain. Nasr et al. [9], suggest that PGNMID-LC is mediated by local APC activation in the glomeruli by the MIg-LC, which then activates downstream inflammatory mediators that promote glomerular proliferation, leukocyte infiltration, and glomerular basement membrane damage and reparative changes leading to MPGN. However, in our case, there is relevant data, such as the absence of hypocomplementemia and MPGN lesions associated with a normal serum FLC ratio, which leads us to think that there may be other mechanisms of glomerular damage mediated by MIg not yet known in this rare variant of PGNMID-LC.

As in other forms of MGRS-related lesions, the treatment strategies are based on chemotherapy that must be adapted to the nature of the cell clone, both lymphocytic or plasma, renal function, and the presence or absence of extrarenal involvement [6]. CLL is a malignancy characterized by clonal proliferation of B-lymphocytes that are often CD20 positive [21]. Therefore, the abnormal lambda LC produced by the malignant clone is responsible for the LC deposition and subsequent proliferation observed in our case with PGNMID-LC. Rituximab (a monoclonal antibody to CD20) produces depletion of B-lymphocytes in patients with CLL [21] and would be expected to reduce the production and deposition of pathogenic MIg-LC. Most previously reported cases only refer to the management of rituximab in patients with CLL and PGNMID-IgG [22, 23]. However, there are no cases describing CLL and PGNMID-LC. Two of the cases of CLL and PGNMID-IgG show ambiguous results. Barbour et al. [22] reported two cases treated with rituximab with reduced proteinuria and improved renal function, in addition to a complete hematologic response. On the other hand, Bhat et al. [23] described 3 patients, 2 of them experienced partial remission of their disease and 1 patient was able to come off hemodialysis therapy after treatment with 7 and 11 biweekly doses of rituximab, 375 mg/m. Both patients subsequently experienced a relapse of their hematologic and renal diseases and eventually progressed to end-stage renal disease and death. A third patient was treated with two 1,000 mg infusions of rituximab separated by 2 weeks, with sustained partial remission at 18 months follow-up. In a small, multicenter, retrospective study of 17 patients with CLL and PGNMID-LC by Nasr et al. [9], plasma cell-targeted chemotherapy (mostly bortezomib-based therapy) resulted in complete or partial renal recovery in 6 of the 10 patients treated, whereas none of 5 patients given nontargeted treatment recovered kidney function. As in other forms of MGRS-related kidney lesions, renal response depended on hematologic response [6]. Our patient was treated with *B*-lymphocyte cell-targeted chemotherapy (mostly Rituximab-based therapy) and experienced partial renal remission and complete hematologic response.

In conclusion, we describe an exceptional case of PGNMID-Lambda LC with CLL. This condition is a rare morphological variant of PGNMID, poorly described in CLL patients. This case provides sheds light on the unknown pathophysiological mechanisms of MIg-mediated glomerular damage in CLL patients and may be helpful for the investigation of a more effective treatment.

Consent

The patient has given their written informed consent to publish their case (including publication of images).

References

[1] D. A. Arber, A. Orazi, R. Hasserjian et al., "The 2016 revision to the world health organization classification of myeloid neoplasms and acute leukemia," *Blood*, vol. 127, no. 20, pp. 2391–2405, 2016.

[2] A. L. Poitou-Verkinder, A. Francois, F. Drieux et al., "The spectrum of kidney pathology in *B*-cell chronic lymphocytic leukemia/small lymphocytic lymphoma: a 25-year multicenter experience," *PLoS One*, vol. 10, no. 3, Article ID e0119156, 2015.

[3] B. Moulin, P. M. Ronco, B. Mougenot, A. Francois, J. P. Fillastre, and F. Mignon, "Glomerulonephritis in chronic lymphocytic leukemia and related *B*-cell lymphomas," *Kidney International*, vol. 42, no. 1, pp. 127–135, 1992.

[4] P. Strati, S. H. Nasr, N. Leung et al., "Renal complications in chronic lymphocytic leukemia and monoclonal *B*-cell lymphocytosis: the mayo clinic experience," *Haematologica*, vol. 100, no. 9, pp. 1180–1188, 2015.

[5] N. Leung, F. Bridoux, V. Batuman et al., "The evaluation of monoclonal gammopathy of renal significance: a consensus report of the international kidney and monoclonal gammopathy research group," *Nature Reviews Nephrology*, vol. 15, no. 1, pp. 45–59, 2019.

[6] N. Leung, F. Bridoux, and S. H. Nasr, "Monoclonal gammopathy of renal significance," *New England Journal of Medicine*, vol. 384, no. 20, pp. 1931–1941, 2021.

[7] S. H. Nasr, A. Satoskar, G. S. Markowitz et al., "Proliferative glomerulonephritis with monoclonal IgG deposits," *Journal of the American Society of Nephrology*, vol. 20, no. 9, pp. 2055–2064, 2009.

[8] G. Bhutani, S. H. Nasr, S. M. Said et al., "Hematologic characteristics of proliferative glomerulonephritides with nonorganized monoclonal immunoglobulin deposits," *Mayo Clinic Proceedings*, vol. 90, no. 5, pp. 587–596, 2015.

[9] S. H. Nasr, C. P. Larsen, C. Sirac et al., "Light chain only variant of proliferative glomerulonephritis with monoclonal immunoglobulin deposits is associated with a high detection rate of the pathogenic plasma cell clone," *Kidney International*, vol. 97, no. 3, pp. 589–601, 2020.

[10] J. Lin, G. S. Markowitz, A. M. Valeri et al., "Renal monoclonal immunoglobulin deposition disease: the disease spectrum," *Journal of the American Society of Nephrology*, vol. 12, no. 7, pp. 1482–1492, 2001.

[11] F. D. Seney, "A review of nephrotic syndrome associated with chronic lymphocytic leukemia," *Archives of Internal Medicine*, vol. 146, no. 1, pp. 137–141, 1986.

[12] J. C. Brouet, J. P. Clauvel, F. Danon, M. Klein, and M. Seligmann, "Biologic and clinical significance of

cryoglobulins," *The American Journal of Medicine*, vol. 57, no. 5, pp. 775–788, 1974.

[13] J. C. De La Flor, M. Alonso, E. Sandoval, A. Marschall, and M. Rodeles, "Monoclonal gammopathy of renal significance with deposits of peculiar morphology and injuries of secondary thrombotic microangiopathy: a case report and review of the literature," *Case Reports in Nephrology*, vol. 2020, Article ID 6679857, 7 pages, 2020.

[14] F. Bridoux, N. Leung, C. A. Hutchison et al., "Diagnosis of monoclonal gammopathy of renal significance," *Kidney International*, vol. 87, no. 4, pp. 698–711, 2015.

[15] S. H. Nasr, G. S. Markowitz, M. B. Stokes et al., "Proliferative glomerulonephritis with monoclonal IgG deposits: a distinct entity mimicking immune-complex glomerulonephritis," *Kidney International*, vol. 65, no. 1, pp. 85–96, 2004.

[16] A. Chang, C. J. Peutz-Kootstra, C. A. Richardson, and C. E. Alpers, "Expanding the pathologic spectrum of light chain deposition disease: a rare variant with clinical follow-up of 7 years," *Modern Pathology*, vol. 18, pp. 998–1004, 2005.

[17] A. Komatsuda, M. Nara, H. Ohtani, T. Nimura, K. Sawada, and H. Wakui, "Proliferative glomerulonephritis with monoclonal immunoglobulin light chain deposits: a rare entity mimicking immune-complex glomerulonephritis," *Internal Medicine*, vol. 51, no. 23, pp. 3273–3276, 2012.

[18] C. E. Alpers, W. H. Tu, J. Hopper, and C. G. Biava, "Single light chain subclass (kappa chain) immunoglobulin deposition in glomerulonephritis," *Human Pathology*, vol. 16, no. 3, pp. 294–304, 1985.

[19] S. Meri, V. Koistinen, A. Miettinen, T. Tornroth, and I. J. Seppala, "Activation of the alternative pathway of complement by monoclonal lambda light chains in membranoproliferative glomerulonephritis," *Journal of Experimental Medicine*, vol. 175, no. 4, pp. 939–950, 1992.

[20] T. S. Jokiranta, A. Solomon, M. K. Pangburn, P. F. Zipfel, and S. Meri, "Nephritogenic lambda light chain dimer: a unique human miniautoantibody against complement factor H," *Journal of Immunology*, vol. 163, no. 8, pp. 4590–4596, 1999.

[21] M. Hallek, B. D. Cheson, D. Catovsky et al., "Guidelines for the diagnosis and treatment of chronic lymphocytic leukemia: a report from the international workshop on chronic lymphocytic leukemia updating the national cancer institute-working group 1996 guidelines," *Blood*, vol. 111, no. 12, pp. 5446–5456, 2008.

[22] S. J. Barbour, M. C. Beaulieu, N. Y. Zalunardo, and A. B. Magil, "Proliferative glomerulonephritis with monoclonal IgG deposits secondary to chronic lymphocytic leukemia report of two cases," *Nephrology Dialysis Transplantation*, vol. 26, no. 8, pp. 2712–2714, 2011.

[23] P. Bhat, S. Weiss, G. B. Appel, and J. Radhakrishnan, "Rituximab treatment of dysproteinemias affecting the kidney: a review of three cases," *American Journal of Kidney Diseases*, vol. 50, no. 4, pp. 641–644, 2007.

37

Deterioration in Clinical Status is not Enough to Suspend Eculizumab: A Genetic Complement-Mediated Atypical Hemolytic Uremic Syndrome Case Report

Luca Calvaruso[1,2] **Alessandro Naticchia,**[1,2] **Pietro Manuel Ferraro**[1,2]
Gisella Vischini,[1,2] **and Stefano Costanzi**[1,2]

[1]*U.O.C. Nefrologia, Fondazione Policlinico Universitario A. Gemelli IRCCS, Rome, Italy*
[2]*Università Cattolica del Sacro Cuore, Rome, Italy*

Correspondence should be addressed to Luca Calvaruso; lucacalvaruso2307@gmail.com

Academic Editor: Yoshihide Fujigaki

Background. Atypical hemolytic uremic syndrome (aHUS) is characterized by microangiopathic hemolytic anemia, thrombocytopenia, and renal failure. Mutations in CFI gene coding for complement regulation factors and in THBD gene coding for endothelial cell receptor thrombomodulin could predispose to the disease and hypertension can trigger the onset. *Case Presentation.* A 51-year-old female patient who had received kidney transplant eighteen years ago presented with hypertensive peak and hemolysis pattern. Normal ADAMTS13 levels as well as negative culture and serology for Shiga-toxin excluded, respectively, thrombotic thrombocytopenic purpura (TTP) and typical HUS caused by Shiga toxin-producing *Escherichia coli* (STEC-HUS). In suspicion of aHUS, we administered eculizumab and hemodialysis sessions were started as the patient showed severe renal failure. After an initial response, the patient developed cerebral hemorrhage. After last eculizumab administration, according to hematological parameters, an unsatisfactory response was observed: given the worsening clinical scenario, we withdrew eculizumab. Pathogenic mutations in CFI and THBD genes were found. After eculizumab reinitiation, looking at hemolysis indexes, we observed a suboptimal response as well as an otherwise adequate renal one: renal graft function was recovered despite persistence of hemolysis signs, after 6 months on regular dialysis. *Conclusion.* For the first time, we report an aHUS case in which a peculiar combination of mutations in CFI and THBD is found. We describe the importance of continuing eculizumab despite deterioration of patient's clinical conditions.

1. Background

Thrombotic microangiopathy (TMA) is characterized by a clinical presentation with thrombocytopenia, microangiopathic hemolytic anemia (MAHA), and organ injury (kidney, CNS, gut, etc.) [1].

Atypical hemolytic-uremic syndrome (aHUS) belonging to the group of TMA is a genetic or acquired ultrarare, life-threatening disease mainly associated with complement dysregulation. aHUS has an incidence of approximately 0.5 per million per year [2].

Mostly, we refer to aHUS as a hereditary complement-mediated disease [3]. The underlying genetic mutations which predispose to aHUS have incomplete penetrance so that a second hit is required for disease manifestation [4].

On the other hand, pathogenic variants responsible for permanent complement dysregulation are detected in about 40 to 60% of patients with aHUS [5].

Since diagnosis can often be challenging, we can adopt a predictive model for the initial diagnosis of TMA based on LDH and platelet count which was found to accurately predict the presence of TMA [6].

In the pre-eculizumab era, aHUS was characterized by significant morbidity and mortality, with 25% of patients dying, 50% progressing toward end-stage renal disease, and 40-80% experiencing disease recurrence after transplantation [7].

To date, four prospective clinical studies conducted in patients with aHUS have shown efficacy of eculizumab, a monoclonal antibody that specifically binds to the terminal complement protein C5, in aHUS treatment [2, 8].

2. Case Presentation

Here, we report a 51-year-old female patient who was referred to our hospital due to hypertensive peak and acute kidney injury (AKI) on a background of chronic kidney disease.

The patient whose primary cause of CKD remains unknown reached ESRD at age of 19. In 1988, she received a cadaveric renal transplantation. The posttransplant therapy included cyclosporine and prednisone. After eighteen years, serum creatinine increased from 132.63 to 707.36 μmol/L [normal laboratory values 44-88 μmol/L]. A kidney biopsy was performed in suspicion of acute rejection and graft failure. The biopsy did not show neither features of cellular rejection nor features of antibody mediated rejection. Furthermore, a suspicion for polyomavirus nephropathy was ruled out as no significant polyomavirus DNA replication was detected on quantitative PCR. No significant lesions related to CNI toxicity such as nodular hyalinosis and striped fibrosis nor isometric vacuolization of tubules were found.

Cyclosporine therapy was suspended, starting therefore immunosuppressive therapy with tacrolimus and prednisone. AKI gradually regressed. Last creatinine baseline value was 158.4 μmol/L.

After three weeks the patient was referred from emergency room to our hospital (February 2nd, 2018) due to hypertensive peak and pulmonary edema.

Basic laboratory investigations showed a pattern of hemolysis: LDH 1,014 IU/L [normal laboratory values <250 IU/L], bilirubin 39.33 μmol/L [normal laboratory values 5.13-20.52 μmol/L], platelets 121,000 per microliter [normal laboratory values 150-450 per microliter], severe anemia (Hb 63 g/L) [normal laboratory values 120–150 g/L], and positive finding of schistocytes on the blood smear. ADAMTS13 activity level was normal (51.9%) [normal laboratory values > 50%] and the Coombs test was negative. No neurological signs were present. Moreover, on the first week of February, the patients showed at baseline CKD stage IV with serum creatinine 290.4 μmol/L, eGFR 15.5 ml/min/1.73m^2, and 24-hour proteinuria 0.84 g.

In suspicion of drug-related TMA, tacrolimus was suspended (tacrolimus blood level was 3.9 ng/ml [normal laboratory values 5–15 ng/mL]) and the dose of mycophenolate mofetil and prednisone was increased. However, no response was observed. The severe anemia (Hb 64 g/L) made blood transfusions necessary.

Given the laboratory and clinical pattern consistent with aHUS, and after having ruled out HUS and secondary causes of TMA, we administered eculizumab 900 mg e.v. after the patient had received meningococcal vaccine and antibiotic prophylaxis using the schedule of 900 mg/weekly for four weeks then 1200 mg starting from the fourth week. Due to worsening AKI with serum creatinine and urea values at 608.33 μmol/L and 21478.5 μmol/L, respectively [urea normal laboratory values 1665.00–3829.50 μmol/L], the patient underwent hemodialysis sessions after positioning a central venous catheter in the femoral vein.

According to hematological parameters, especially platelet count, a quick response to eculizumab was observed two days after administration (Figure 1).

Platelet count increased up to 217,000 per microliter, Hb remained stable in the normal range, and haptoglobin levels and clinical conditions improved.

A second administration of eculizumab was given seven days later. We started observing a poor response to therapy: LDH levels remained out of normal range (686 IU/L) as schistocytes were still present on blood smear.

Due to fever onset, blood cultures were performed and resulted negative, while urine culture showed 366 JC Polyomavirus genome copies per mL whose value gradually decreased to normal range over time of hospital stay. Immunosuppressive therapy with mycophenolate was tapered to 500 mg/die. Research for BK Polyomavirus genome turned out to be negative both in urine and in blood.

Three days later, the patient showed tonic-clonic seizures. On the CT scan, a parietal cortical-subcortical hemorrhage was found. The patient was then transferred to intensive care of our hospital where her clinical picture gradually improved.

During stay at intensive care, atrial fibrillation onset was observed and enoxaparin 2000 UI twice a day was started. Eculizumab was administered twice more with a one-week interval. After the last administration, we observed an unsatisfactory hematological response (low levels of haptoglobin, high levels of LDH, and reticulocyte count) and at the same time oligoanuria, tendency to dyspnea, and ponderal increase so that dialysis sessions were repeated regularly every other day. Given the worsening clinical picture, we suspended eculizumab, despite eculizumab induction therapy being incomplete and CH 50 level being low (<15 Ueq/ml [normal value < 70 Ueq/ml]).

As clinical conditions were gradually getting better, the patient was discharged from our hospital.

On follow-up, we observed a partial resolution of the hemolysis pattern: no schistocyte was found, LDH levels showed a decreasing trend, and anemia and thrombocytopenia were no longer observed. (Figure 2)

The patient kept on being dialysis-dependent until September.

Genomic analysis of the patient's CFH, MCP/CD46, CFI, C3, CFB, THBD, DGKE, CFHR1, CFHR3, and CFRH5 genes by next generation sequencing (NGS) revealed a pathogenic heterozygous mutation in CFI gene (c.292A>G (p.Thr98Ala)) as well as a heterozygous variant in THBD gene (c.1502C>T (p.Pro501Leu)). The clinical diagnosis of aHUS was confirmed.

On September, in consideration of the mutations found and in order to prevent aHUS relapse, we restarted eculizumab therapy with a fixed dose of 1200 mg every two weeks. After the first administration, we observed a clear improvement of renal function and diuresis as the patient stopped being dialysis-dependent. Nevertheless, according to hematological parameters, the response to therapy had never been complete. Haptoglobin levels, indeed, never rose to normal range after eculizumab administration.

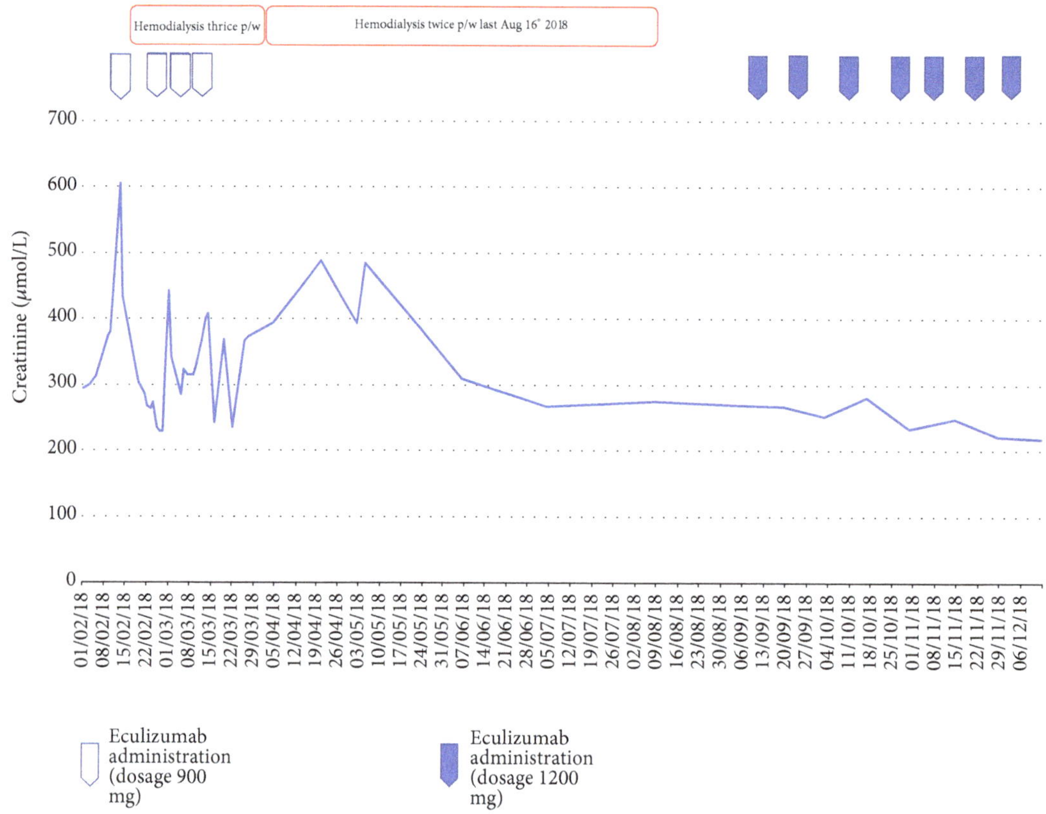

Figure 1: Parameters of serum creatinine across study timeline.

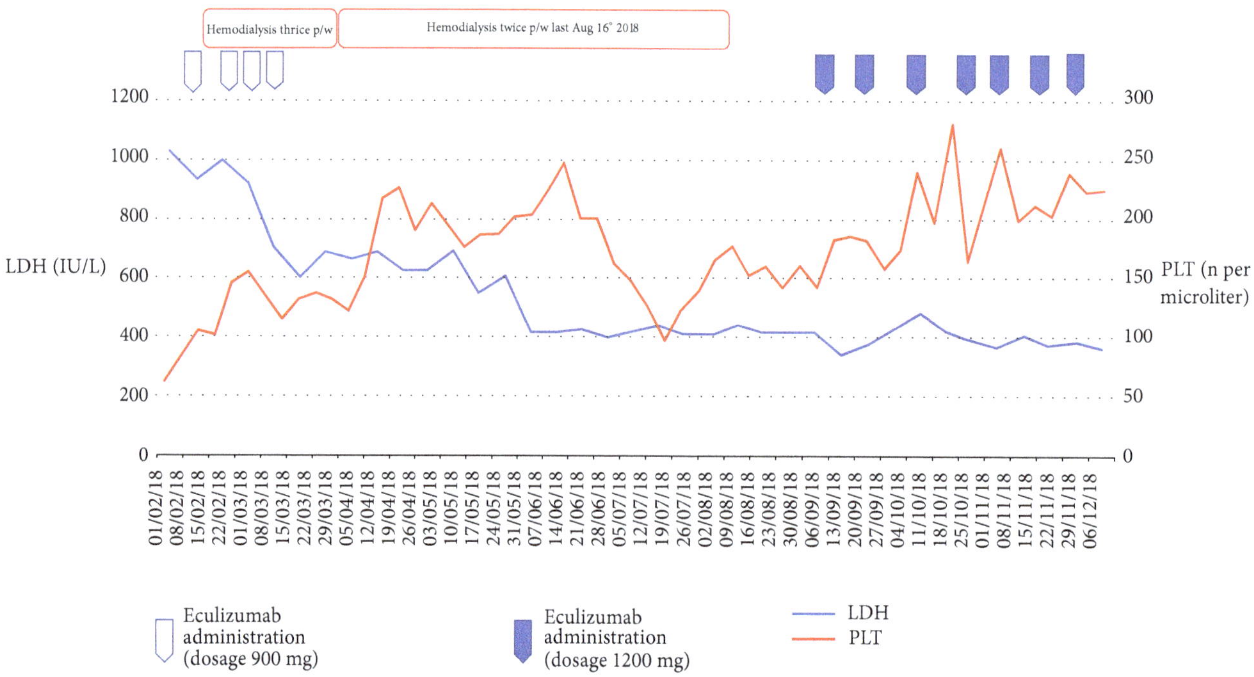

Figure 2: LDH and platelet count across study timeline.

3. Discussion

Thrombotic microangiopathies (TMA) are a group of disorders characterized by intravascular microangiopathic hemolytic anemia, thrombocytopenia, and vascular thrombosis. [9]

The currently accepted classification by George et al. describes primary TMAs (known as either acquired or inherited), secondary TMAs, and infection-associated TMAs.

aHUS with complement gene mutation could belong either to hereditary subgroup or to acquired subgroup as, for instance, in the case of aHUS mediated by antibody anticomplement factor H [1].

Several lines of evidence indicate that genetic mutations in the alternative pathway are found in up to half of patients with a clinical diagnosis of aHUS [10].

Finding more than one mutation related to aHUS is rare as around 3% of hereditary complement-mediated aHUS patients have more than one mutation, with increased penetrance per additional mutation [3].

In our case, the patient presented mutations in CFI and THBD genes. As many authors previously reported, CFI mutations do not directly cause TMA, but rather predispose to it [11].

CFI is a factor involved in the downregulation of the alternative pathway. CFI, cooperating with other factors such as CFH and MCP, accelerates the decay of convertase C3bBb, a cornerstone in membrane attack complex activation [12].

As Bresin et al. suggested, CFI seems to have a low pathogenic potential since a mutation of CFI requires another genetic abnormality to induce aHUS. Indeed, several CFI mutations were only found combined with mutations in other genes [13].

Thrombomodulin (TM) regulates coagulation, innate immunity, and complement activation. TM is a transmembrane-type 1-glycoprotein expressed on the vascular endothelium which suppresses clot formation by accelerating thrombin-mediated activation of protein C. Otherwise, thrombomodulin inactivates complement-derived anaphylatoxins C3a and C5a enhancing thrombin-mediated activation of plasma procarboxypeptidase B (thrombin activatable fibrinolysis inhibitor [TAFI]), an inhibitor of fibrinolysis. Mutations in the gene coding for thrombomodulin were previously revealed to be associated with diminished capacity to inactivate C3b [14, 15].

Delvaeye et al. found mutations that jeopardize thrombomodulin function in about 5% of patients with aHUS [15].

Many authors hypothesize that variants of the gene encoding thrombomodulin (THBD) confer a predisposition to endothelial injury that could manifest beside aHUS [14].

In our case, the clinical onset was characterized by hypertensive peak which we can speculate had possibly played the role of TMA trigger. Furthermore, a mutation in THBD was found (c.1502C>T (p.Pro501Leu)).

Van Laeche et al. reported a case of a 33-year-old woman who presented with malignant hypertension and aHUS: the same mutation on the gene coding for TM (C.1502C>T) we noticed was found [16].

The patient showed tonic-clonic seizures and on CT imaging parietal cortical-subcortical hemorrhage. Neurologic involvement is frequently reported. Recently, Schaefer et al. in an analysis of patients with aHUS from the Global aHUS Registry found neurologic involvement in 24% of pediatric and 25% of adult patients, compared with 16% and 8% of children and adults with aHUS previously reported [5, 17].

Eculizumab, a recombinant IgG2/4κ humanized monoclonal antibody, was shown to be effective and safe in aHUS treatment. It blocks the cleavage of C5, hindering formation of the proinflammatory peptide C5a and the cytotoxic membrane attack complex C5b-9 [18–20].

The patient discontinued eculizumab therapy due to lack of response and evolving towards end-stage renal disease. Although the main rationale for discontinuing eculizumab therapy is to protect patients from the risk of side effects of meningococcal infection [21, 22] as well as to have a smaller impact on patient's quality of life and on health costs, we took into account the patient's clinical conditions which have been worsening over time. This raises the question if eculizumab should be administered anyway despite the clinical scenario.

As Olson et al. recently stated in a review, several lines of evidence corroborate that risk of relapse after eculizumab discontinuation is high (30%) with unpredictable timing [9].

Some authors observed a relationship between type of complement mutation and the subsequent risk of TMA manifestation [23].

It has also previously been demonstrated that patients with mutations in CFH or THBD genes had the earliest onset of aHUS and the highest mortality [23].

It is worth emphasizing though that, in our case, initial eculizumab induction was not complete: this could explain the above-mentioned suboptimal response as well.

We observed a peculiar clinical presentation as the patient's response to therapy shifted from optimal to unsatisfactory in between the first and the last eculizumab administrations. As the genetic diagnosis was revealed, we restarted eculizumab and obtained an almost complete renal remission. The patient became dialysis-independent. Only serum haptoglobin levels remained low until last observation.

Although the clinical scenario could affect the compliance to eculizumab therapy as well as the risk for meningococcal infection, the response we observed after restart of the drug seems to advocate that eculizumab should not be suspended despite a deterioration of clinical conditions.

In order to provide reliable risk stratification tools and individualize treatment, the development of biomarkers to monitor eculizumab response is mandatory in the future.

To the best of our knowledge, this is the first genetic complement-mediated aHUS case in which such combined mutation in CFI and THBD genes is found and is associated with a suboptimal response to eculizumab.

Abbreviations

ADAMTS13: A disintegrin and metalloproteinase with a thrombospondin type 1 motif, member 13 (also known as von Willebrand factor-cleaving protease)

aHUS: Atypical hemolytic uremic syndrome
AKI: Acute kidney injury
CFH: Complement factor H
CFI: Complement factor I
MAHA: Microangiopathic hemolytic anemia
NGS: Next generation sequencing
STEC-HUS: Typical HUS caused by Shiga toxin-producing *Escherichia coli*
THBD: Thrombomodulin
TMA: Thrombotic microangiopathy
TTP: Thrombotic thrombocytopenic purpura.

Authors' Contributions

All authors read and approved the final manuscript. Luca Calvaruso and Alessandro Naticchia contributed equally to this work.

References

[1] J. N. George and C. M. Nester, "Syndromes of thrombotic microangiopathy," *The New England Journal of Medicine*, vol. 371, no. 7, pp. 654–666, 2014.

[2] C. M. Legendre, C. Licht, P. Muus et al., "Terminal complement inhibitor eculizumab in atypical hemolytic-uremic syndrome," *The New England Journal of Medicine*, vol. 368, no. 23, pp. 2169–2181, 2013.

[3] V. Brocklebank, K. M. Wood, and D. Kavanagh, "Thrombotic microangiopathy and the kidney," *Clinical Journal of the American Society of Nephrology*, vol. 13, no. 2, pp. 300–317, 2018.

[4] S. A. M. E. G. Timmermans, M. A. Abdul-Amid, J. Vanderlocht et al., "Patients with hypertension-associated thrombotic microangiopathy may present with complement abnormalities," *Kidney International*, vol. 91, no. 6, pp. 1420–1425, 2017.

[5] V. Fremeaux-Bacchi, F. Fakhouri, A. Garnier et al., "Genetics and outcome of atypical hemolytic uremic syndrome: a nationwide french series comparing children and adults," *Clinical Journal of the American Society of Nephrology*, vol. 8, no. 4, pp. 554–562, 2013.

[6] P. M. Ferraro, G. Lombardi, A. Naticchia et al., "A STARD-compliant prediction model for diagnosing thrombotic microangiopathies," *Journal of Nephrology*, vol. 31, no. 3, pp. 405–410, 2018.

[7] M. Noris and G. Remuzzi, "Atypical hemolytic-uremic syndrome," *The New England Journal of Medicine*, vol. 361, no. 17, pp. 1676–1687, 2009.

[8] J. Zuber, F. Fakhouri, L. T. Roumenina, C. Loirat, and V. Frémeaux-Bacchi, "Use of eculizumab for atypical haemolytic uraemic syndrome and C3 glomerulopathies," *Nature Reviews Nephrology*, vol. 8, no. 11, pp. 643–657, 2012.

[9] S. Olson, E. Lu, E. Sulpizio, J. Shatzel, J. Rueda, and T. DeLoughery, "When to stop eculizumab in complement-mediated thrombotic microangiopathies," *American Journal of Nephrology*, vol. 48, no. 2, pp. 96–107, 2018.

[10] D. Kavanagh, T. H. Goodship, and A. Richards, "Atypical hemolytic uremic syndrome," *Seminars in Nephrology*, vol. 33, no. 6, pp. 508–530, 2013.

[11] D. Kavanagh, E. J. Kemp, E. Mayland et al., "Mutations in complement factor I predispose to development of atypical hemolytic uremic syndrome," *Journal of the American Society of Nephrology*, vol. 16, no. 7, pp. 2150–2155, 2005.

[12] V. Fremeaux-Bacchi, M.-A. Dragon-Durey, J. Blouin et al., "Complement factor I: a susceptibility gene for atypical haemolytic uraemic syndrome," *Journal of Medical Genetics*, vol. 41, no. 6, p. e84, 2018.

[13] E. Bresin, E. Rurali, J. Caprioli et al., "Combined complement gene mutations in atypical hemolytic uremic syndrome influence clinical phenotype," *Journal of the American Society of Nephrology*, vol. 24, no. 3, pp. 475–486, 2013.

[14] M. Demeulenaere, K. Devreese, H. Vanbelleghem et al., "Thrombomodulin and endothelial dysfunction: a disease-modifier shared between malignant hypertension and atypical hemolytic uremic syndrome," *Nephron*, vol. 140, no. 1, pp. 63–73, 2018.

[15] M. Delvaeye, M. Noris, A. de Vriese et al., "Thrombomodulin mutations in atypical hemolytic-uremic syndrome," *The New England Journal of Medicine*, vol. 361, no. 4, pp. 345–357, 2009.

[16] S. Van Laecke and W. Van Biesen, "Severe hypertension with renal thrombotic microangiopathy: what happened to the usual suspect?" *Kidney International*, vol. 91, no. 6, pp. 1271–1274, 2017.

[17] F. Schaefer, G. Ardissino, G. Ariceta, F. Fakhouri, M. Scully, N. Isbel et al., "Clinical and genetic predictors of atypical hemolytic uremic syndrome phenotype and outcome," *Kidney International*, vol. 94, no. 2, pp. 408–418, 2018.

[18] C. Loirat and V. Frémeaux-Bacchi, "Atypical hemolytic uremic syndrome," *Orphanet Journal of Rare Diseases*, vol. 6, no. 60, 2011.

[19] C. Licht, L. A. Greenbaum, P. Muus et al., "Efficacy and safety of eculizumab in atypical hemolytic uremic syndrome from 2-year extensions of phase 2 studies," *Kidney International*, vol. 87, no. 5, pp. 1061–1073, 2015.

[20] F. Fakhouri, M. Hourmant, J. M. Campistol et al., "Terminal complement inhibitor eculizumab in adult patients with atypical hemolytic uremic syndrome: a single-arm, open-label trial," *American Journal of Kidney Diseases*, vol. 68, no. 1, pp. 84–93, 2016.

[21] G. H. Struijk, A. H. M. Bouts, G. T. Rijkers, E. A. C. Kuin, I. J. M. Ten Berge, and F. J. Bemelman, "Meningococcal sepsis complicating eculizumab treatment despite prior vaccination," *American Journal of Transplantation*, vol. 13, no. 3, pp. 819-820, 2013.

[22] E. Rodriguez, C. Barrios, and M. J. Soler, "Should eculizumab be discontinued in patients with atypical hemolytic uremic syndrome?" *Clinical Kidney Journal*, vol. 10, no. 3, pp. 320–322, 2017.

[23] M. Noris, J. Caprioli, E. Bresin et al., "Relative role of genetic complement abnormalities in sporadic and familial aHUS and their impact on clinical phenotype," *Clinical Journal of the American Society of Nephrology*, vol. 5, no. 10, pp. 1844–1859, 2010.

38

The Association of TNF-Alpha Inhibitors and Development of IgA Nephropathy in Patients with Rheumatoid Arthritis and Diabetes

Vedran Premužić,[1] Ivan Padjen,[2] Mislav Cerovec,[2] Marijana Ćorić,[3] Bojan Jelaković,[1] and Branimir Anić[2]

[1]*Department of Nephrology, Hypertension, Dialysis and Transplantation, University Hospital Centre Zagreb, Kispaticeva 12, Zagreb 10 000, Croatia*
[2]*Department of Immunology and Rheumatology, University Hospital Centre Zagreb, Kispaticeva 12, Zagreb 10 000, Croatia*
[3]*Department of Pathology, University Hospital Centre Zagreb, Kispaticeva 12, Zagreb 10 000, Croatia*

Correspondence should be addressed to Vedran Premužić; vpremuzic@gmail.com

Academic Editor: Anja Haase-Fielitz

IgA nephropathy (IgAN) is a rather uncommon complication of TNF-alpha inhibition with a range of findings such as asymptomatic microscopic/macroscopic hematuria or different degrees of proteinuria and could progress to end-stage renal disease. We are reporting three patients with longstanding rheumatoid arthritis (RA), which developed IgAN while receiving TNF-alpha inhibitors. All off our three patients had RA, which lasted 2–4 years, and none of them had a prior history of chronic kidney disease. Two patients were treated with adalimumab while one patient was treated with golimumab. Discontinuation of anti-TNF-alpha therapy and initiation of immunosuppressive therapy led to improvement in serologic abnormalities and renal function in two patients, while the third patient's 24-hour proteinuria was only partially reduced, which supports previous reports on TNF-alpha inhibitor induced autoimmunity. Two of our patients had previously been diagnosed with type 2 diabetes mellitus while the third patient developed diabetes years after the onset of IgAN. This is in line with the previously described association of IgAN and diabetes mellitus. To our best knowledge, this is the first report to analyze the development of IgAN as a potential consequence of anti-TNF-alpha therapy and its possible association with pretreatment or posttreatment diabetes.

1. Introduction

Introduction of TNF-alpha inhibitors has tremendously improved outcomes in patients with rheumatoid arthritis (RA). However, TNF-alpha inhibition in RA has been associated with various renal diseases including (proliferative lupus glomerulonephritis, pauci-immune necrotizing and crescentic glomerulonephritis, membranous glomerulonephritis, and renal vasculitis) [1–3]. Several centers have reported cases of IgA nephropathy (IgAN) related to treatment with TNF-alpha inhibitors [4–6]: the diagnosis of IgAN was based on typical pathohistological findings indistinguishable from idiopathic IgAN and/or nephritis associated with IgA vasculitis. Onset of IgAN associated with initiation of an anti-TNF-alpha agent and regression of renal impairment after drug withdrawal seem to be useful clues for diagnosing this entity. Current evidence on the mechanisms and predictors of development of IgAN in RA patients treated with TNF-alpha inhibitors is insufficient. The main reason is the paucity of data due to the low incidence of IgAN in the population of RA patients treated with this class of agents, as well the population of RA patients in general.

We report on three RA patients that developed IgAN during the course of treatment with TNF-alpha inhibitor.

1.1. Case 1. A 33-year-old man was referred to our rheumatology department in 2003 because of low back pain accompanied by tenderness of the knees and small joints of the wrists. Since the axial pattern of affection dominated the clinical presentation at that time and the patient was HLA B27 positive, he was diagnosed with ankylosing spondylitis with accompanying peripheral arthritis. Low-dose glucocorticoids and methotrexate (15 mg weekly) were introduced, leading to significant improvement of signs and symptoms, as well as decline in the number of swollen and tender peripheral joints within the following months. Basal blood pressure values were normal (128/76 mmHg) while the estimated glomerular filtration rate (eGFR) was 99.8 mL/min/1.73 m^2.

Despite initial improvement, the following time course was marked by aggravation of signs and symptoms consistent with peripheral polyarthritis, leading to a diagnosis of seronegative RA in 2005, fulfilling the 1987 classification criteria [7]. Methotrexate was continued, now in combination with sulfasalazine (2 grams daily) being replaced with leflunomide (20 mg daily) after several months. Despite combined treatment with conventional disease-modifying agents (DMARDs) and concomitant use of low-dose glucocorticoids, the patient suffered from a persistently active disease with a 28-joint disease activity score calculated using the erythrocyte sedimentation rate, ESR (DAS28-ESR) of 5.52. This prompted the initiation of adalimumab (40 mg subcutaneous every other week), while methotrexate was continued at a lower dose (10 mg weekly). This treatment strategy led to a satisfactory clinical response and reduction of DAS28-ESR to 2.66.

In 2006, the patient developed a psoriatic rash of the palms and soles, which was successfully treated with topical therapy. In the same year, the patient developed arterial hypertension (175/94 mmHg), for which an ACE inhibitor was introduced.

In 2011, the patient was still in stabile remission of his rheumatic condition (s) while continuously taking the biological drug; however, routine urinalysis unexpectedly revealed microscopic hematuria (urine sediment E 20–30 erythrocytes and 66–73% dysmorphic erythrocytes), accompanied by non-nephrotic proteinuria (2.25 g in daily urine, dU) with eGFR of 56 mL/min/1.73 m^2. Urine cytology revealed no urothelial atypia, and urine was negative for *M. tuberculosis*. The erythrocyte sedimentation rate (ESR) was increased (64 mm/h) as well as the C-reactive protein (CRP) level (18.3 mg/L). The complete blood count was unremarkable, as well as blood urea nitrogen (BUN) (5.0 mg/dl) and serum electrolytes. Serum creatinine was increased (137 μmol/l), as well as total cholesterol (5.7 mmol/L), LDL-cholesterol (3.52 mmol/L), and triglycerides (2.78 mmol/L). Antinuclear, anti-neutrophil cytoplasmic, and anti-glomerular basement membrane antibodies (ANA, ANCA, and GBM, respectively) were negative. Serum protein electrophoresis, immunoelectrophoresis, and immunofixation were normal as well as serum complement levels (C3 and C4). Screening for hepatitis B, hepatitis C, and HIV (human immunodeficiency virus) were negative. On ultrasonography, both kidneys were of normal size with hyperechogenic parenchyma.

Percutaneous kidney biopsy was performed, and its results are shown in Figures 1(a) and 1(b).

On light microscopy, diffuse mesangial hypercellularity was observed in all glomeruli, whereas global sclerosis was established in 1 of 15 glomeruli (6.66%). The tubules demonstrated degenerative changes while there were no changes on arteries. A moderate mononuclear infiltrate and mild fibrosis was noted in the interstitium. Immunofluorescence microscopy revealed mild mesangioproliferative changes. Electronic microscopy showed eosinophil infiltrates mostly in the mesangium, while several subendothelial and subepithelial eosinophil deposits were seen in the capillaries. In some glomeruli, there were signs of podocyte loss. Electronic microscopy also revealed glomerulonephritis with diffuse mesangial deposits and several subendothelial and subepithelial deposits compliant with glomerulonephritis caused by circulating immune complexes. The findings were in concert with the diagnosis of IgAN. There were no elements of diabetic nephropathy. The patient's MEST-C score was M1, E0, S1, T2, and C0.

Treatment with adalimumab and medium-dose glucocorticoids (prednisone 20 mg) was continued as well as an ACE inhibitor. Over the next two years, the patient was in a state of low disease activity (DAS28 3.08) of his RA, with progression of chronic kidney disease (eGFR 35.3 mL/min/1.73 m^2) and persistent proteinuria (2.26 g/dU). This prompted discontinuation of adalimumab and a further increase in the dose of glucocorticoids (prednisone 60 mg), with the intention to control the renal disease.

Due to the increased prednisone dose, the patient gradually developed cushingoid features including type 2 diabetes mellitus; he was diagnosed in 2014. A slight improvement in kidney function (eGFR 44.1 mL/min/1.73 m^2) and proteinuria (1.60 g/dU) allowed for a reduction of the prednisone dose to 40 mg. Of note, the patient's blood pressure was unremarkable, often being 120/80 mmHg or even less.

In 2015, the patient's kidney function was without further deterioration (eGFR 42.2 mL/min/1.73 m^2) and without progression of proteinuria. Diabetes was not adequately controlled, and the patient also experienced a relapse of his RA; so, rituximab was introduced in 2016. Unfortunately, the drug had to be discontinued after three cycles due to lacking efficacy and an increase in proteinuria from 0.78 to 2.04 g/dU. After discontinuation of rituximab, a decision was made to commence treatment with baricitinib, an oral selective JAK inhibitor. This finally led to the achievement of a low disease activity state of RA. However, the patient still continued to have persistent proteinuria of 1.9 g/dU, with no further decline in the eGFR.

1.2. Case 2. A 27-year-old woman was referred in 2007 to our rheumatology department because she had tenderness of her feet and knees with normal levels of acute phase parameters. Nine years before this referral, she was diagnosed with diabetes type 1 with consequent mild retinopathy and neuropathy.

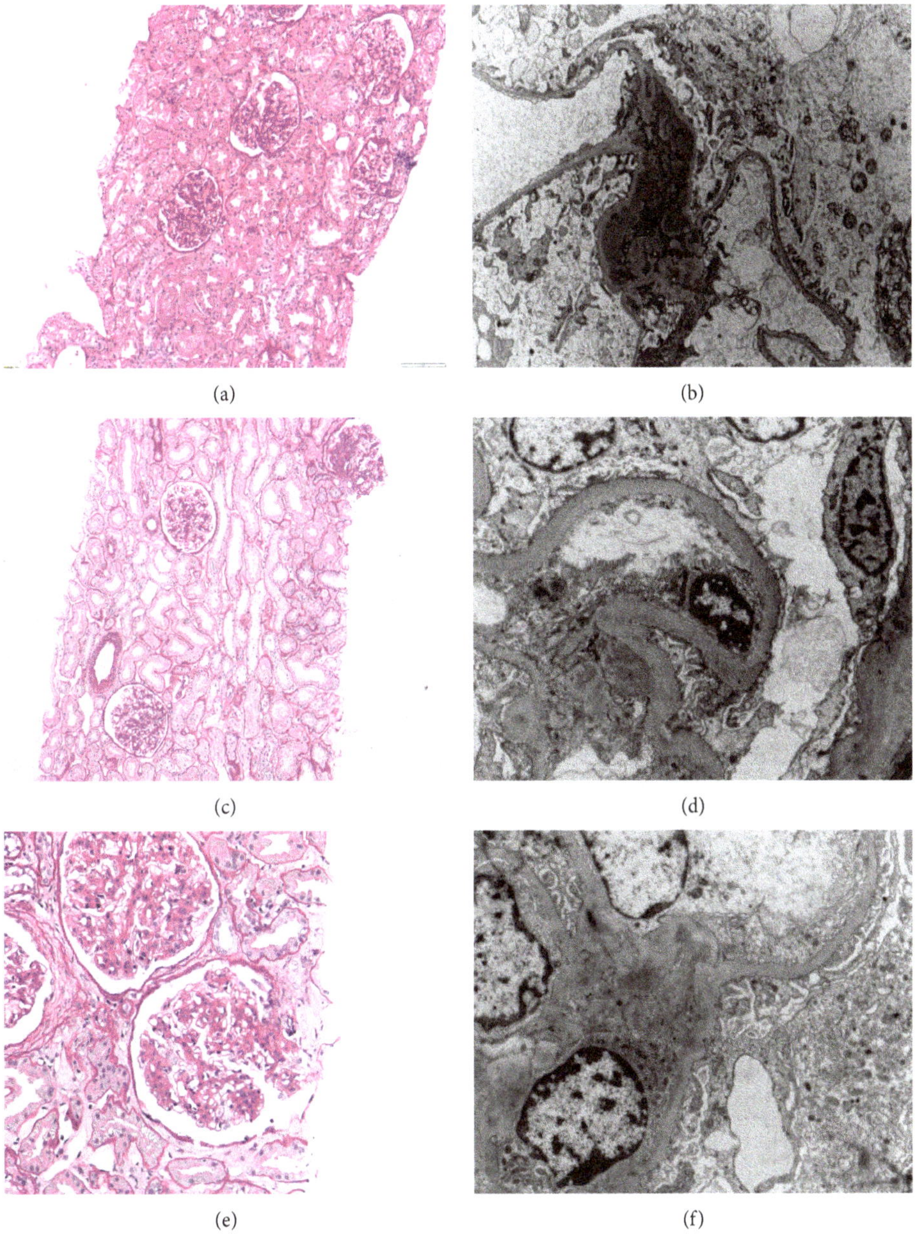

FIGURE 1: Kidney pathology of three cases. Case 1: (a) glomeruls with normal appearance (PSA stain × 100); (b) diffuse mesangial immune deposits (electron microscopy × 2800). Case 2: (c) one glomeruls with perihilar segmental sclerosis (PSA stain × 100); (d) mesangial immune deposits (electron microscopy × 5600). Case 3: (e) glomeruls with diffuse mesangial hypercellularity (PSA stain × 200); (f) mesangial immune deposits (electron microscopy × 7500).

Given that she had no swollen joint, an expectative approach was initially taken, and she was treated with NSAIDs. However, in early 2009, she developed symmetrical peripheral polyarthritis consistent with a diagnosis of seronegative RA, and she was put on low-dose methylprednisolone (8 mg qd) and weekly methotrexate (15 mg). Due to suboptimal response, sulfasalazine (2 grams daily) was added to the aforementioned regimen. Her blood pressure values were normal (122/64 mmHg), while her estimated glomerular filtration rate (eGFR) was 103.2 mL/min/1.73 m^2. Although low disease activity was achieved in the following months, she again started to develop active disease with swollen and tender joints of her hands, feet, and knees. A pattern of persistently active disease with a DAS28-ESR exceeding 5.00 led to the decision to start the patient on golimumab (50 mg subcutaneously, once monthly) in 2012. Achievement of sustained clinical remission allowed the discontinuation of glucocorticoids, while the dose of methotrexate was also gradually tapered, and the drug was finally stopped in 2013. Around that time, the patient developed arterial hypertension (160/90 mmHg), with an intact renal function.

In 2015, the patient was still in persistent remission of her rheumatic disease. Routine screening of her 24 h urine revealed albuminuria of 420.53 mg/dU and proteinuria of 0.47 g/dU. The findings were accompanied by a history of oscillatory hypertension and occasional ankle oedema. Laboratory tests revealed the following: hemoglobin: 11.7 g/dl, hematocrit: 37%, white blood cell count: 7.1×10^9/L, platelet count: 247×10^9/L, BUN: 4.9 mg/dl, serum creatinine: 61 μmol/L, eGFR 112.8 mL/min/1.73 m^2, albumin: 34.6 g/L, cholesterol: 4.6 mmol/L, triglycerides 0.61 mmol/L, and LDL-cholesterol: 2.36 mmol/L. Serum electrolytes were within normal limits. The erythrocyte sedimentation rate (ESR) was 20 mm/h, while the level of C-reactive protein (CRP) was normal. Serum protein electrophoresis and classes of immunoglobulins (IgG, IgA, and IgM) were within normal limits. Immunological screening (comprised of complement components C3 and C4, anti-neutrophil cytoplasmic antibodies, antinuclear antibodies including extractable nuclear antigens, and anti-glomerular basement membrane antibodies) was also unremarkable. Screening for hepatitis B and C, as well as HIV) was negative. On ultrasonography, both kidneys were of normal size, with a hyperechogenic parenchyma.

Percutaneous kidney biopsy was performed, and the pathohistological findings are shown in Figures 1(c) and 1(d).

On light microscopy, diffuse mesangial hypercellularity was demonstrated in all glomeruli, whereas a perihilar segment of sclerosis was established in 1 of 17 glomeruli (5.88%). Degenerative changes were seen in the tubules, while segmental intimal deposits were described in the arteries. There were no signs suggestive of interstitial inflammation and/or fibrosis.

Immunofluorescence microscopy showed diffuse IgA, moderate C3, and lambda light chains, and low IgM and kappa light chains deposits in the mesangium while there were no IgG, C1q, and fibrin deposits. Moderate C3 deposits were described in the arteries. Electronic microscopy revealed eosinophil infiltrates mostly in the mesangium and several subendothelial and subepithelial eosinophil deposits in the capillaries. Loss of podocytes was described in some of the glomeruli. There were no elements of diabetic nephropathy. The biopsy findings were consistent with IgAN class II, with a MEST-C score being M1, E1, S1, T2, and C0.

Given the remarkable and sustained response of RA to golimumab, the biological drug was continued, with the addition of an ACE inhibitor. During 2016, the patient was still in clinical remission of her RA with a stabile kidney function (eGFR 60.2 mL/min/1.73 m^2), but proteinuria increased to 3.0 g/dU. This led to the decision to discontinue golimumab and start the patient on oral cyclophosphamide (50 mg bid) with 40 mg of prednisone. Three months later after introduction of Endoxan, proteinuria dropped to 1.03 g/dU (partial remission); thus, cyclophosphamide was replaced with azathioprine (50 mg bid), with gradual tapering of prednisone. It is noteworthy that the kidney function did not decline over the follow-up period (eGFR 62.5 mL/min/1.73 m^2), while proteinuria continued to gradually improve (to 0.65 g/dU), despite inadequately controlled glycemia (provoked due to relatively high doses of prednisone). Such an improvement allowed for a further tapering of prednisone. In the following year, rituximab was introduced as a biological disease-modifying agent to control rheumatoid arthritis (1 gram on days 0 and 14, repeated every 6 months). Given that it was found reasonable to expect that rituximab may serve as a sound option for the maintenance of remission of the patient's renal disease, azathioprine was discontinued. In the following course (after three cycles of rituximab), the patient continued to be in clinical remission of her RA, but also achieved a complete decline in proteinuria to 0.09 g/dU with normal kidney function (eGFR was 73.3 mL/min/1.73 m^2) and good blood pressure control (<130/90 mmHg).

1.3. Case 3. A 48-year-old woman was referred to our rheumatology department in 2004 due to tenderness of her small joints of the wrists and knees, accompanied by morning stiffness of the lower back. Four years prior to the first visit, she was diagnosed with diabetes type 2. After initial workup, she was diagnosed as undifferentiated polyarthritis and was treated with NSAIDs and medium- to low-dose prednisone with good response and relief of symptoms. In 2009, she was finally diagnosed as seropositive rheumatoid arthritis with high titers of both RF and anti-CCP antibodies. She was put on 15 mg of methotrexate weekly, as well as sulfasalazine 2 grams daily.

In 2011, RA was still clinically active with increased inflammatory parameters and high DAS28-ESR of 7.09, so methotrexate was increased to 25 mg once a week but without considerable clinical effect. Therefore, a TNF-α inhibitor was introduced; she was started on adalimumab (40 mg subcutaneous every other week) with methotrexate 25 mg once weekly. She continued to take low-dose prednisone (up to 7.5 mg daily), achieving a satisfactory clinical response and reduction of DAS28-ESR to 2.28.

However, in 2015, she again started developing clinically active disease, but with normal inflammatory parameters. In 2016, she developed increased inflammatory markers with development of puffy pretibial edema and microcytic anemia. Laboratory tests showed hemoglobin: 10.5 g/dl, hematocrit: 33%, mean corpuscular volume: 73.2 fL, white blood cell count: 13.3×10^9/L, platelet count: 297×10^9/L, BUN: 8.5 mg/dl, serum creatinine: 81 μmol/l, eGFR: 68 mL/min/1.73 m^2, albumin: 31.0 g/L, cholesterol: 5.6 mmol/L, triglyceride: 1.65 mmol/L, and LDL-cholesterol: 3.59 mmol/L. Serum electrolytes were within normal limits. Proteinuria was 4.55 g/dU. Erythrocyte sedimentation rate (ESR) was 100 mm/h, CRP 45.9 mg/L. Serum complement levels (C3 and C4), ANA, ANCA, and anti-glomerular basement membrane (GBM) antibodies were all unremarkable. Serum protein electrophoresis revealed polyclonal hypergammaglobulinemia while immunofixation was normal. Screening for hepatitis B, hepatitis C, and HIV was negative. On ultrasonography, both kidneys were of normal size, with hyperechogenic parenchyma.

Percutaneous kidney biopsy was performed; results of the histopathological analyses are shown in Figures 1(e) and 1(f).

Light microscopy revealed diffuse mesangial hypercellularity with segmental formation of nodules in all glomeruli, whereas global sclerosis was established in 5 of 22 glomeruli (22.7%). Degenerative changes were demonstrated in the tubules, while the findings in the arterioles included concentric intimal hyalinosis and moderate intimal fibrosis with elastosis. There was no mononuclear infiltrate but fibrosis was present in interstitium.

Immunofluorescence microscopy showed diffuse IgA, moderate C3 and lambda light chains, and low IgM and kappa light chain deposits in the mesangium while there were no IgG and C1q deposits. Moderate C3 deposits were detected in the arteries. Electronic microscopy showed osmiophilic deposits mostly in the mesangium and paramesangium deposits. Glomerular basal membranes were a bit thicker without osmiophilic deposits, with stationary thicker internal lamina rara. Podocyte loss was described in some of the glomeruli. Therefore, a diagnosis of diabetic nephropathy with superimposed IgAN was established, prompting the decision to discontinue adalimumab. The patient's MEST-C score was M1, E1, S1, T2, and C0. The cause of microcytic anemia was two polyps of the colon which were removed. At that time, the patient developed arterial hypertension (170/90 mmHg) and an ACE inhibitor was introduced, with the aim to control hypertension and to control the proteinuria. Arthritis was suboptimally controlled with low-dose steroids. The patient continued to have nephrotic-range proteinuria, as well as high disease activity of her RA. This prompted the decision to target both patient's conditions with a single agent, rituximab, administered in 4 cycles. This led to remission of arthritis, as well as a pronounced decline in proteinuria to 0.13 g/dU, with a stabile kidney function, which was sustained through the following period (eGFR 65 mL/min/1.73 m^2).

2. Discussion

TNF-alpha inhibition in patients with RA may lead to the development of new-onset renal disease [4, 8]. IgAN is a rather uncommon complication of TNF-alpha inhibition with a range of findings such as asymptomatic microscopic/macroscopic hematuria or different degrees of proteinuria and could progress to end-stage renal disease [8, 9]. Renal biopsy reveals classical features with or without C3 activation, which discriminates classic from crescentic IgAN. It is worth noting that neither the complement components nor immunoglobulins were detected in kidney biopsies of our patients.

The exact pathophysiological mechanism for the development of IgAN in patients treated with TNF-alpha inhibitors has not yet been determined. Anti-TNF-alpha agents may lead to autoantibody formation including antinuclear, anti-double stranded DNA (anti-dsDNA), and anticardiolipin antibodies [10, 11]. Binding of anti-TNF-alpha on immune cells could induce a release of immunogenic nucleosomal antigens, which promote the production of anti-dsDNA antibodies. Recently, a correlation between elevated concentrations of circulating TNF-alpha and renal progression in IgAN has been reported [12]. The activation of alternative complement pathway including C3 and formation of deposits could be responsible for IgAN development. Therefore, biological therapy could induce an immune response with the production of IgA and IgM antibodies against TNF-alpha inhibitors.

We are reporting three patients with longstanding RA, which developed IgAN while receiving TNF-alpha inhibitors. All of our three patients had RA, which lasted 2–4 years, and none of them had a prior history of chronic kidney disease (Table 1). Two patients were treated with adalimumab, while one patient was treated with golimumab (treatment duration: 36–70 months, median: 55 months). The development of IgAN occurred after months of therapy and included pathologic and serologic findings specific for the pathogenic role of TNF-alpha inhibitors. Discontinuation of anti-TNF-alpha therapy and initiation of immunosuppressive therapy led to improvement in serologic abnormalities and renal function in two patients, while the third patient's 24-hour proteinuria was only partially reduced (Table 2 and Figures 2(a)–2(c)), which supports previous reports on TNF-alpha inhibitor induced autoimmunity. Since all of our patients developed IgAN while on TNF-alpha inhibiting treatment, it is plausible to assume that IgAN developed as a consequence of the biological treatment. It is less likely that IgAN was triggered by rheumatoid arthritis, given that the rheumatic disease was adequately controlled (i.e. in remission or low disease activity) following the institution of a TNF-alpha inhibiting drug. Furthermore, none of the presented patients exhibited features of renal affection prior to the institution of the respective TNF-alpha inhibitor. Although cases of IgAN were reported in groups of patients with RA, it is worth noting that a cause-effect relationship between RA and IgAN has never been confirmed and that it is likely that these observations were coincidental. Moreover, the finding of a relatively high percentage (12%) of IgAN in a Japanese group of 100 patients has not been replicated ever since [13]. This observation should be interpreted with caution because the patients included in the respective study originate from an era when RA had been commonly recognized at a more established stage. Additionally, therapeutic approaches used at the time when the study was conducted did not meet today's stringent standards and aims.

Interestingly, two of our patients had previously been diagnosed with type 2 diabetes mellitus, while the third patient developed diabetes years after the onset of IgAN. This is in line with the previously described association of IgAN and diabetes mellitus [14]. Given that type 2 diabetes mellitus has already been associated with other immune-mediated entities such as celiac disease and dermatitis herpetiformis, it may be reasonable to suggest that the occurrence of IgAN in diabetic patients is not a mere coincidence. Some studies reported that patients with diabetes had higher values of IgA when compared to healthy controls [14, 15]. This may be a consequence of enhanced antigen stimulation as an immune response to advanced glycosylation end products and diabetic metabolic disturbance, finally leading to nonenzymatic glycation of immunoglobulins, especially IgA.

TABLE 1: Clinical characteristics of three RA patients with IgA glomerulonephritis following anti-TNF-α therapy.

	Case 1	Case 2	Case 3
Months from first visit to diagnosis of RA	22	24	57
Steroids in months	22	5	51
Methotrexate in months	3	36	23
Prior diabetes	No	Yes	Yes
Prior arterial hypertension	No	No	No
Months from diagnosis of RA to introduction of biologic treatment	48	34	27
DAS28 at biologic treatment introduction	5.52	6.30	7.09
DAS28 after biologic treatment introduction	2.66	2.09	2.28
TNF-α inhibitor	Adalimumab	Golimumab	Adalimumab
Months from introduction of biologic treatment to kidney biopsy	59	36	70
Peripheral oedema	No	Yes	Yes
24 h urine proteinuria (g/dU)	2.25	0.47	4.55
Erithrocyturia	Yes	No	No
Serum creatinine (μmol/L)	137	61	81
eGFR (mL/min/1.73 m^2)	54.8	112.8	68.0
Blood pressure (mmHg)	175/94	160/90	170/90
Arterial hypertension	Yes	Yes	Yes
Hemoglobin (g/dl)	13.1	11.7	10.5
White blood cell count ($\times 10^9$/L)	7.8	7.1	13.3
Cholesterol (mmol/L)	5.7	4.6	5.6
Triglycerides (mmol/L)	2.78	0.61	1.65
Erythrocyte sedimentation rate (mm/h)	64	20	100
C-reactive protein (mg/L)	18.3	1.7	45.9

RA-rheumatoid arthritis; eGFR-estimated glomerular filtration rate.

TABLE 2: Clinical characteristics and renal survival of three RA patients with IgA glomerulonephritis following kidney biopsy.

METS-C score	Case 1 M1, E0, S1, T2, C0	Case 2 M1, E1, S1, T2, C0	Case 3 M1, E1, S1, T2, C0
Therapy after kidney biopsy			
Steroids in months	24	24	24
Methotrexate in months	—	—	24
Original TNF-α inhibitor in months	24	19	—
Rituximab (number of cycles)	3	3	4
Endoxan/Azathioprine	No	Yes	No
DAS28 one year after biopsy	3.08	2.76	4.54
Renal survival after biopsy	2 years	1 year	1 year
24 h urine proteinuria (g/dU)	2.26	3.00	0.68
Serum creatinine (μmol/L)	195	103	88
eGFR (mL/min/1.73 m^2)	35.3	60.2	61.1
Renal survival after biopsy	4 years	2 years	2 years
24 h urine proteinuria (g/dU)	1.57	0.09	0.13
Serum creatinine (μmol/L)	166	87	83
eGFR (mL/min/1.73 m^2)	42.2	73.3	65.1

eGFR-estimated glomerular filtration rate.

IgA levels are further increased in patients with IgAN superimposed to diabetes. To our best knowledge, this is the first report to analyze the development of IgAN as a potential consequence of anti-TNF-alpha therapy and its possible association with pretreatment or posttreatment diabetes. Taking into account already elevated IgA levels in diabetic patients, the administration of biologic treatment could hasten the development of IgAN, although TNF-alpha inhibitors are of IgG class. A strategy of biologic drug discontinuation combined with initiation of an immunosuppressive drug led to IgAN remission in two patients. The third patient still had significant proteinuria and stationary chronic kidney disease, although he had received two biologic drugs. A possible explanation could be the development of diabetes after initial biologic treatment and persistently elevated IgA levels. Switching to the patient's current treatment with baricitinib (a Janus kinase inhibitor) unfortunately did not yield a significant reduction in proteinuria. Combining the MEST-C score with clinical data at biopsy has the same predictive value as monitoring clinical findings for two years [16]. The score takes into account four features: mesangial and endocapillary cellularity, segmental sclerosis, and interstitial fibrosis/tubular atrophy. The scoring of each biopsy sample (for instance M1, E0, S1, and T1) gives us a predicted rate of decline in renal function over a follow-up

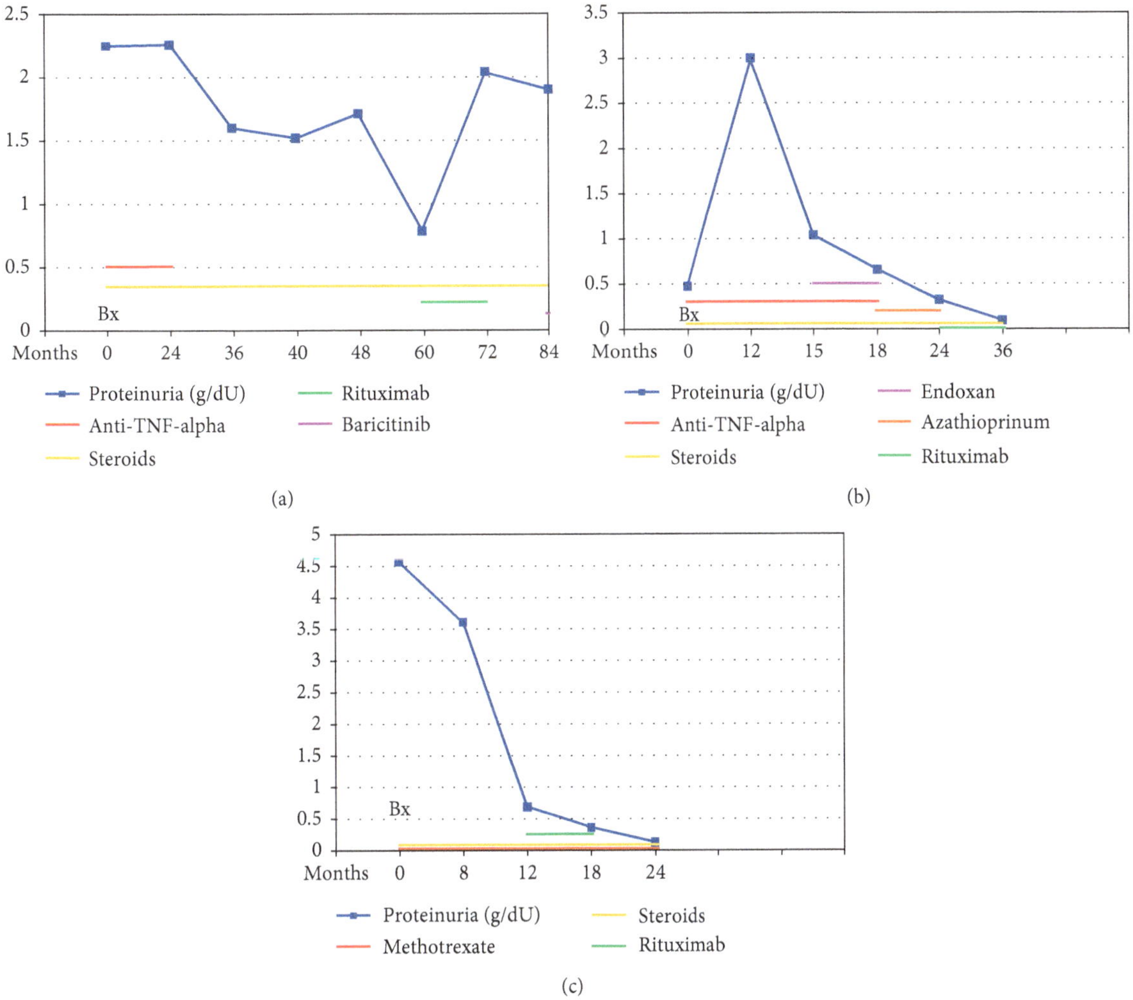

FIGURE 2: Proteinuria and therapy after kidney biopsy. Case 1 (a); Case 2 (b); Case 3 (c).

period of 59 months where 12% patients progressed to ESRD. Two of our patients did not have a decline in renal function despite their MEST-C score being M1, E0, S1, T2, and C0. The third patient had a reduced glomerular filtration rate but without progression in a four-year follow-up period. Our findings confirmed previous reports on the development of IgAN after biologic treatment with TNF-alpha inhibitors. Although this is a report on only three patients, it could be speculated that the presence of diabetes may act as a risk factor for the development of IgAN in patients with RA treated with TNF-alpha inhibitors. Determining serum IgA levels could have a prognostic importance in predicting the development of IgA nephropathy superimposed on diabetes mellitus in patients with RA. We suggest that RA patients, especially those with high risk of developing renal disorders should be prescribed TNF-alpha inhibitors cautiously and should be closely monitored over an extended period of time.

References

[1] N. Mohan, E. T. Edwards, T. R. Cupps et al., "Leukocytoclastic vasculitis associated with tumor necrosis factor-alpha blocking agents," *Journal of Rheumatology*, vol. 31, no. 10, pp. 1955–1958, 2004.

[2] T. W. R. Doulton, B. Tucker, J. Reardon, and N. Velasco, "Antineutrophil cytoplasmic antibody-associated necrotizing crescentic glomerulonephritis in a patient receiving treatment with etanercept for severe rheumatoid arthritis," *Clinical Nephrology*, vol. 62, no. 9, pp. 234–238, 2004.

[3] N. Shakoor, M. Michalska, C. A. Harris, and J. A. Block, "Drug-induced systemic lupus erythematosus associated with etanercept therapy," *The Lancet*, vol. 359, no. 9306, pp. 579-580, 2002.

[4] X. Li, J. Ma, Y. Zhao, H.-Y. Wang, and X.-M. Li, "Development of crescentic immunoglobulin A nephritis and multiple autoantibodies in a patient during adalimumab treatment for rheumatoid arthritis," *Chinese Medical Journal*, vol. 128, no. 18, pp. 2555-2556, 2015.

[5] M. B. Stokes, K. Foster, G. S. Markowitz et al., "Development of glomerulonephritis during anti-TNF-α therapy for rheumatoid arthritis," *Nephrology Dialysis Transplantation*, vol. 20, no. 7, pp. 1400–1406, 2005.

[6] A. A. den Broeder, K. J. Assmann, P. L. van Riel, and J. F. Wetzels, "Nephrotic syndrome as a complication of anti-TNFalpha in a patient with rheumatoid arthritis," *The Netherlands Journal of Medicine*, vol. 61, no. 4, pp. 137–141, 2003.

[7] F. C. Arnett, S. M. Edworthy, D. A. Bloch et al., "The american rheumatism association 1987 revised criteria for the classification of rheumatoid arthritis," *Arthritis & Rheumatism*, vol. 31, no. 3, pp. 315–324, 1988.

[8] S. S. Wei and R. Sinniah, "Adalimumab (TNF inhibitor) therapy exacerbates IgA glomerulonephritis acute renal injury and induces lupus autoantibodies in a psoriasis patient," *Case Reports in Nephrology*, vol. 2013, Article ID 812781, 4 pages, 2013.

[9] E. Kemp, H. Nielsen, L. J. Petersen et al., "Newer immunomodulating drugs in rheumatoid arthritis may precipitate glomerulonephritis," *Clinical Nephrology*, vol. 55, no. 1, pp. 87-88, 2001.

[10] T. Jonsdottir, J. Forslid, A. van Vollenhoven et al., "Treatment with tumour necrosis factor antagonists in patients with rheumatoid arthritis induces anticardiolipin antibodies," *Annals of the Rheumatic Diseases*, vol. 63, no. 9, pp. 1075–1078, 2004.

[11] M. Piga, E. Chessa, V. Ibba et al., "Biologics-induced autoimmune renal disorders in chronic inflammatory rheumatic diseases: systematic literature review and analysis of a monocentric cohort," *Autoimmunity Reviews*, vol. 13, no. 8, pp. 873–879, 2014.

[12] D. Khanna, M. McMahon, and D. E. Furst, "Safety of tumour necrosis factor-alpha antagonists," *Drug Safety*, vol. 27, no. 5, pp. 307–324, 2004.

[13] H. Makino, Y. Yoshinaga, Y. Yamasaki, Y. Morita, H. Hashimoto, and M. Yamamura, "Renal involvement in rheumatoid arthritis: analysis of renal biopsy specimens from 100 patients," *Modern Rheumatology*, vol. 12, no. 2, pp. 148–154, 2002.

[14] R. O. B. Gans, Y. Ueda, S. Ito et al., "The occurrence of IgA-nephropathy in patients with diabetes mellitus may not Be coincidental: a report of five cases," *American Journal of Kidney Diseases*, vol. 20, no. 3, pp. 255–260, 1992.

[15] M. Kanauchi, T. Kawano, and K. Dohi, "Serum IgA levels in patients with diabetic nephropathy and IgA nephropathy superimposed on diabetes mellitus," *Diabetes Research and Clinical Practice*, vol. 48, no. 2, pp. 113–118, 2000.

[16] H. Trimarchi, J. Barratt, D. C. Cattran et al., "Oxford classification of IgA nephropathy 2016: an update from the IgA nephropathy classification working group," *Kidney International*, vol. 91, no. 5, pp. 1014–1021, 2017.

39

Gadolinium-Induced Acute Graft Pancreatitis in a Simultaneous Pancreas-Kidney Transplant Recipient

Chiang Sheng Lee,[1,2] Rachel Yi Ping Tan,[1,2] and Nitesh N. Rao[1,3,4]

[1]*Renal Unit, Flinders Medical Centre, Flinders Drive, Bedford Park, South Australia, Australia*
[2]*College of Medicine and Public Health, Flinders University, Bedford Park, South Australia, Australia*
[3]*Renal Unit, Lyell McEwin Hospital, Haydown Road, Elizabeth Vale, Adelaide, South Australia, Australia*
[4]*Adelaide Medical School, University of Adelaide, Adelaide, South Australia, Australia*

Correspondence should be addressed to Chiang Sheng Lee; chiangsheng88@gmail.com

Academic Editor: David Mudge

Gadolinium-induced acute pancreatitis is a rare phenomenon associated with the administration of gadolinium-based contrast agents. Only five cases of gadolinium-induced acute pancreatitis have been reported worldwide in patients with native pancreas and none with a pancreatic graft. We present a 32-year-old woman with prior history of simultaneous pancreas-kidney transplant who presented with generalized abdominal pain associated with systemic inflammatory response syndrome requiring admission to the intensive care unit. This occurred within 48 hours after having a magnetic resonance imaging (MRI) with gadolinium for investigation of subacute left optic atrophy. She was noted to have a marked rise in serum lipase, and the computed tomography findings were consistent with acute graft pancreatitis. Other causes of pancreatitis were ruled out, and she was managed conservatively with aggressive hydration, bowel rest, and analgesia with good recovery. This is the first reported case of gadolinium-induced acute graft pancreatitis occurring in a simultaneous pancreas-kidney transplant recipient. Clinicians should consider this rare differential diagnosis as a cause of graft pancreatitis in patients who have received gadolinium-based contrast agents.

1. Introduction

Gadolinium-based contrast agents (GBCAs) have been increasingly used in magnetic resonance imaging (MRI) to aid clinicians' diagnostic ability in neurological and inflammatory disorders. It is occasionally used in patients who are not suitable for iodinated contrast agents in computed tomography (CT) imaging [1]. Contrary to the well-described adverse effect of nephrogenic systemic fibrosis caused by GBCAs, little is known about gadolinium-induced acute pancreatitis with only five cases reported worldwide in patients with native pancreas. We describe the first case of gadolinium-induced acute pancreatitis occurring in a simultaneous pancreas-kidney transplant recipient. This is an entity which should be differentiated from transplant graft rejection as the management differs.

2. Case Presentation

A 32-year-old woman, who was two years post simultaneous pancreas-kidney (SPK) transplant for type I diabetes, presented to the Emergency Department with sudden onset generalized abdominal pain. The pain was constant and dull in nature. It did not radiate, and there were no exacerbating or relieving factors. It was associated with fever, nausea, and vomiting, but there was no alteration in bowel habits leading up to this sudden abdominal pain. She denied any recent trauma, abnormal bowel movements, or urinary symptoms. She denied any illicit drug or alcohol use. The only relevant history was a recent magnetic resonance imaging (MRI) brain with gadolinium-based contrast agent (GBCA), gadobutrol

(*Gadovist*), 48 hours prior to investigate for subacute left optic atrophy.

As for her SPK transplant, it was a 3/6 human leukocyte antigen mismatch with positive angiotensin II receptor type 1 antibody of 33.7 IU/ml. Her baseline renal graft function was 85 μmol/L. There was no history of pancreatic graft rejection or acute pancreatitis.

Her other past medical history included migraine, recurrent urinary tract infections, and recent investigation for left vision loss. Regular medications included mycophenolate mofetil 750 mg twice daily, tacrolimus 3 mg twice daily, prednisolone 10 mg daily, pantoprazole 40 mg daily, trimethoprim-sulfamethoxazole 160/800 mg twice weekly, candesartan 8 mg daily, atorvastatin 20 mg daily, aspirin 100 mg daily, and amitriptyline 25 mg daily.

On arrival to the Emergency Department, she was observed to be in shock with cool peripheries and recorded blood pressure of 90/29 mmHg. She was tachycardic at 100 beats per minute and hypothermic at 34.3°C. The blood glucose level was 6.5 mmol/L. Examination was remarkable for abdominal tenderness over the pancreatic graft. Renal graft was non-tender and there was no bruit audible.

Initial arterial blood gas demonstrated lactate acidosis with pH of 7.24, pO_2 of 106 mmHg, pCO_2 of 44 mmHg, HCO_3 of 18 mmol/L, and lactate of 3.2 mmol/L. Urine analysis showed trace of ketones. Urinary beta-human chorionic gonadotropin was negative. Initial investigations demonstrated white cell count of 22.34×10^9/L, haemoglobin of 141 g/L, platelet count of 409×10^9/L, acute renal injury with serum creatinine of 159 μmol/L (baseline of 85 umol/L), urea of 12.4 mmol/L, sodium of 145 mmol/L, and potassium of 4.6 mmol/L. Blood glucose was 8.4 mmol/L. Serum lipase was elevated at 3368 U/L (normal range: 0–60 U/L). Liver function test was unremarkable, and C-reactive protein was not elevated. 12-hour tacrolimus trough level was 6.2 ug/L (Table 1). Donor specific antibody was negative.

Resuscitation was undertaken with intravenous fluids, and antibiotics for presumed intraabdominal sepsis were initiated. Computed tomography (CT) of her abdomen demonstrated inflammatory changes of transplanted pancreatic graft with poor enhancement suggestive of graft pancreatitis (Figure 1). There was an absence of bladder distension, hydroureter, or hydronephrosis of the transplanted kidney graft. Cytomegalovirus polymerase chain reaction (PCR) was negative. Blood and urine cultures were unremarkable, and antibiotics were discontinued within 48 hours. Pancreatic graft rejection was considered less probable given the improvement in clinical condition, normal fasting C-peptide level of 915 pmol/L, normal blood glucose levels, and therapeutic drug levels (Table 1). After excluding other causes of allograft pancreatitis, she was treated for gadolinium-induced acute pancreatitis. She improved with conservative management and was discharged after 3 days. She has had no further episodes of acute pancreatitis upon follow-up for 12 months.

3. Discussion

Gadolinium-induced acute pancreatitis (gadolinium-induced AP) is a rare phenomenon. Despite the safety and tolerability of GBCAs, there are five cases which reported gadolinium-induced AP in patients with native pancreases [2–6]. It has been described to develop between three to six hours after administration of GBCAs including gadodiamide (Omniscan) [2, 6], gadolinium-diethylenetriamine pentaacetic acid (Gd-DTPA) [4], gadobenate dimeglumine (MultiHance) [3], and gadoterate meglumine [5].

Multiple mechanisms of GBCA toxicity have been proposed. In a recent review [7], they suggest the main factor for GBCA toxicity is the dissociation of gadolinium ion (Gd^{3+}) from chelated complexes leading to non-chelated Gd^{3+} being retained in organ tissues. Other studies also proposed that free Gd^{3+} leads to cytokine stimulation, macrophagic activation, and attraction of fibroblasts. However, none of the animal studies recorded the effects of GBCA on the pancreas.

There are no formalized criteria for gadolinium-induced AP. It is a clinical diagnosis that correlates with the development of acute pancreatitis following the administration of gadolinium. The diagnosis of acute pancreatitis itself is based on the revised Atlanta Classification which requires at least 2 of the 3 characteristics: abdominal pain consistent with pancreatitis, serum lipase value 3 times the upper limit of normal, and supportive imaging findings [5]. CT findings suggestive of acute pancreatitis include pancreatic enhancement with increased attenuation in peripancreatic fat, peripancreatic fluid collection, or pancreatic necrosis in severe cases [8]. Our patient fulfilled all criteria. She was low risk for severe pancreatitis based on the modified Glasgow system [9] (Table 1).

There are three main differences compared to the other cases reported. Firstly, this is the first case of acute pancreatitis due to gadobutrol occurring in a pancreatic graft. She also developed symptoms after 48 hours of GBCA administration. Given the temporal relationship of GBCA administration and development of graft pancreatitis with no further recurrence during subsequent follow-ups while being on the same immunosuppressants, drug-induced pancreatitis attributed to her regular medications was deemed less likely as per the Mallory and Kern criteria [10].

Another challenging aspect for our patient was to differentiate between other causes of transplant graft pancreatitis including pancreatic graft rejection. Transplant graft pancreatitis is the second most common complication after vascular thrombosis [11]. Reported risk factors for graft pancreatitis include exocrine bladder drainage, mechanical stricture, direct mechanical pressure to the graft, intraparenchymal microvascular thrombosis, recurrent infection surrounding graft, occlusion of Oddi's sphincter due to rejection, and cytomegalovirus infection [11].

Similarly, pancreatic graft rejection can manifest as acute pancreatitis with elevated serum lipase with or without accompanying graft tenderness as the graft itself is insensate [12]. The evaluation of pancreatic graft rejection should be accompanied by other features such as elevated glycated haemoglobin, hyperglycaemia, low fasting C-peptide, and exclusion of other structural pancreatic pathology by imaging. A core needle biopsy of the graft pancreas is the gold standard for diagnosis and should be considered if graft rejection is suspected. This will distinguish between antibody

TABLE 1: Relevant laboratory parameters during the patient's hospital admission (the 8 criteria included in the modified Glasgow system to predict the severity of acute pancreatitis at 48 hours include age, white cell count, partial pressure of oxygen, serum calcium, urea, lactate dehydrogenase, serum albumin, and blood glucose [9]).

Test	3 months prior	Day 0	Day 1	Day 2	Day 3	Normal Range
Haemoglobin (g/L)	146	141	123	116	122	115–155
White cell count ($\times 10^9$/L)	8.98	22.34	15.66	13.73	13.95	4–11
Absolute neutrophil count ($\times 10^9$/L)	6.70	12.96	14.50	10.40	11.20	1.8–7.5
Platelet count ($\times 10^9$/L)	304	409	285	252	250	150–450
C-Reactive protein (mg/L)		12.4	—	98.8	—	0–8
Urea (mmol/L)	8.6	12.4	10.8	7.6	4.4	2.7–8.0
Creatinine (umol/L)	97	159	115	108	86	45–90
Serum calcium (mmol/L)	—	2.33	2.21	2.02	2.11	2.10–2.60
Blood glucose (mmol/L)		8.4	7.2	4.8	4.7	3.2–5.5
Lipase (U/L)	20	3368	541	115	30	0–60
C-Peptide (pmol/L)		915	—	—	—	166–1466
Lactate dehydrogenase (U/L)		249	418	414	382	120–250
Alanine aminotransferase (U/L)		31	38	32	20	0–55
Total cholesterol (mmol/L)		3.4	—	—	—	
Triglyceride (mmol/L)		0.5	—	—	—	
Tacrolimus level (ug/L)		5.0	—	—	6.2	5–15

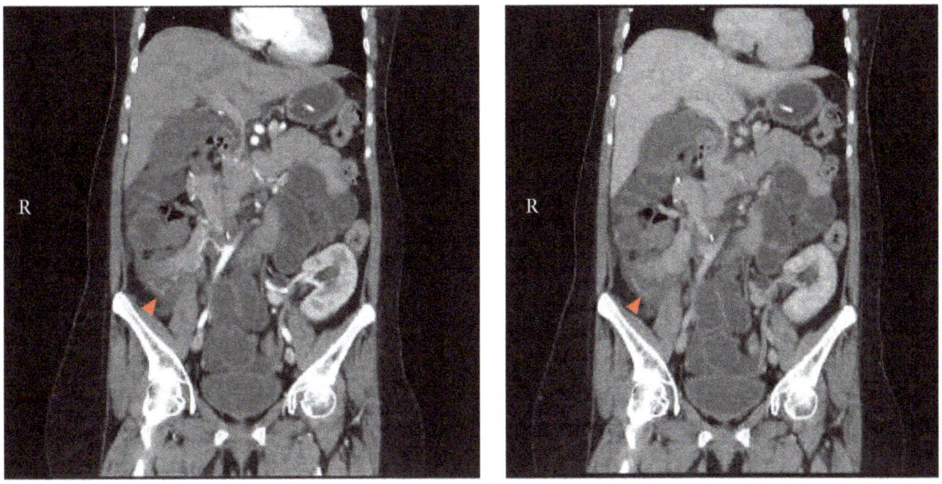

(a) (b)

FIGURE 1: Computed tomography of the abdomen in coronal view. (a) Arterial phase demonstrates satisfactory enhancement of pancreatic artery (red arrow). (b) Venous phase demonstrates poor enhancement of pancreatic tail with surrounding inflammatory changes (red arrow).

mediated rejection from acute cellular rejection based on the Banff classification. The presence of DSA can also aid in the diagnosis of graft rejection as it is an independent predictor of graft failure [12]. In our case, pancreatic graft biopsy was not undertaken as there was rapid improvement in her clinical parameters in addition to having normal blood glucose and C-peptide levels and negative DSAs.

While both entities can lead to elevated amylase or lipase levels, graft pancreatitis would have a significantly higher reading compared to pancreatic graft rejection. Imaging adjacent to pancreatic allograft showing pancreatic infiltration, oedema, and peripancreatic fluid would also favour graft pancreatitis [11].

To our knowledge, this is the first case report of gadolinium-induced acute graft pancreatitis in a patient with simultaneous pancreas-kidney transplant. While this is a rare occurrence, physicians should consider gadolinium-induced pancreatitis as a differential diagnosis for pancreatic graft pancreatitis.

Consent

Written informed consent was obtained from the patient by the authors.

Disclosure

This case report was presented in the Australia and New Zealand Society of Nephrology (ANZSN) 2021 Annual

Scientific Meeting as a lightning talk and abstracts were included in supplementary journal in Nephrology [13].

Authors' Contributions

All authors were involved in the preparation of this work. CSL contributed by obtaining consent, collecting data, and writing and revising the manuscript. RYPT and NNR contributed to writing and revision of manuscript.

References

[1] A. Falk Delgado, D. Van Westen, M. Nilsson et al., "Diagnostic value of alternative techniques to gadolinium-based contrast agents in MR neuroimaging—a comprehensive overview," *Insights Imaging*, vol. 10, no. 1, p. 84, 2019.

[2] C. Erenoglu, A. H. Uluutku, C. Top, M. L. Akin, and T. Celenk, "Do MRI agents cause or worsen acute pancreatitis?" *Turkish Journal of Trauma & Emergency Surgery*, vol. 13, no. 1, pp. 78-79, 2007.

[3] H. Blasco-Perrin, B. Glaser, M. Pienkowski, J. Peron, and J. Payen, "Gadolinium induced recurrent acute pancreatitis," *Pancreatology*, vol. 13, no. 1, pp. 88-89, 2013.

[4] C. Terzi and S. Sokmen, "Acute pancreatitis induced by magnetic-resonance-imaging contrast agent," *The Lancet*, vol. 354, no. 9192, pp. 1789-1790, 1999.

[5] D. Morse, N. Kumar, and G. Aisenberg, "Gadolinium-induced acute pancreatitis," *Gastroenterol Consult*, vol. 58, no. 9, pp. 257-258, 2018.

[6] M. P. Schenker, J. A. Solomon, and D. A. Roberts, "Gadolinium arteriography complicated by acute pancreatitis and acute renal failure," *Journal of Vascular and Interventional Radiology*, vol. 12, no. 3, p. 393, 2001.

[7] M. Rogosnitzky and S. Branch, "Gadolinium-based contrast agent toxicity: a review of known and proposed mechanisms," *Biometals*, vol. 29, no. 3, pp. 365–376, 2016.

[8] O. J. O'Connor, S. McWilliams, and M. M. Maher, "Imaging of acute pancreatitis," *American Journal of Roentgenology*, vol. 197, no. 2, pp. 221–225, 2011.

[9] S. L. Blamey, C. W. Imrie, J. O'Neill, W. H. Gilmour, and D. C. Carter, "Prognostic factors in acute pancreatitis," *Gut*, vol. 25, no. 12, pp. 1340–1346, 1984 Dec.

[10] A. Mallory and F. Kern Jr, "Drug-induced pancreatitis: a critical review," *Gastroenterology*, vol. 78, no. 4, pp. 813–820, 1980.

[11] S. Nadalin, P. Girotti, and A. Konigsrainer, "Risk factors for and management of graft pancreatitis," *Current Opinion in Organ Transplantation*, vol. 18, no. 1, pp. 89–96, 2013.

[12] R. R. Redfield, D. B. Kaufman, and J. S. Odorico, "Diagnosis and treatment of pancreas rejection," *Current Transplantation Reports*, vol. 2, pp. 169–175, 2015.

[13] C. S. Lee and N. Rao, "Gadolinium induced pancreatitis in a simultaneous pancreas kidney transplant recipient," *Nephrology*, vol. 26, no. 2, pp. 33–45, 2021.

40

Exacerbation of Congenital Hydronephrosis as the First Presentation of COVID-19 Infection in Children

Masoumeh Mohkam,[1] Mahnaz Jamee,[1] Farshid Kompani,[2] Mitra Khalili,[3] Atena Seifi,[1] and Leily Mohajerzadeh[4]

[1]*Pediatric Nephrology Research Center, Research Institute for Children's Health, Shahid Beheshti University of Medical Sciences, Tehran, Iran*
[2]*Department of Pediatric Nephrology, Golestan University of Medical Sciences, Golestan, Iran*
[3]*Department of Pediatric Radiology, Mofid Children's Hospital, Shahid Beheshti University of Medical Sciences, Tehran, Iran*
[4]*Pediatric Surgery Research Center, Institute for Children's Health, Shahid Beheshti University of Medical Sciences, Tehran, Iran*

Correspondence should be addressed to Mahnaz Jamee; mahnaz.jamee@gmail.com

Academic Editor: Anja Haase-Fielitz

Background. Congenital hydronephrosis is one of the most common abnormalities of the upper urinary tract, which can be exacerbated by a variety of intrinsic or extrinsic triggers. The urinary tract system is one of the major organs complicated by COVID-19 infection. *Case Presentations.* Here, we report five patients with an established diagnosis of congenital hydronephrosis, who presented with acute abdominal pain and fever and an abrupt increase in the anteroposterior pelvic diameter (APD). Patients had a previous stable course and were under regular follow-up with serial ultrasonographic studies. They underwent surgery or supportive treatment due to the later exacerbation of hydronephrosis. Based on the clinical and imaging findings, no plausible etiologies for these exacerbation episodes, including infection, nephrolithiasis, or abdominal masses, could be postulated. The common aspect in all these patients was the evidence of a COVID-19 infection. *Conclusions.* Infection with COVID-19 in children with antenatal hydronephrosis may exacerbate the degree of hydronephrosis and renal APD in ultrasonography, which itself may be mediated by the increase in inflammatory mediators.

1. Background

Congenital hydronephrosis is one of the most common abnormalities of the upper urinary tract diagnosed by prenatal ultrasonography. Hydronephrosis, as defined by a renal pelvic diameter of more than 5 mm according to the Bristol group, is found in approximately 1–5% of all pregnancies [1]. Now, it has become clear that 70–98% of the mild isolated congenital hydronephrosis cases improve spontaneously during follow-up without any need for surgical intervention [2].

More than forty percent of congenital hydronephrosis cases are due to transient etiologies [3]; physiologic etiologies comprise 15%, ureteropelvic junction obstruction (UPJO) 11%, and vesicoureteral reflex 9% of etiologies, while other etiologies are encountered less frequently [4]. Based on the anteroposterior pelvic diameter (APD) grading system (classified as grades 1 to 4 over a scale of 5 mm), hydronephrosis grades 1 to 4 are found to resolve in 80.0%, 41.2%, 13.1%, and 2.5% of patients over a 4-year-period, respectively [5].

The most common types of postnatal hydronephrosis are the transient and physiologic ones in which a close follow-up with serial ultrasonographic studies is required if the first renal function tests are normal and no unitary tract infection (UTI) or hypertension is present.

Antibiotic prophylaxis is recommended especially in moderate to severe cases of hydronephrosis [4] and may be associated with an improvement rate of 47% in a 12-month follow-up [6].

An acute increase in the APD sometimes occurs with accompanying complications in mild to moderate cases of hydronephrosis following infections, urolithiasis, blood clots, trauma, abdominal masses, fibrosis, retroperitoneal lymphadenopathy, and malignancies.

In the present era of widespread COVID-19 infection, a heterogeneous spectrum of manifestations is plausible in the setting of COVID-19. The renal manifestations of COVID-19 in the acute phase usually range from mild proteinuria, leukocyturia, or asymptomatic hematuria to severe acute kidney injury and blood pressure changes [7, 8].

Herein, we aim to report the presentation of severe hydronephrosis in children with a previous stable mild postnatal hydronephrosis, complicated by COVID-19 infection.

2. Case Presentations

2.1. Case 1. A 6-year-old male was referred to the Emergency Department of Mofid Children's Hospital with complaints of abdominal pain and vomiting in the 2020 late spring.

The case was under follow-up due to congenital hydronephrosis in our nephrology clinic. On neonatal ultrasonography, the APD of the renal pelvis was 13 mm on the right and 12 mm on the left. The blood pressure, renal function tests, urinalysis, and voiding cystourethrography (VCUG) were normal. The APD had gradually decreased to 6 mm on the right and 5 mm on the left at 5 years of age (6 months before the last admission) in our serial follow-ups together with a normal bladder appearance and postvoiding residual volume.

On admission, the weight was 22 kg (65% percentile) and blood pressure was 100/60 mmHg. On physical examination, there was mild generalized abdominal and right costovertebral angle tenderness and there was no fever or evidence of a respiratory or another gastrointestinal problem.

The hemoglobin level was 12.8 g/dl and C-reactive protein (CRP) was in the normal range and urinalysis showed 3-4 RBCs with no WBC or protein.

Abdominal ultrasonography was performed on the first day of admission which showed the size of the kidneys to be 108 mm on the right and 80 mm on the left and severe hydronephrosis on the right with the APD of 35 mm. The APD of the left kidney and the echogenicity of both kidneys were normal. The ultrasonography of the urinary tract was repeated after 2 days and on the last imaging, the APD increased to 45 mm while clinically abdominal pain persisted without any localized tenderness during this time.

Spiral abdominopelvic computerized tomography (CT) scan showed the same findings on ultrasonography without detection of urolithiasis. TC-99m diethylenetriamine pentaacetate (DTPA) scan showed obstructive hydronephrosis in the right kidney.

The patient underwent surgery due to symptomatic obstruction and the findings during surgery were moderate obstruction and marked inflammation at the ureteropelvic junction (UPJ) without complete obstruction. He became febrile the day following the surgery, and the evaluations showed a positive CRP and also a positive polymerase chain reaction (PCR) test for the SARS-CoV-2 virus.

The chest CT scan showed the characteristic pulmonary involvement in favor of COVID-19 infection. The patient was transferred to the COVID-19 ward and was discharged after one week with a good general condition.

On the day of discharge, the ultrasonography showed mild hydronephrosis with an RPD of 8 mm and also normal laboratory tests and blood pressure.

The patient was followed quarterly for one year and showed no abnormal clinical or laboratory findings.

2.2. Case 2. A 13-month-old female was referred to the outpatient clinic of our hospital with complaints of mild fever and abdominal pain in February 2020. Urinalysis and urine culture were performed due to a prior history of prenatal mild hydronephrosis with a stable clinical course. Urine analysis showed pyuria, and oral cefixime was prescribed with a presumed urinary tract infection diagnosis. The patient became afebrile within two days and began to develop diarrhea and vomiting. Further evaluations showed a positive PCR test for COVID-19. The patient underwent abdominal ultrasonography which reported a severe degree of hydronephrosis.

The patient underwent pyeloplasty due to the uptake defect on the DMSA (dimercaptosuccinic acid) scan, signs of obstruction in the DTPA scan, and exacerbation of hydronephrosis after the recovery period of COVID-19 infection.

2.3. Case 3. A 3-year-old female was followed up due to a history of mild hydronephrosis and antireflux surgery at one year of age. She had no history of UTI and was quite stable clinically with only mild unilateral hydronephrosis on renal ultrasonography two months before referral in July 2020.

She was referred due to fever for a few days and was admitted with a presumed diagnosis of UTI due to pyuria and proteinuria in urinalysis. On repeat ultrasonography, severe hydronephrosis was detected in the ipsilateral kidney, and on the DMSA scan, a severe uptake defect of the hydronephrotic kidney was detected. In recent history, the child had exposure to a case of COVID-19 one week before admission. The patient is now well and in stable health condition.

2.4. Case 4. The patient was a 6-year-old female who was under follow-up due to prenatal hydronephrosis and one episode of UTI. There was no evidence of vesicoureteral reflux in her infantile evaluation.

Pyeloplasty was performed at one year of age due to the obstructive pattern on the DTPA scan. At her postsurgical follow-up, the APD in renal ultrasonography was normal and the clinical course was stable.

Three months after the last visit (in November 2020), she was referred to our outpatient clinic due to occasional complaints of abdominal pain and anorexia. In the first evaluation, urinalysis was normal and on ultrasonography, a severe degree of hydronephrosis was reported. The past medical history revealed infection with COVID-19 a week before referral.

The DTPA scan showed a nonobstructive pattern despite the severe hydronephrosis.

The patient is now under follow-up with decreasing APD in serial ultrasonography and normal clinical and laboratory data.

2.5. Case 5. The case was a 5-year-old male who was under follow-up due to bilateral hydronephrosis from birth. There was no history of UTI and no evidence of vesicoureteral reflux in the neonatal evaluation. Her evaluation in infancy showed a nonobstructive pattern on DTPA scan and serial follow-up revealed improving course bilaterally.

Six months before the last visit, renal function tests, urinalysis, and blood pressure were normal and the renal ultrasonography showed an improving trend of hydronephrosis.

On the last visit in May 2021, kidney ultrasonography showed a marked bilateral increase in the APD despite a stable clinical course and the history revealed infection with COVID-19 virus one month before referral. A DTPA scan was ordered and is being awaited.

3. Conclusions

Ureteropelvic junction obstruction (UPJO), classified as congenital anomalies of the kidney and urinary tract (CAKUT) with an obstructive pattern, constitutes the most important etiology of hydronephrosis and also one of the common causes of chronic kidney disease (CKD) in children. Severe UPJO is associated with obstruction to urine flow from the renal pelvis to the ureter and can result in ultimately complete loss of the involved kidney [9].

In childhood, UPJO is usually congenital and can be diagnosed by the prenatal kidney and urinary tract ultrasonography (usually in the 3rd trimester). The acquired cases of UPJO are divided into intrinsic and extrinsic etiologies. The extrinsic causes are associated with outside pressure to the ureteropelvic junction or proximal ureters elicited by fibrosis, mass, or retroperitoneal lymphadenopathy.

The intrinsic causes of UPJO result from urolithiasis, radiation, or chronic inflammation, which cause scars in the ureteral wall or paraureteral region. According to some studies, one of the important etiologies for exacerbation of UPJO is urolithiasis, especially in the COVID-19 pandemic. In a recent study in Turkey on 149 patients with ureteral stones, it was shown that the number of emergency cases with admission during the COVID-19 epidemic increased by 3-fold in comparison with the time before the epidemic. This finding together with the simultaneous higher incidence of severe hydronephrosis in these patients can be the result of the delay in referral to the clinic as a result of personal isolation. This delayed referral can also explain some cases with a higher creatinine level [10].

The inflammatory mechanisms can be a predisposing factor for UPJO among the different abovementioned etiologies. Moreover, UPJO itself can trigger the production of vasoactive peptides and cytokines such as interleukin-5 and eotaxin-2 which recruit leukocytes and form inflammatory cell infiltrate [11].

Several studies have been conducted to evaluate the relationship between inflammatory mechanisms and UPJO over the last decades. In a study by Chiou et al. in 2005, the pathology of 24 ureteropelvic junction segments of 24 patients was evaluated. They noted an increased expression of IL-5, and eotaxin, and increased urothelial mast cell degranulation. The study showed increased levels of IL-5, γ-interferon, and eotaxin in the kidneys with an obstructed system, among which IL-5 and γ-interferon were highly ($p < 0.05$) associated with the severity of obstructive uropathy [12]. In an animal-model study by Chen et al., it was shown that the establishment of unilateral ureteral obstruction is associated with increased expression of IL-33 in vimentin-positive cells of medullary layers, cortex, and UPJ stroma. They proposed that the IL-33/ST2 axis may mediate the activation of innate immune responses and results in urothelial hyperplasia [13].

Infection with SARS-CoV-2 may result in persistent endothelial inflammation in different organs such as the lung, heart, and kidneys [14]. According to different studies, there is a marked increase in proinflammatory cytokines like ILIB, IL-6, IL-12, IFN-γ, IP-10, and MCP-1 in the serum of infected patients [15].

We think this marked and generalized increase in the inflammatory state may predispose patients to the exacerbation of UPJO as was observed in our patients with prior histories of COVID-19 infection.

Infection with SARS-CoV-2 in children with antenatal hydronephrosis may exacerbate the degree of hydronephrosis and renal APD in ultrasonography which itself may be mediated by the increase in inflammatory mediators.

This study has several limitations that should be considered, including lack of PCR test results, histopathologic evaluation of renal biopsies, and renal DTPA/DMSA scans for all patients. However, this is the first study that suggests COVID-19 infection as a predisposing factor for hydronephrosis exacerbation in the pediatric population. Further studies are required to confirm these clinical observations and identify the underlying pathomechanisms.

Abbreviations

APD: Anteroposterior pelvic diameter
CAKUT: Congenital anomalies of the kidney and urinary tract
CKD: Chronic kidney disease
CRP: C-reactive protein
CT: Computerized tomography
DMSA: Dimercaptosuccinic acid
DTPA: Diethylenetriamine pentaacetate
IL: Interleukin
PCR: Polymerase chain reaction
UPJO: Ureteropelvic junction obstruction
UTI: Unitary tract infection
VCUG: Voiding cystourethrography.

Consent

Written informed consent for publication was obtained from the parents of the patients prior to being included in the study.

Disclosure

The earlier version of this manuscript was previously presented as a preprint [16].

Authors' Contributions

MM and MJ contributed to the conceptualization, data curation, supervision, and writing the original draft. MM and FK examined and managed the patients. MKH performed the imaging. MM, MJ, AS, and LM gathered patient's data. All authors read and approved the final manuscript.

Acknowledgments

The authors thank the patients and their families for their participation in this study.

References

[1] H. T. Nguyen, C. A. Herndon, C. Cooper et al., "The Society for Fetal Urology consensus statement on the evaluation and management of antenatal hydronephrosis," *Journal of Pediatric Urology*, vol. 6, no. 3, pp. 212–231, 2010.

[2] F. Yalçınkaya and Z. B. Özçakar, "Management of antenatal hydronephrosis," *Pediatric Nephrology*, vol. 35, no. 12, pp. 2231–2239, 2020.

[3] J. A. Kari, S. Habiballah, S. A. Alsaedi et al., "Incidence and outcomes of antenatally detected congenital hydronephrosis," *Annals of Saudi Medicine*, vol. 33, no. 3, pp. 260–264, 2013.

[4] M. Woodward and D. Frank, "Postnatal management of antenatal hydronephrosis," *BJU International*, vol. 89, no. 2, pp. 149–156, 2002.

[5] J. Jung, J. H. Lee, K. S. Kim, and Y. S. Park, "Utility of society for fetal urology and anteroposterior pelvic diameter grading systems for estimating time to resolution of isolated hydronephrosis: a single center study," *The Journal of Urology*, vol. 204, no. 5, pp. 1048–1053, 2020.

[6] J. A. Dudley, J. M. Haworth, M. E. McGraw, J. D. Frank, and E. J. Tizard, "Clinical relevance and implications of antenatal hydronephrosis," *Archives of Disease in Childhood - Fetal and Neonatal Edition*, vol. 76, no. 1, pp. F31–F34, 1997.

[7] Y. Cheng, R. Luo, K. Wang et al., "Kidney disease is associated with in-hospital death of patients with COVID-19," *Kidney International*, vol. 97, no. 5, pp. 829–838, 2020.

[8] M. Mohkam, M. Mirzaee, F. Abdollah Gorgi et al., "Renal involvement in COVID-19 among Iranian children," *Archives Pediatric Infectious Diseases*, vol. 9, no. 1, Article ID e106597, 2021.

[9] I. Bilge, "Symptomatology and clinic of hydronephrosis associated with uretero pelvic junction anomalies," *Front Pediatr*, vol. 8, p. 520, 2020.

[10] M. Gul, M. Kaynar, M. Yildiz et al., "The increased risk of complicated ureteral stones in the era of COVID-19 pandemic," *Journal of Endourology*, vol. 34, no. 8, pp. 882–886, 2020.

[11] M. S. Al Aaraj and A. M. Badreldin, "Ureteropelvic junction obstruction," *StatPearls*, StatPearls Publishing LLC, Treasure Island, FL, USA, 2021.

[12] Y. Y. Chiou, C. C. Shieh, H. L. Cheng, and M. J. Tang, "Intrinsic expression of Th2 cytokines in urothelium of congenital ureteropelvic junction obstruction," *Kidney International*, vol. 67, no. 2, pp. 638–646, 2005.

[13] W. Y. Chen, J. L. Yang, Y. H. Wu et al., "IL-33/ST2 axis mediates hyperplasia of intrarenal urothelium in obstructive renal injury," *Experimental and Molecular Medicine*, vol. 50, no. 4, pp. 1–11, 2018.

[14] S. K. Patel, J. A. Juno, W. S. Lee et al., "Plasma ACE2 activity is persistently elevated following SARS-CoV-2 infection: implications for COVID-19 pathogenesis and consequences," *European Respiratory Journal*, vol. 57, no. 5, Article ID 2003730, 2021.

[15] C. Huang, Y. Wang, X. Li et al., "Clinical features of patients infected with 2019 novel coronavirus in Wuhan, China," *The Lancet*, vol. 395, no. 10223, pp. 497–506, 2020.

[16] M. Masoumeh, J. Mahnaz, K. Farshid, K. Mitra, S. Atena, and M. Leily, "Exacerbation of congenital hydronephrosis as the first presentation of covid-19 infection in children: a case series," *Research Square*, 2021.

41

Angiosarcoma of an Arteriovenous Fistula for Hemodialysis in a Kidney Transplant Recipient Affected by Lowe's Syndrome

V. D'Ambrosio,[1] P. Silvestri,[2] F. Aureli,[2] A. Sturniolo,[2] G. Grandaliano,[1,2] and P. M. Ferraro[1,2]

[1]*Università Cattolica del Sacro Cuore, Rome, Italy*
[2]*U.O.C. Nefrologia, Fondazione Policlinico Universitario A. Gemelli IRCCS, Rome, Italy*

Correspondence should be addressed to P. M. Ferraro; pietromanuel.ferraro@unicatt.it

Academic Editor: Manel Vera

Objective/Background. To describe an uncommon, life-threatening condition such as angiosarcoma of a fistula for hemodialysis occurring in a transplant recipient affected by Lowe's syndrome. *Summary.* We present the case of a 56-year-old male kidney transplant recipient affected by Lowe's syndrome, also known as oculocerebrorenal syndrome, a rare X-linked disorder characterized by congenital cataracts, hypotonia, intellectual disability, and Fanconi-like renal tubular dysfunction, who was diagnosed with angiosarcoma of a functioning arteriovenous fistula for hemodialysis. *Conclusion.* Angiosarcoma is a rare soft tissue tumor, and only 22 cases of angiosarcoma of arteriovenous fistulae were described so far; although a correlation between Lowe's syndrome and a higher risk of tumor compared to the general population has not been described so far, the mechanisms of disease causation could be an interesting starting point for future studies on a possible connection between the two events.

1. Introduction

Angiosarcomas (AS) arising from arteriovenous fistulas (AVFs) for hemodialysis are rare events. Oskrochi et al. in a recent review described 22 cases, 19 of which were post-transplant recipients and 18 were on immunosuppression therapy [1]. Multiple possible pathogenic mechanisms, such as immunosuppressive therapy and altered lymphatic flow, are already described in the literature, although a certain etiology has not been established yet.

We present the case of a 56-year-old male kidney transplant recipient affected by Lowe's syndrome, also known as oculocerebrorenal syndrome, a rare X-linked disorder characterized by congenital cataracts, hypotonia, intellectual disability, and Fanconi-like renal tubular dysfunction, who was diagnosed with angiosarcoma of a functioning arteriovenous fistula for hemodialysis. There is no evidence of an increased risk of tumor in these patients except for subcutaneous benign fibromas; however, the disease's molecular pathogenesis could potentially play a role.

2. Case Report

A 56-year-old male kidney transplant recipient affected by Lowe's syndrome was admitted to our hospital for a hematoma on his left forearm.

The patient had a history of end-stage renal disease (ESRD) and had undergone hemodialysis for 11 years through a distal AVF on his left forearm. In 2013, the patient received a deceased-donor kidney transplant and has been treated with immunosuppressive therapy with tacrolimus 1 mg + 0.5 mg daily ever since. He also had a recent history of ischemic stroke and accidental fall at home which caused a trauma of his left wrist.

A week before the admission, the patient was evaluated by the surgical team of our department because of a painful and swelling mass on his left forearm where the AVF for hemodialysis was originally created.

The enlarging mass first appeared two months before and was treated in another hospital as a complicated AVF, and thus the vascular access was closed.

During the hospitalization in our Nephrology Department, the patient underwent surgical revision of the hematoma and ligation of the distal radial artery. A left wrist radiogram was also performed which showed an area of diaphyseal osteolysis of the radius surrounded by a voluminous soft-tissue swelling. After a few days, the radial artery required ligation right after its origin from the brachial artery because of enlarging hematoma.

After a short time of apparent stability, the patient was admitted once again to our emergency department because of active bleeding from the surgical site which required urgent evacuation of the hematoma. Although the specific source of the hematoma was undetectable, the hemostasis was achieved using surgical glue devices. A surgical reduction of the brachial artery's diameter was also necessary. The hospitalization was complicated by two events of severe anemia which required blood transfusions.

During the follow-up, because of chronic anemia and worsening of the forearm lesion, the patient was readmitted to our department. A Doppler US was performed; however, detailed characterization of the mass required further imaging with computed tomography (CT). Because of high suspicion of malignancy (spread vascular enhancement and pathologic fracture of the radius), a bone biopsy of the fractured radius was required, which then confirmed the presence of epithelioid sarcoma. A total-body CT scan was performed with evidence of enlarged ipsilateral axillary lymph nodes.

After a consultation with the oncologist and the radiotherapist, considering the extension of the lesion, comorbidities, and scarce compliance of the patient, chemo and radiotherapy were ruled out and a surgical approach was favored. The patient was then submitted for left arm amputation (above elbow). The hospitalization was complicated by *Clostridium difficile* infection treated with oral vancomycin and *Proteus mirabilis* urinary tract infection treated with intravenous meropenem. Four months following amputation, the patient was found to have metastatic disease to both lungs, the left iliac wing, and the duodenum. Five months later, the patient died.

3. Discussion

Angiosarcoma is a rare yet very aggressive tumor that arises from endothelial tissue. AS arising from AVFs are even rarer events. Steal syndrome, aneurysms, ischemia, and thrombosis are well-known blood-flow related complications of AVFs. Malignancies such as angiosarcomas may occur in both functioning and nonfunctioning fistulae, and although they can occur spontaneously, multiple risk factors have been identified. Chronic lymphedema may play an important role; as a matter of fact, when creating an AVF, not only the blood flow is altered but the lymphoid dynamics of soft tissues surrounding the AVF itself changes as well. This mechanism leads to the creation of a localized immunosuppressed environment which contributes to AS occurrence [2, 3]. AVF creation and altered blood flow also lead to hypoxia and wall shear stress, both strong proinflammatory stimuli. Hypoxic and ischemic injury promote inflammation, angiogenesis, and proliferation by stimulating the release of cytokines such as hypoxia-inducible factor-1 alpha (HIF-1α), immediate-early responsive gene (IEX-1), vascular endothelial growth factor (VEGF), interleukin-1 beta (IL-1β), tumor necrosis factor alpha (TNFα), and interferon gamma (IFγ) from endothelial cells. These cytokines function both as proliferation stimuli and leukocyte attractant, ultimately resulting in intima hyperplasia and blood flow-related complications of AVFs, but could also potentially play a role in AS pathogenesis [4]. In transplant recipients or patients undergoing immunosuppressive therapy for other reasons, an important risk factor for malignancy occurrence is immunosuppression; it is well known that immunosuppressed populations have a double incidence rate of all malignancies compared to the normal population [5, 6].

Our patient had many risk factors that could have been potentially implicated in the pathogenesis of AS of the fistula, including being affected by a rare disease whose molecular pathogenesis interferes with cellular migration and differentiation of many cell types.

Lowe's syndrome (oculocerebrorenal syndrome) is a rare X-linked disorder characterized by involvement of the eyes, central nervous system, and kidneys.

Dense congenital cataract is the most common and earliest eye manifestation; nystagmus, microphthalmos, enophthalmos, severe glaucoma, strabismus, retinal dystrophy, secondary corneal scarring, and calcific band keratopathy with keloid formation may be present and worsen visual damage, ultimately progressing to blindness.

In almost all affected males, generalized hypotonia is present soon after birth (absent deep tendon reflexes, poor head control, sucking and swallowing problems leading to feeding difficulties, and delayed growth), but it may improve with age. Seizures and behavior problems are frequent, as much as intellectual impairment.

Renal pathology is characterized by proximal renal tubular dysfunction resulting in an abnormal loss of bicarbonate, sodium, potassium, amino acids, organic acids, albumin, calcium, and L-carnitine in the urine.

Low-molecular-weight proteinuria (LMW proteinuria) and albuminuria are present as first clinical manifestations, followed by polyuria and renal tubular acidosis. Some patients may develop full-spectrum renal Fanconi syndrome (bicarbonaturia and renal tubular acidosis, phosphaturia with hypophosphatemia and renal rickets, sodiuria and potassiuria, glycosuria, polyuria, and apparent urine-concentrating defect), and others may develop LMW proteinuria, hypercalciuria with nephrocalcinosis, and nephrolithiasis similar to Dent's disease. Chronic tubular injury eventually leads to glomerulosclerosis and thus to a decline in glomerular filtration rate (GFR). End-stage renal disease (ESRD) usually occurs between the second and the fourth decade of life.

Other clinical manifestations may be short stature, feeding difficulties and gastrointestinal problems such as gastroesophageal reflux and chronic constipation, scoliosis, arthritis, tenosynovitis and subcutaneous benign fibromas, cryptorchidism, and dental malformations. Superficial cysts are also frequent, especially on the skin and in the mouth, but they can also occur in the kidneys and brain. Lowe patients may also have an intrinsic platelet defect leading to prolonged bleeding time [7].

Almost all of the disease's manifestations may be explained by its molecular pathogenesis. Lowe's syndrome is caused by a hemizygous pathogenic variant in OCRL, a gene located on the X chromosome (locus q26.1) decoding for inositol polyphosphate 5-phosphatase or phosphoinositide 5-phosphatase OCRL-1/INPP5F. The same gene is also involved in type 2 Dent's disease, a disease characterized by LMW proteinuria, hypercalciuria, nephrolithiasis, nephrocalcinosis, and progressive renal failure [8].

There are 10 different isozymes of phosphoinositide 5-phosphatase (PI 5-phosphatase/INPP5P) [9], and each protein is expressed in specific cell types and interacts with specific pathways by regulating intracellular concentrations of their substrates. All PI 5-phosphatase, except for INPP5A, catalyze the dephosphorylation of two lipids: PI-(3,4,5)-trisphosphate (PI-(3,4,5)-P3) and PI-(4,5)-bisphosphate (PI-(4,5)-P2) [10, 11]. They therefore act as potential tumor suppressors in tumor cells by reducing the intracellular concentrations of PI-(3,4,5)-P3 [12] and by increasing intracellular concentrations of PI-(3,4)-P2.

Reduced or absent activity of PI 5-phosphatases leads to intracellular accumulation of their substrate. In Lowe's syndrome, OCRL-1/INPP5F codes for a very specific phosphatase and its altered function lead to phosphatidylinositol (4,5) bisphosphate [PtdIns (4,5) P2] increase [13], a molecule that has many signaling functions in endocytosis, exocytosis, migration, and adhesion by interacting with cellular compounds such as scaffold proteins, ion channels, and cytoskeleton proteins [14]. PtdIns (4,5) P2 thus interferes with many cellular processes such as differentiation and cell migration by altering cell membrane composition, cytoskeletal organization, and ciliary function, which could partially explain the ophthalmologic complications. Recent evidence demonstrates that PtdIns (4,5) P2 is involved in endocytosis and lysosomal-autophagic pathway and its accumulation may alter intracellular protein trafficking and tubular transport. This mechanism could explain LMW proteinuria and tubular defects [10].

Although the tumor promotor versus tumor suppressor role of 5-phosphatases has been discussed in the literature, correlating some of them to cancer (e.g., overexpression of SYNJ2 is correlated with breast cancer growth and metastases) [15], there is no association between OCRL-1/INPP5F and cancer [16].

However, in Lowe's syndrome, the intracellular alterations cited above are present in many different cell types, from kidney, brain, lung, ovary, and testis cells to fibroblasts which share their mesenchymal origin with endothelial cells.

4. Conclusion

Among the many risk factors that contributed to the development of AS from our patient's fistula, Lowe's syndrome could potentially play a role, although a direct link between the two events has not been described yet.

Because of the poor prognosis of AS, an early diagnosis is crucial to a successful treatment or at least to a prolonged survival. When bleeding or painful masses arise from the site of AVFs in transplant recipients, angiosarcomas must be ruled out among the differential diagnoses, especially in patients with other comorbidities.

References

[1] Y. Oskrochi, K. Razi, J. Stebbing, and J. Crane, "Angiosarcoma and dialysis-related arteriovenous fistulae: a comprehensive review," *European Journal of Vascular and Endovascular Surgery*, vol. 51, no. 1, pp. 127–133, 2016.

[2] C. Bordea, M. Cortina-Borja, F. Wojnarowska, and P. J. Morris, "Distribution of upper limb skin cancers in relation to arteriovenous fistula side in renal transplant recipients," *Transplantation*, vol. 71, pp. 143–145, 2001.

[3] P. J. Conlon, T. Daly, G. Doyle, and M. Carmody, "Angiosarcoma at the site of a ligated arteriovenous fistula in a renal transplant recipient," *Nephrology Dialysis Transplantation*, vol. 8, pp. 259–262, 1993.

[4] M. K. Fitts, D. B. Pike, K. Anderson, and Y.-T. Shiu, "Hemodynamic shear stress and endothelial dysfunction in hemodialysis access," *The Open Urology & Nephrology Journal*, vol. 7, no. 1, pp. 33–44, 2014.

[5] E. A. Engels, R. M. Pfeiffer, and J. F. Fraumeni, "Spectrum of cancer risk among US solid organ transplant recipients," *JAMA*, vol. 306, p. 1891, 2011.

[6] A. E. Grulich, M. T. van Leeuwen, M. O. Falster, and C. M. Vajdic, "Incidence of cancers in people with HIV/AIDS compared with immunosuppressed transplant recipients: a meta-analysis," *The Lancet*, vol. 370, no. 9581, pp. 59–67, 2007.

[7] R. A. Lewis, R. L. Nussbaum, and E. D. Brewer, "Lowe syndrome," in *GeneReviews®*, M. P. Adam, H. H. Ardinger, R. A. Pagon et al., Eds., University of Washington, Seattle, WA, USA, 1993.

[8] O. Devuyst and R. V. Thakker, "Dent's disease," *Orphanet Journal of Rare Diseases*, vol. 5, no. 28, 2010.

[9] D. Blero, B. Payrastre, S. Schurmans, and C. Erneux, "Phosphoinositide phosphatases in a network of signalling reactions," *Pflügers Archiv—European Journal of Physiology*, vol. 455, no. 1, pp. 31–44, 2007.

[10] C. Erneux, W. s. E. Edimo, L. Deneubourg, and I. Pirson, "SHIP2 multiple functions: a balance between a negative control of PtdIns(3,4,5)P3level, a positive control of PtdIns(3,4)P2production, and intrinsic docking properties," *Journal of Cellular Biochemistry*, vol. 112, no. 9, pp. 2203–2209, 2011.

[11] C. Erneux, S. Ghosh, A. Raquel Ramos, and W. s. Elong Edimo, "New functions of the inositol polyphosphate 5-phosphatases in cancer," *Current Pharmaceutical Design*, vol. 22, no. 16, pp. 2309–2314, 2016.

[12] A. Toker and L. Rameh, "PIPPing on AKT1: how many phosphatases does it take to turn off PI3K?" *Cancer Cell*, vol. 28, no. 2, pp. 143–145, 2015.

[13] X. Zhang, P. A. Hartz, E. Philip, L. C. Racusen, and P. W. Majerus, "Cell lines from kidney proximal tubules of a patient with Lowe syndrome lack OCRL inositol polyphosphate 5-phosphatase and accumulate phosphatidylinositol 4,5-

bisphosphate," *Journal of Biological Chemistry*, vol. 273, no. 3, pp. 1574–1582, 1998.

[14] A. R. Ramos, W. Elong Edimo, and C. Erneux, "Phosphoinositide 5-phosphatase activities control cell motility in glioblastoma: two phosphoinositides PI(4,5)P2 and PI(3,4)P2 are involved," *Advances in Biological Regulation*, vol. 67, no. 40–48, 2018.

[15] N. Ben-Chetrit, D. Chetrit, R. Russell et al., "Synaptojanin 2 is a druggable mediator of metastasis and the gene is overexpressed and amplified in breast cancer," *Science Signaling*, vol. 8, p. ra7, 2015.

[16] S. A. Rudge and M. J. O. Wakelam, "Phosphatidylinositolphosphate phosphatase activities and cancer," *Journal of Lipid Research*, vol. 57, no. 2, pp. 176–192, 2016.

42

Very Early Severe Posttransplant Recurrent Antineutrophil Cytoplasmic Antibody-Associated Glomerulonephritis after Kidney Transplantation: Two Case Reports

Reda Laamech,[1] Hamza Naciri-Bennani,[1] Diane Giovannini,[2,3] Johan Noble,[1,2] Bénédicte Janbon,[1] Paolo Malvezzi,[1] Thomas Jouve,[1,2] and Lionel Rostaing[1,2]

[1]*Nephrology, Hemodialysis, Apheresis and Kidney Transplantation Department, Grenoble University Hospital, Grenoble, France*
[2]*Grenoble Alpes University, Grenoble, France*
[3]*Laboratory of Pathology, Grenoble University Hospital, Grenoble, France*

Correspondence should be addressed to Lionel Rostaing; lrostaing@chu-grenoble.fr

Academic Editor: Rumeyza Kazancioglu

Successful kidney transplantation (KTx) in patients with antineutrophil cytoplasmic antibody-associated vasculitis (AAV) has been reported with excellent patient and graft survival rates. The recurrence of AAV in transplant recipients is rare, and its mechanisms of action are not clearly known. The optimum time for KTx and the relevance of ANCA titer at the time of transplantation remain controversial. We report two cases of extremely rapid recurrent AAV after renal transplantation; both were still ANCA-positive at the time of transplantation, which led us to question the pathogenesis of ANCA antibodies in recurrence in a kidney allograft. Apheresis plus immunosuppressive therapies were ineffective in the first case and the patient became dialysis-dependent, whereas in the second case methylprednisone pulses plus rituximab infusions resulted in long-lasting remission.

1. Introduction

End-stage kidney disease (ESKD) associated with anti-neutrophil cytoplasmic autoantibody-associated vasculitis (AAV) is considered an indication for renal transplantation. It improves the quality of life and life expectancy in patients with ESKD. Indeed, kidney transplantation (KTx) has been successfully performed in AAV patients [1, 2], and several studies confirm the survival benefits of renal transplantation compared to maintenance dialysis [3]. Nonetheless, AAV relapses have been reported many times; in pooled analyses from multiple studies, between 5 and 6% of transplant recipients suffer a relapse [4], which often affects allograft outcomes. These cases display different mechanisms and risk factors, such as the timing of renal transplantation after AAV diagnosis, the role of immunosuppressive maintenance in patients during chronic dialysis period, and antineutrophil cytoplasmic antibody (ANCA) titers at the time of transplantation. However, a link between ANCA titers and allograft failure has not been clearly established, although there is a trend showing a link between ANCA titers at the time of transplantation and the risk of relapse and overall graft survival [5].

Direct and indirect involvement of ANCA antibodies in AAV disease has been widely discussed. Herein, we report two cases of patients presenting with AAV and having high ANCA titers at the time of transplantation; they also had rapid AAV recurrence on the allograft kidney with a primary failure in one case.

2. Case Report/Case Presentation

The case presentations were conducted ethically in accordance with the World Medical Association Declaration of Helsinki.

2.1. Case 1. A 54-year-old man was admitted for a kidney transplant. He had been on hemodialysis for 21 months because of ANCA-associated ESKD; he was almost anuric. When he was diagnosed, he was treated with pulses of methylprednisolone and two IV injections (one month apart) of cyclophosphamide 0.6 g/m^2, but there was no improvement. No maintenance immunosuppressive treatment was introduced. He received a living-related ABO and HLA-compatible KTx on July 9, 2020. He was fully matched for class II HLA antigens and was not HLA sensitized at pretransplant. He received induction therapy with antithymocyte globulins (ATG), in addition to tacrolimus, mycophenolate mofetil (MMF), and steroids, i.e., methylprednisone 500 mg preoperatively and then 500 mg on days 1 and 2. He recovered immediate diuresis and serum creatinine began to decrease 12 hours after surgery (from 6.9 to 5.4 mg/dL). However, urine output suddenly decreased on day 1 after transplantation. Serum creatinine (sCr) then rose from 5.4 to 6.9 mg/dL.

On day 1, posttransplant serum ANCA titer was >1280 UI/mL with an MPO specificity of >740 UI/mL. No ANCA serum titer was performed immediately before kidney transplantation.

On day 2, Doppler ultrasound evaluation of the kidney allograft was normal. Surgery was performed in search of a vascular plication, but no explanation for allograft failure was found. A biopsy realized on day 7 after transplantation revealed necrotizing vasculitis with fibrinoid necrosis and extracapillary proliferation, confirming AAV relapse (shown in Figures 1 and 2). Proteinuria was dosed at 1.7 g/L; there was no associated hematuria. We implemented plasmapheresis sessions (nine over a 14-day period), plus three methylprednisolone pulses (10 mg/kg each) and rituximab (375 mg/m^2) on postop days 9, 17, 24, and 37. This resulted in a sharp decrease in the anti-MPO titer (from >740 to 80 U/mL). However, the patient remained dialysis-dependent.

Allograft biopsies on postop days 15 and 21 were scored according to Banff classification as i1, t1, g1 ptc2, and C4d0 and revealed persisting fibrinoid necrosis and extracapillary proliferation, with no histological improvement (D21 vs. previous biopsies). On postop day 60, we observed a rebound in ANCA titer to >1280 UI/mL and in anti-MPO titer of 317.8 U/mL with a patient still dialysis-dependent. We therefore decided to implement seven semispecific immunoadsorption (IA) using a Globaffin® immunoadsorber. Maintenance immunosuppression was based on MMF 500 mg bid, prednisone 20 mg/d, and tacrolimus in order to achieve trough levels between 6 and 8 ng/mL. A follow-up kidney biopsy was performed at 3 months postop showing no improvement in extracapillary proliferation or fibrinoid necrosis, but there were no signs of allograft rejection. We then decided to perform two IA sessions for 2 weeks. However, unfortunately, the patient remained dialysis-dependent with predialytic serum creatinine remaining at >5 mg/dL, even though ANCAs with MPO specificity remained low at 55–70 UI/mL. The relevant biological markers for evolution are shown in Figure 3.

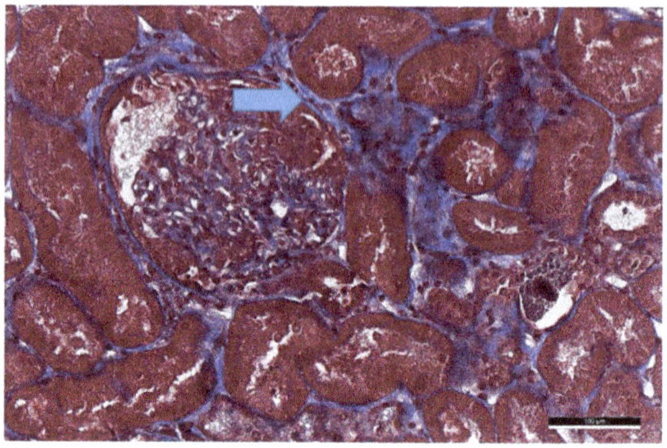

FIGURE 1: One glomerulus highlighted a cellular crescent—blue arrow (blue trichrome, high power field).

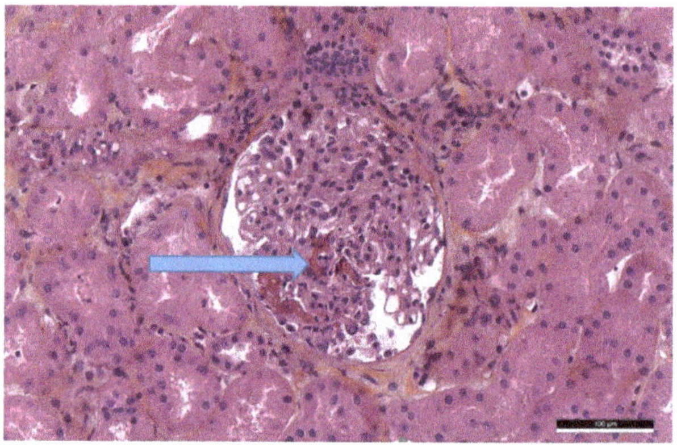

FIGURE 2: Another glomerulus highlighted a fibrinoid necrosis—blue arrow (PAS staining, high power field).

One month later, i.e., postop day 120, there was no improvement in kidney function. We decided that further therapeutic approaches were not possible. The patient remained dialysis-dependent; MMF was stopped, tacrolimus (trough levels 5–6 ng/mL) and prednisone (10 mg/d) were maintained; unfortunately, he died of septic shock at 6 months after transplantation. His brother (the kidney donor) has given written informed consent to publish the case.

2.2. Case 2. An 84-year-old man with chronic kidney disease of unknown origin had an episode of acute kidney injury. The estimated glomerular filtration rate (eGFR) declined from 30 to 10 ml/min/1.73 m^2 in one month. No kidney biopsy was performed. He went onto maintenance dialysis in May 2018. The first assessments showed high levels of anti-MPO titers, at 640 UI/L. The first kidney biopsy (January 4, 2018) showed diffuse thickening of the glomerular basement membrane (GBM) throughout all the glomeruli without hypercellularity. Immunofluorescence microscopy revealed a diffuse granular pattern of immunoglobulin G without C3 staining along the GBM. PLA2R antibodies were negative. There were no signs of AAV on the kidney biopsy; thus, membranous nephropathy was diagnosed. He received no immunosuppressive therapy for that condition.

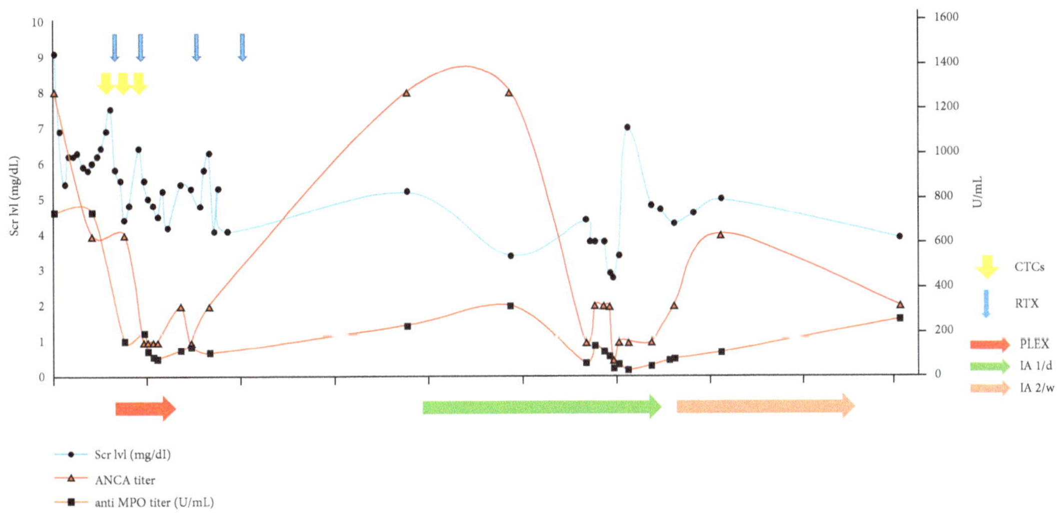

FIGURE 3: Case 1: serum creatinine level, ANCA titer, and anti-MPO level evolution over time. Scr lvl, serum creatinine level; CTCs, methylprednisone pulse; RTX, rituximab; PLEX, plasmapheresis; IA 1/d, immunoadsorption one per day; IA 2/w, immunoadsorption, two per week; ANCA, antineutrophil cytoplasmic antibody; MPO, myeloperoxidase.

He received a transplant on October 24, 2019, from a deceased donor. He had no anti-HLA antibodies at pretransplant. He was given induction therapy with ATG, along with tacrolimus, everolimus, and prednisone. The patient initially had a good urine output of >1 L/day and serum creatinine decreased to 3.7 mg/dL on postoperative day 8. At 2 weeks, serum creatinine stabilized at 3.95 mg/dL. An allograft biopsy, realized on postop day 11, revealed necrotizing vasculitis compatible with relapsing AAV and/or cellular rejection grade 3. Histological injuries included glomerular and arteriolar thrombotic microangiopathy, acute tubular necrosis, g1, cg2, ptc1, C4d0, t1 + i0, FIAT1, v0, cv3, ah3, and aah0 (shown in Figure 4). Biology revealed ANCA positivity with MPO specificity reaching 285 UI/mL at the time of kidney transplantation. Treatment included pulses of methylprednisone (500 mg daily dose for 5 days), two injections of rituximab (375 mg/m^2 on postop days 12 and 26): it provided good efficacy, i.e., serum creatinine was reduced to 2.8 mg/dL and ANCA titer was decreased to 80 UI/mL. The relevant biological markers for evolution are shown in Figure 5.

Maintenance therapy included perfusions of rituximab (375 mg/m^2 every 6 months). Allograft function was stabilized with eGFR at 20 mL/min/1.73 m^2. At postop 9 months, serum creatinine level was 2.38 mg/dL and proteinuria was 0.5 g/L, with no anti-HLA alloantibodies. Anti-MPO was 70.7 UI/L and a biopsy showed tubulointerstitial inflammation without any signs of AAV. By the end of 2020 (postop month 14), the patient was admitted into the hospital for SARS-CoV-2 infection and died of SARS-CoV-2-related pneumopathy. His late wife has given written informed consent to publish the case.

3. Discussion

In pooled analyses from multiple studies, 5.4% of AAV patients with a transplant have a relapse. The relapse rate after transplantation seems to have declined over the last few years, with rates of 0.01–0.10 per patient/year reported in studies older than 10 years compared to rates of 0.01–0.03 per patient/year in more recent studies. Although the frequency of AAV recurrence after kidney transplantation is rare, there is a one-in-three risk of graft loss within 5 years [6].

The timing of KTx in patients with AAV is still being discussed. Little et al. [5] found that the strongest predictor for graft loss and mortality in AAV patients was when transplantation was conducted shortly (<1 year) after the induction of a remission. ANCA positivity per se, at the time of transplantation, was not associated with adverse graft survival. The finding of severe vascular lesions on a transplant biopsy was the only factor significantly associated with graft failure. However, the impact of ANCA is not definitive from the study of Little et al., as graft failure could have been induced by several other factors.

Gera et al. [7] in their single-center experience reported that AAV needs to be in clinical remission at the time of transplantation. Both the 2012 Kidney Disease Improving Global Outcomes Guidelines for Glomerulonephritis (KDIGO) and the 2005 Canadian Society of Transplantation Consensus Guidelines recommend a period of 1 year of clinical remission prior to transplantation.

The necessity of ANCA testing before proceeding with KTx is less fully agreed upon. ANCA positivity alone is not a contraindication for transplantation. However, Gera et al. [7] reported a trend towards a higher relapse rate among patients that had a positive ANCA test just before KTx; that is, 13% vs. 5% in those having no longer detectable ANCA at the time of transplantation.

Nonetheless, rapid relapse and allograft failure are rarely reported in the literature. The time to relapse is highly variable, ranging from weeks to more than 10 years, with a mean time of 26.5 months posttransplant [8]. For example, the average time to relapse was 30.9 months (range: 4–84 months) in the pooled analysis performed by Nachman et al.

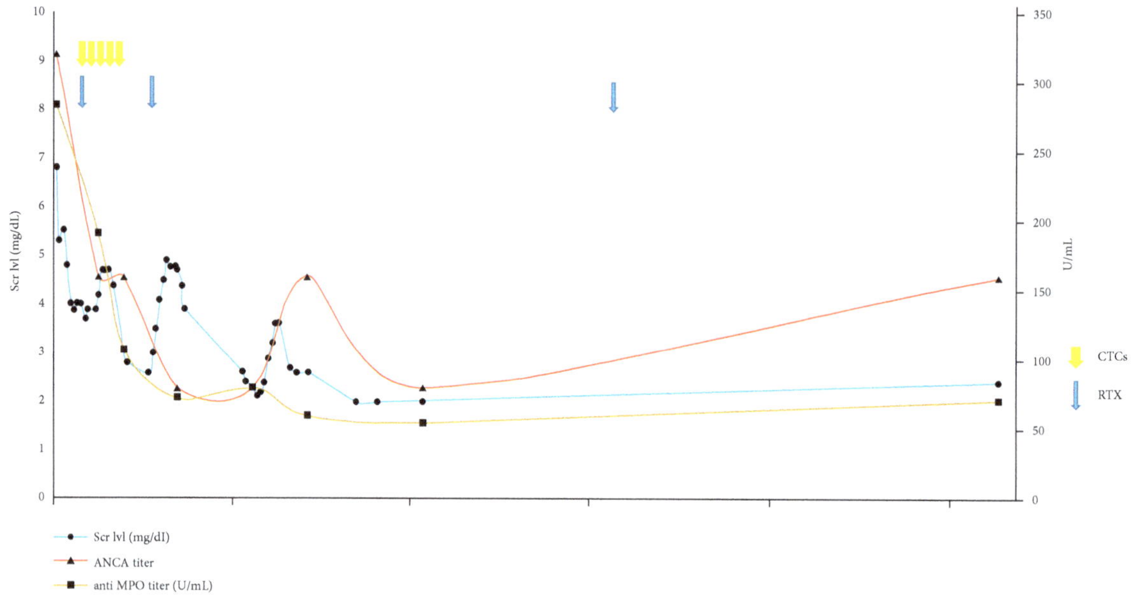

Figure 4: Case 2: serum creatinine level, ANCA titer, and anti-MPO level evolution over time. Scr lvl, serum creatinine level; CTCs, methylprednisone pulse; RTX, rituximab; ANCA, antineutrophil cytoplasmic antibody; MPO, myeloperoxidase.

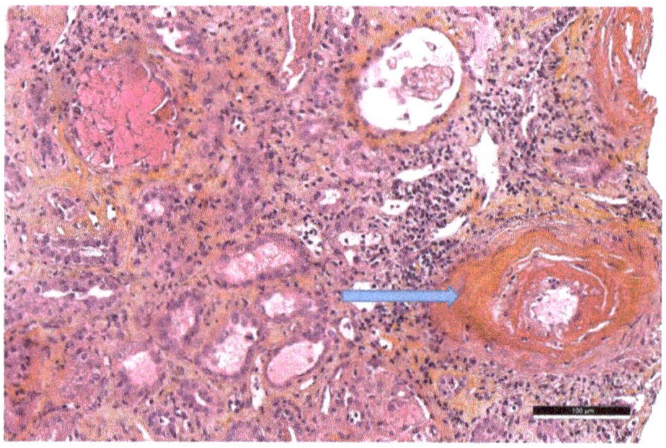

Figure 5: HES high power field: an apoplectic glomerulus and two medium-sized arteries presenting with fibrinoid necrosis (blue arrow).

[9]. Lobbedez et al. [10] reported a recurrence of ANCA-positive glomerulonephritis immediately after renal transplantation. The renal biopsy (performed on postoperative day 6) showed crescentic necrotizing glomerulonephritis and the p-ANCA titer was positive at 1 : 400 on the day of renal transplantation. This relapse was successfully treated with cyclophosphamide, intravenous immunoglobulins (IVIg), steroid pulses, cyclosporine, and plasmapheresis sessions. The ANCA titer became negative by the end of the treatment.

Kai Ming Chow et al. [11] reported a case of rapid (1 month post-KTx) recurrence of ANCA-negative glomerulonephritis after KTx. Five sessions of plasmapheresis with cyclophosphamide did not improve renal function, and the patient remained dialysis-dependent.

These findings along with ours led us to question the pathogenesis of ANCA antibodies. Several animal models of AAV have been established [12]. This shows that ANCAs not only serve as a biomarker for AAV but also have pathogenic potential in themselves. But ANCA titers do not necessarily reflect disease activity. The lack of a correlation between ANCA titers and the activity of vasculitis disease could be explained by differences in epitopes and the affinity of ANCAs [12].

Also, ANCAs cannot be detected in some patients with clinical manifestations of MPO-AAV; laboratory tests can give false-negative results because fragments of ceruloplasmin can bind to the ANCAs in the serum. The absence of ANCAs in necrotizing lesions can be explained by the presence of neutrophil extracellular traps (NETs), which induce digestion of immunoglobulins by neutrophil elastase derived from NET-forming neutrophils. All these elements make the underlying mechanisms hard to elucidate and demonstrate the pathogenesis of the ANCA complex [13].

Such rapid recurrences among patients receiving a kidney allograft, with positive ANCA titers at the time of transplantation, have led us to discuss the pathogenesis of ANCA and the importance of finding a biomarker for disease activity (still not yet available). This could inform us of the pertinence and safety of renal transplantation in AAV patients, as well as the prognosis of AAV in kidney-transplant recipients.

4. Conclusion

We report two cases of AAV in recipients of allograft kidneys. Both cases presented with very early posttransplant allograft dysfunction in the setting of a high titer level of ANCAs and MPO specificity at the time of kidney transplantation. Pathogenicity of ANCAs has been a subject of controversy as no evidence has been provided since its discovery in the 1980s of cases where it has occurred on native kidneys, allograft relapses, or in de novo post-KTx, where immunosuppressive therapy is thought to avoid outcomes. Further exploration of the mechanisms behind this phenomenon should be made.

Authors' Contributions

RL collected the data. HNB performed the apheresis sessions. RL wrote the manuscript under the supervision of HNB and JN. DG interpreted the kidney biopsies. BJ, PM, and TJ looked after the patients (inpatient and outpatient clinics). LR supervised the work and edited the manuscript.

References

[1] M. S. Sagmeister, M. Grigorescu, and U. Schönermarck, "Kidney transplantation in ANCA-associated vasculitis," *Journal of Nephrology*, vol. 32, no. 6, pp. 919–926, 2019.

[2] W. H. Schmitt and F. J. Van Der Woude, "Organ transplantation in the vasculitides," *Current Opinion in Rheumatology*, vol. 15, no. 1, pp. 22–28, 2003.

[3] R. A. Wolfe, V. B. Ashby, E. L. Milford et al., "Comparison of mortality in all patients on dialysis, patients on dialysis awaiting transplantation, and recipients of a first cadaveric transplant," *New England Journal of Medicine*, vol. 341, no. 23, pp. 1725-1730, 1999.

[4] E. M. Briganti, G. R. Russ, J. J. McNeil, R. C. Atkins, and S. J. Chadban, "Risk of renal allograft loss from recurrent glomerulonephritis," *New England Journal of Medicine*, vol. 347, no. 2, pp. 103–109, 2002.

[5] M. A. Little, B. Hassan, S. Jacques et al., "Renal transplantation in systemic vasculitis: when is it safe?" *Nephrology Dialysis Transplantation*, vol. 24, no. 10, pp. 3219–3225, 2009.

[6] A. Göçeroğlu, C. Rahmattulla, A. E. Berden, M. E. J. Reinders, R. Wolterbeek, and E. J. Steenbergen, "The Dutch transplantation in vasculitis (DUTRAVAS) study: outcome of renal transplantation in antineutrophil cytoplasmic antibody-associated glomerulonephritis," *Transplantation*, vol. 100, no. 4, pp. 916–924, 2016.

[7] M. Gera, M.-D. Griffin, U. Specks, N. Leung, M.-D. Stegall, and F.-C. Fervenza, "Recurrence of ANCA-associated vasculitis following renal transplantation in the modern era of immunosupression," *Kidney International*, vol. 71, no. 12, pp. 1296–1301, 2007.

[8] H. Marco, E. Mirapeix, E. Arcos et al., "Long-term outcome of antineutrophil cytoplasmic antibody-associated small vessel vasculitis after renal transplantation," *Clinical Transplantation*, vol. 27, no. 3, pp. 338–347, 2013.

[9] P. H. Nachman, M. Segelmark, K. Westman et al., "Recurrent ANCA-associated small vessel vasculitis after transplantation: a pooled analysis," *Kidney International*, vol. 56, no. 4, pp. 1544–1550, 1999.

[10] T. Lobbedez, F. Comoz, E. Renaudineau, M. Pujo, J. P. Ryckelynck, and B. Hurault de Ligny, "Recurrence of ANCA-positive glomerulonephritis immediately after renal transplantation," *American Journal of Kidney Diseases*, vol. 42, no. 4, pp. E2–E6, 2003.

[11] K. M. Chow, A. Y. Wang, F. Mac-Moune Lai, T. Y. Wong, and P. K. Li, "Rapid recurrence of ANCA-negative pauci-immune vasculitis after cadaveric renal transplantation," *American Journal of Kidney Diseases*, vol. 38, no. 1, p. E3, 2001.

[12] D. Nakazawa, S. Masuda, U. Tomaru, and A. Ishizu, "Pathogenesis and therapeutic interventions for ANCA-associated vasculitis," *Nature Reviews Rheumatology*, vol. 15, no. 2, pp. 91–101, 2019.

[13] A. J. Roth, J. D. Ooi, J. J. Hess et al., "Epitope specificity determines pathogenicity and detectability in ANCA-associated vasculitis," *Journal of Clinical Investigation*, vol. 123, no. 4, pp. 1773–1783, 2013.

Permissions

All chapters in this book were first published by Hindawi Publishing Corporation; hereby published with permission under the Creative Commons Attribution License or equivalent. Every chapter published in this book has been scrutinized by our experts. Their significance has been extensively debated. The topics covered herein carry significant findings which will fuel the growth of the discipline. They may even be implemented as practical applications or may be referred to as a beginning point for another development.

The contributors of this book come from diverse backgrounds, making this book a truly international effort. This book will bring forth new frontiers with its revolutionizing research information and detailed analysis of the nascent developments around the world.

We would like to thank all the contributing authors for lending their expertise to make the book truly unique. They have played a crucial role in the development of this book. Without their invaluable contributions this book wouldn't have been possible. They have made vital efforts to compile up to date information on the varied aspects of this subject to make this book a valuable addition to the collection of many professionals and students.

This book was conceptualized with the vision of imparting up-to-date information and advanced data in this field. To ensure the same, a matchless editorial board was set up. Every individual on the board went through rigorous rounds of assessment to prove their worth. After which they invested a large part of their time researching and compiling the most relevant data for our readers.

The editorial board has been involved in producing this book since its inception. They have spent rigorous hours researching and exploring the diverse topics which have resulted in the successful publishing of this book. They have passed on their knowledge of decades through this book. To expedite this challenging task, the publisher supported the team at every step. A small team of assistant editors was also appointed to further simplify the editing procedure and attain best results for the readers.

Apart from the editorial board, the designing team has also invested a significant amount of their time in understanding the subject and creating the most relevant covers. They scrutinized every image to scout for the most suitable representation of the subject and create an appropriate cover for the book.

The publishing team has been an ardent support to the editorial, designing and production team. Their endless efforts to recruit the best for this project, has resulted in the accomplishment of this book. They are a veteran in the field of academics and their pool of knowledge is as vast as their experience in printing. Their expertise and guidance has proved useful at every step. Their uncompromising quality standards have made this book an exceptional effort. Their encouragement from time to time has been an inspiration for everyone.

The publisher and the editorial board hope that this book will prove to be a valuable piece of knowledge for researchers, students, practitioners and scholars across the globe.

List of Contributors

Shreeyukta Bhattarai, Stephen Pupillo and Gulshan Man Singh Dangol
Northeast Ohio Medical University, Department of Medicine, Rootstown, Ohio, USA
St. Elizabeth Youngstown Hospital, Department of Internal Medicine, Youngstown, Ohio, USA

Erdal Sarac
Northeast Ohio Medical University, Department of Medicine, Rootstown, Ohio, USA
St. Elizabeth Youngstown Hospital, Department of Internal Medicine, Youngstown, Ohio, USA
Lake Erie College of Osteopathic Medicine, Erie, Pennsylvania, USA
Ohio University Heritage College of Osteopathic Medicine, Athens, Ohio, USA

Kosaku Nitta
Department of Nephrology, Tokyo Women's Medical University, Tokyo, Japan

Mayuko Yamazaki, Hidekazu Sugiura, Yosuke Iwatani, Mizuki Kyoda, Hirohiko Nokiba and Nobuyuki Amemiya
Department of Nephrology, Division of Medicine, Saiseikai Kurihashi Hospital, Saitama, Japan
Department of Nephrology, Tokyo Women's Medical University, Tokyo, Japan

Ken Tsuchiya
Department of Nephrology, Tokyo Women's Medical University, Tokyo, Japan
Department of Blood Purification, Kidney Center, Tokyo Women's Medical University Tokyo, Japan

Mika Kondo, Hideaki Oka, Taro Kamimura and Atsumi Harada
Kidney Center, Matsuyama Red Cross Hospital, Japan

Shunsuke Yamada, Toshiaki Nakano and Takanari Kitazono
Department of Medicine and Clinical Science, Graduate School of Medical Sciences, Kyushu University, Fukuoka, Japan

Kazuhiko Tsuruya
Department of Nephrology, Nara Medical University, Nara, Japan

Seishi Aihara
Kidney Center, Matsuyama Red Cross Hospital, Japan
Department of Medicine and Clinical Science, Graduate School of Medical Sciences, Kyushu University, Fukuoka, Japan

Varun Mamidi, Manikantan Shekar, Jaiju James Chakola, Vamsi Krishna Makkena and Jayakumar Matcha
Department of Nephrology, Sri Ramachandra Institute of Higher Education and Research, Chennai, India

Fumika Honma, Yoshihide Fujigaki, Yoshikazu Nemoto, Hirotoshi Kikuchi, Michito Nagura, Shigeyuki Arai, Kenichi Ishizawa, Osamu Yamazaki, Yoshifuru Tamura, Shunya Uchida and Shigeru Shibata
Department of Internal Medicine, Teikyo University School of Medicine, Itabashi-ku, Tokyo, Japan

Fukuo Kondo
Department of Pathology, Teikyo University Hospital, Itabashi-ku, Tokyo, Japan

Ryuji Ohashi
Department of Diagnostic Pathology, Nippon Medical School Musashikosugi Hospital, Kawasaki, Kanagawa, Japan

Sebastián Jaurretche
Physiology Department, School of Medicine, Instituto Universitario Italiano de Rosario, Rosario, Argentina
Los Manantiales, Neurosciences Center, Rosario, Argentina

Germán R. Perez
School of Biochemical and Pharmaceutical Sciences, National University of Rosario, Rosario, Argentina
Gammalab Grupo Gamma, Rosario, Argentina

Graciela Venera
Research Department, School of Medicine, Instituto Universitario Italiano de Rosario, Rosario, Argentina

ZayMyo Htet and Mahzuz Karim
Department of Renal Medicine, Norfolk and Norwich University Hospital, Norwich, UK

Cesar Gomez
Department of Haematology, Norfolk and Norwich University Hospital, Norwich, UK

Ahsan Ali
Department of Cellular Pathology, Norfolk and Norwich University Hospital, Norwich, UK

Sunil Nair
Department of Cardiology, Norfolk and Norwich University Hospital, Norwich, UK

I. Spozio Züst and H. R. Räz
Division of Nephology, Kantonsspital Baden, Switzerland

F. Burkhalter
Clinic for Transplant Immunology and Nephrology, University Hospital Basel, Switzerland

Ankur Gupta, Susan Lavoie, Mohan Biyani and Brendan B. McCormick
Division of Nephrology, Department of Medicine, University of Ottawa andThe Ottawa Hospital, Canada
Kidney Research Centre, University of Ottawa, Canada

Brian Blew
Department of Surgery, University of Ottawa and the Ottawa Hospital, Canada

J. Coutinho, R. S. Chorão and C. R. Santos
Hospital Amato Lusitano, Castelo Branco, Portugal

M. Oliveira
Centro Hospitalar Cova da Beira, Covilhã, Portugal

Hamza Naciri Bennani, Paolo Malvezzi and Rachel Tetaz
Service de Néphrologie, Hémodialyse, Aphérèses et Transplantation Rénale, CHU Grenoble-Alpes, Grenoble, France

Thomas Jouve, Johan Noble and Lionel Rostaing
Service de Néphrologie, Hémodialyse, Aphérèses et Transplantation Rénale, CHU Grenoble-Alpes, Grenoble, France
Université Grenoble Alpes, Grenoble, France

Edgar Dehesa-López
Department of Internal Medicine and Nephrology, Hospital Civil de Culiacán, Culiacán, Mexico
Centro de Investigación y Docencia en Ciencias de la Salud, Universidad Autónoma de Sinaloa, Culiacán, Mexico
Instituto Mexicano del Seguro Social (IMSS), Mexico

Rolando Claure-Del Granado
Division of Nephrology, Hospital Obrero #2 - C.N.S., Cochabamba, Bolivia

Rafael Valdez-Ortiz
Department of Nephrology, Hospital General de México, Mexico City, Mexico

Sergio Saul Irizar-Santana
Department of Internal Medicine and Nephrology, Hospital Civil de Culiacán, Culiacán, Mexico
Centro de Investigación y Docencia en Ciencias de la Salud, Universidad Autónoma de Sinaloa, Culiacán, Mexico

Ashley Rose and Samuel Slone
Internal Medicine, University of South Florida, Tampa, FL 33602, USA

Eric Padron
Malignant Hematology, H. Lee Moffitt Cancer Center and Research Institute, Tampa, FL 33602, USA

Sangeeta Mutnuri, Hania Kassem and John Badalamenti
Department of Internal Medicine, University of Texas Medical Branch, Galveston, TX, USA

You-Wen Qian and Christopher Marquez
Department of Pathology, University of Texas Medical Branch, Galveston, TX, USA

Marjan Afrouzian
Department of Internal Medicine, University of Texas Medical Branch, Galveston, TX, USA
Department of Pathology, University of Texas Medical Branch, Galveston, TX, USA

Mohamedanwar Ghandour, Yahya Malik-Osman and Zeenat Y. Bhat
Department of Internal Medicine WSU SOM, Division of Nephrology Wayne State University, Detroit, MI, USA

Heba Osman
Department of Internal Medicine/Pediatrics, Wayne State University/Detroit Medical Center, Detroit, MI, USA

Samer Alkassis, Alix Charles, Kristina Zalewski and Jarrett Weinberger
Department of Internal Medicine WSU SOM, Wayne State University, Detroit, MI, USA

Amol M. Patel, Lily Anne Romero Karam, Stephanie C. Fuentes Rojas and Warren E. Redfearn
Department of Internal Medicine, Houston Methodist Hospital, Houston, TX, USA

Luan D. Truong
Department of Pathology and Genomic Medicine, Houston Methodist Hospital, Houston, TX, USA

Juan M. Gonzalez
Department of Internal Medicine, Division of Nephrology, Houston, TX, USA

Ali Oullaï, Edouard Cubilier, Mohamed Tayeb Salaouatchi, Maxime Taghavi, Yasmin Zouggari, Joëlle Nortier and Maria Do Carmo Filomena Mesquita
Department of Nephrology, Brugmann University Hospital, Université Libre de Bruxelles, Brussels, Belgium

Yannick Nlandu, Franck Pourcine, Ly van phach Vong, Jonathan Chelly, Sebastien Jochmans, Sandie Mazerand and Mehran Monchi
Groupe Hospitalier Sud Ile-De-France, Centre Hospitalier de Melun, 77000 Melun, France

Théodore-Junior M. Sakaji, Karel Van Echkout, Jean-Pierre M. Kanku, Golan Kalifa and Rodolphe Ahmed
Intensive Care Unit, Centre Médical de Kinshasa, Kinshasa, Democratic Republic of the Congo

Yannick M. Nlandu, Yannick M. Engole, Marie-France I. Mboliassa and Justine B. Bukabau
Intensive Care Unit, Centre Médical de Kinshasa, Kinshasa, Democratic Republic of the Congo
Nephrology Unit, Kinshasa University Hospital, Kinshasa, Democratic Republic of the Congo

Patrick U. Kobo, Patrick M. Boloko, Pally K. Mafuta and Joseph P. Tsangu
Intensive Care Unit, Centre Médical de Kinshasa, Kinshasa, Democratic Republic of the Congo
Intensive Care Unit, Kinshasa University Hospital, Kinshasa, Democratic Republic of the Congo

Faten Aqeel and Duvuru Geetha
Division of Nephrology, Johns Hopkins Hospital, Baltimore, MD, USA

Serena M. Bagnasco
Department of Pathology, Johns Hopkins Hospital, Baltimore, MD, USA

Kei Nagai
Department of Nephrology, Hitachi General Hospital, 2-1-1 Jonan-cho, Hitachi, Ibaraki 317-0077, Japan
Department of Nephrology, Faculty of Medicine, University of Tsukuba, 1-1-1 Tennodai, Tsukuba, Ibaraki 305-8575, Japan

Kohei Inoue and Atsushi Ueda
Department of Nephrology, Hitachi General Hospital, 2-1-1 Jonan-cho, Hitachi, Ibaraki 317-0077, Japan

Hiroaki Tachi
Department of Respiratory Medicine, Hitachi General Hospital, 2-1-1 Jonan-cho, Hitachi, Ibaraki 317-0077, Japan

D. Lai
Baylor College of Medicine, Houston, TX 77030, USA
Department of Medicine, Baylor College of Medicine, Houston, TX 77030, USA

N. Dave and R. Raghavan
Baylor College of Medicine, Houston, TX 77030, USA
Department of Medicine, Baylor College of Medicine, Houston, TX 77030, USA
Selzman Institute for Kidney Health, Baylor College of Medicine, Houston, TX 77030, USA

Zhuo Lin Yu
Stony Brook University Hospital, 101 Nicolls Rd, Stony Brook, NY 11794, USA

Lisa Fisher
Northport VA Medical Center, 79 Middleville Rd, Northport, NY 11768, USA

Minh Huan Dang, Mathew Mathew and Rajesh Raj
Department of Nephrology, Launceston General Hospital, Launceston, Tasmania, Australia

Anna Curtis, Hussain Rao and Andrew Williams
School of Medicine, University of Missouri-Kansas City, Kansas City, MO 64108, USA

Christian Lamb
Department of Medicine, Brooke Army Medical Center, San Antonio, TX 78234, USA

Amit Patel
Department of Medicine—Division of Nephrology, Truman Medical Center, Kansas City, MO 64108, USA

Abdul Mughees Rana, Kannan Mansoor, Mahmoud Abouzid, Iheanyichukwu Ogu and Ghassan Salim Issa Bandak
Department of Internal Medicine University Huntington, 1249 15th Street Suite 2000, Huntington, WV 25514, USA

Salman Assad
Department of Neurology Marshall University Joan C. Edwards School of Medicine, 1600 Medical Center Drive Office B561, Huntington, WV, USA

Voordeckers
Palliative Care Unit, Centre Hospitalier Universitaire, Hospital Brugmann, Brussels, Belgium

J. Noels
Urology Clinic, Centre Hospitalier Universitaire, Hospital Brugmann, Brussels, Belgium

M. Brognet, M. T. Salaouatchi and M. Mesquita
Department of Internal Medecine, Clinics of Nephrology and Dialysis, Hospital Brugmann, Brussels, Belgium

Ariel A. Chung and Patricia R. Millner
Department of Family Medicine, Tripler Army Medical Center, Honolulu, HI 96859, USA

H. Trimarchi
Nephrology Service, Hospital Británico de Buenos Aires, Buenos Aires, Argentina

Chaudhry Adeel Ebad, Nabeehah Moollan, Adeel Rafi Ahmed and Colm Magee
Department of Nephrology, Beaumont Hospital, Dublin, Ireland

Anthony Dorman
Department of Pathology, Beaumont Hospital, Dublin, Ireland
Royal College of Surgeons Ireland (RCSI), Dublin, Ireland

Akshee Batra, Shatha Herz Allah and Bijin Thajudeen
Department of Nephrology, Banner University of Arizona Medical Center, 1501 North Campbell Ave, Tucson, AZ, USA

Auris Huen and Madeleine Duvic
Department of Dermatology, e University of Texas MD Anderson Cancer Center, Houston, TX, USA

Jessica Tran
Department of Dermatology, e University of Texas MD Anderson Cancer Center, Houston, TX, USA
Baylor College of Medicine, Houston, TX, USA

Amaresh R. Vanga
Division of Nephrology, Department of Internal Medicine, Eastern Virginia Medical School, Norfolk, VA, USA

Samantha A. Schrier Vergano
Division of Medical Genetics and Metabolism, Children's Hospital of the King's Daughters, Norfolk, VA, USA
Department of Pediatrics, Eastern Virginia Medical School, Norfolk, VA, USA

Jolanta Kowalewska
Department of Pathology and Anatomy, Eastern Virginia Medical School, Norfolk, VA, USA

Thomas R. McCune
Division of Nephrology, Department of Internal Medicine, Eastern Virginia Medical School, Norfolk, VA, USA
Center for Congenital Kidney Diseases, Eastern Virginia Medical School, Norfolk, VA, USA

Letizia Zeni
University of Campania Luigi Vanvitelli, Naples, Italy
Fondazione Policlinico Universitario A. Gemelli IRCCS, O. U. of Nephrology, Rome, Italy

Chiara Manenti, Federica Verzeletti and Mario Gaggiotti
3O. U. of Nephrology, ASST Spedali Civili Brescia, Brescia, Italy

Simona Fisogni
Nephrology, Department of Medical and Surgical Specialties, Radiological Science and Public Health, University of Brescia, Brescia, Italy

Vincenzo Terlizzi and Giovanni Cancarini
O. U. of Nephrology, ASST Spedali Civili Brescia, Brescia, Italy
Nephrology, Department of Medical and Surgical Specialties, Radiological Science and Public Health, University of Brescia, Brescia, Italy

GulshanMan Singh Dangol and Hilmer Negrete
Department of Internal Medicine, St. Elizabeth Health Center, Youngstown, Ohio, USA
Department of Internal Medicine, Northeastern Ohio Medical University, Rootstown, Ohio, USA

José C. De La Flor, Tania Linares and Elisa Ruiz
Department of Nephrology, Hospital Central Defense Gomez Ulla, Madrid, Spain

Jacqueline Apaza
Department of Nephrology, Hospital Fuenlabrada, Madrid, Spain

Francisco Díaz and Patricia Núñez
Department of Anatomic Pathology, Hospital Gregorio Marañon, Madrid, Spain

Edna Sandoval
Department of Hematology, Hospital Central Defense Gomez Ulla, Madrid, Spain

Alexander Marschall
Department of Cardiology, Hospital Central Defense Gomez Ulla, Madrid, Spain

Andrea Cecilia Rivas-Nieto
Department of Nephrology, Hospital Cayetano Heredia, Lima, Peru

Luca Calvaruso, Alessandro Naticchia, Pietro Manuel Ferraro, Gisella Vischini and Stefano Costanzi
U.O.C. Nefrologia, Fondazione Policlinico Universitario A. Gemelli IRCCS, Rome, Italy
Università Cattolica del Sacro Cuore, Rome, Italy

Vedran Premužić and Bojan Jelaković
Department of Nephrology, Hypertension, Dialysis and Transplantation, University Hospital Centre Zagreb, Kispaticeva 12, Zagreb 10 000, Croatia

Ivan Padjen, Mislav Cerovec and Branimir Anić
Department of Immunology and Rheumatology, University Hospital Centre Zagreb, Kispaticeva 12, Zagreb 10 000, Croatia

Marijana Ćorić
Department of Pathology, University Hospital Centre Zagreb, Kispaticeva 12, Zagreb 10 000, Croatia

Chiang Sheng Lee and Rachel Yi Ping Tan
Renal Unit, Flinders Medical Centre, Flinders Drive, Bedford Park, South Australia, Australia
College of Medicine and Public Health, Flinders University, Bedford Park, South Australia, Australia

Nitesh N. Rao
Renal Unit, Flinders Medical Centre, Flinders Drive, Bedford Park, South Australia, Australia
Renal Unit, Lyell McEwin Hospital, Haydown Road, Elizabeth Vale, Adelaide, South Australia, Australia
Adelaide Medical School, University of Adelaide, Adelaide, South Australia, Australia

Masoumeh Mohkam, Mahnaz Jamee and Atena Seifi
Pediatric Nephrology Research Center, Research Institute for Children's Health, Shahid Beheshti University of Medical Sciences, Tehran, Iran

Farshid Kompani
Department of Pediatric Nephrology, Golestan University of Medical Sciences, Golestan, Iran

Mitra Khalili
Department of Pediatric Radiology, Mofid Children's Hospital, Shahid Beheshti University of Medical Sciences, Tehran, Iran

Leily Mohajerzadeh
Pediatric Surgery Research Center, Institute for Children's Health, Shahid Beheshti University of Medical Sciences, Tehran, Iran

V. D'Ambrosio
Università Cattolica del Sacro Cuore, Rome, Italy

P. Silvestri, F. Aureli and A. Sturniolo
U.O.C. Nefrologia, Fondazione Policlinico Universitario A. Gemelli IRCCS, Rome, Italy

G. Grandaliano and P. M. Ferraro
Università Cattolica del Sacro Cuore, Rome, Italy
U.O.C. Nefrologia, Fondazione Policlinico Universitario A. Gemelli IRCCS, Rome, Italy

Reda Laamech, Hamza Naciri-Bennani and Bénédicte Janbon
Nephrology, Hemodialysis, Apheresis and Kidney Transplantation Department, Grenoble University Hospital, Grenoble, France

Diane Giovannini
Grenoble Alpes University, Grenoble, France
Laboratory of Pathology, Grenoble University Hospital, Grenoble, France

Index

www.ingramcontent.com/pod-product-compliance
Lightning Source LLC
LaVergne TN
LVHW082231200926
848484LV00008B/2336
9798887406305